Drug Treatments for
Inflammatory Bowel Diseases

Drug Treatments for Inflammatory Bowel Diseases

Editors

Anderson Luiz-Ferreira
Carmine Stolfi

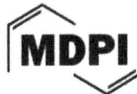 Basel • Beijing • Wuhan • Barcelona • Belgrade • Novi Sad • Cluj • Manchester

Editors
Anderson Luiz-Ferreira
Biological Sciences
Federal University of Catalão
Catalão
Brazil

Carmine Stolfi
Systems Medicine
University of Rome "Tor Vergata"
Rome
Italy

Editorial Office
MDPI
St. Alban-Anlage 66
4052 Basel, Switzerland

This is a reprint of articles from the Special Issue published online in the open access journal *Pharmaceuticals* (ISSN 1424-8247) (available at: www.mdpi.com/journal/pharmaceuticals/special_issues/drug_colitis).

For citation purposes, cite each article independently as indicated on the article page online and as indicated below:

Lastname, A.A.; Lastname, B.B. Article Title. *Journal Name* **Year**, *Volume Number*, Page Range.

ISBN 978-3-0365-9976-2 (Hbk)
ISBN 978-3-0365-9975-5 (PDF)
doi.org/10.3390/books978-3-0365-9975-5

© 2024 by the authors. Articles in this book are Open Access and distributed under the Creative Commons Attribution (CC BY) license. The book as a whole is distributed by MDPI under the terms and conditions of the Creative Commons Attribution-NonCommercial-NoDerivs (CC BY-NC-ND) license.

Contents

About the Editors vii

Preface ix

Anderson Luiz-Ferreira and Carmine Stolfi
Special Issue "Drug Treatments for Inflammatory Bowel Diseases"
Reprinted from: *Pharmaceuticals* **2023**, *17*, 59, doi:10.3390/ph17010059 1

Chin-Hsiao Tseng
Rosiglitazone Does Not Affect the Risk of Inflammatory Bowel Disease: A Retrospective Cohort Study in Taiwanese Type 2 Diabetes Patients
Reprinted from: *Pharmaceuticals* **2023**, *16*, 679, doi:10.3390/ph16050679 6

Chin-Hsiao Tseng
Pioglitazone Has a Null Association with Inflammatory Bowel Disease in Patients with Type 2 Diabetes Mellitus
Reprinted from: *Pharmaceuticals* **2022**, *15*, 1538, doi:10.3390/ph15121538 22

Sumaiah J. Alarfaj, Sally Abdallah Mostafa, Walaa A. Negm, Thanaa A. El-Masry, Marwa Kamal and Mohamed Elsaeed et al.
Mucosal Genes Expression in Inflammatory Bowel Disease Patients: New Insights
Reprinted from: *Pharmaceuticals* **2023**, *16*, 324, doi:10.3390/ph16020324 33

Vlasta Oršić Frič, Vladimir Borzan, Ines Šahinović, Andrej Borzan and Sven Kurbel
Real-World Study on Vedolizumab Serum Concentration, Efficacy, and Safety after the Transition from Intravenous to Subcutaneous Vedolizumab in Inflammatory Bowel Disease Patients: Single-Center Experience
Reprinted from: *Pharmaceuticals* **2023**, *16*, 239, doi:10.3390/ph16020239 46

Eric J. Lebish, Natalie J. Morgan, John F. Valentine and Ellen J. Beswick
MK2 Inhibitors as a Potential Crohn's Disease Treatment Approach for Regulating MMP Expression, Cleavage of Checkpoint Molecules and T Cell Activity
Reprinted from: *Pharmaceuticals* **2022**, *15*, 1508, doi:10.3390/ph15121508 56

Sameh Saber, Mohannad Mohammad S. Alamri, Jaber Alfaifi, Lobna A. Saleh, Sameh Abdel-Ghany and Adel Mohamed Aboregela et al.
(R,R)-BD-AcAc2 Mitigates Chronic Colitis in Rats: A Promising Multi-Pronged Approach Modulating Inflammasome Activity, Autophagy, and Pyroptosis
Reprinted from: *Pharmaceuticals* **2023**, *16*, 953, doi:10.3390/ph16070953 69

Naoto Tsujimura, Takayuki Ogino, Masayuki Hiraki, Taisei Kai, Hiroyuki Yamamoto and Haruka Hirose et al.
Super Carbonate Apatite-miR-497a-5p Complex Is a Promising Therapeutic Option against Inflammatory Bowel Disease
Reprinted from: *Pharmaceuticals* **2023**, *16*, 618, doi:10.3390/ph16040618 97

Ni Jin, Yao Liu, Peiyu Xiong, Yiyi Zhang, Jingwen Mo and Xiushen Huang et al.
Exploring the Underlying Mechanism of Ren-Shen-Bai-Du Powder for Treating Inflammatory Bowel Disease Based on Network Pharmacology and Molecular Docking
Reprinted from: *Pharmaceuticals* **2022**, *15*, 1038, doi:10.3390/ph15091038 116

Alexander V. Blagov, Varvara A. Orekhova, Vasily N. Sukhorukov, Alexandra A. Melnichenko and Alexander N. Orekhov
Potential Use of Antioxidant Compounds for the Treatment of Inflammatory Bowel Disease
Reprinted from: *Pharmaceuticals* **2023**, *16*, 1150, doi:10.3390/ph16081150 . . . . **134**

Yijie Song, Man Yuan, Yu Xu and Hongxi Xu
Tackling Inflammatory Bowel Diseases: Targeting Proinflammatory Cytokines and Lymphocyte Homing
Reprinted from: *Pharmaceuticals* **2022**, *15*, 1080, doi:10.3390/ph15091080 . . . . **149**

Marcello Imbrizi, Fernando Magro and Claudio Saddy Rodrigues Coy
Pharmacological Therapy in Inflammatory Bowel Diseases: A Narrative Review of the Past 90 Years
Reprinted from: *Pharmaceuticals* **2023**, *16*, 1272, doi:10.3390/ph16091272 . . . . **171**

About the Editors

Anderson Luiz-Ferreira

Anderson Luiz-Ferreira is an associate professor at the Institute of Biotechnology at the Federal University of Catalão, Brazil. He has a PhD in Functional and Molecular Biology and has been the head of the Research Laboratory for Inflammatory Bowel Diseases since 2012, working to enhance the space and resources allocated to experimental research and strengthen research with experimental and epidemiological models of gastrointestinal inflammatory diseases. His research interests include studies on the pathophysiological mechanisms involved in gastric ulcers and inflammatory bowel diseases. The results of his research, related to mentorships and partnerships, have been published in peer-reviewed international journals, totaling more than 40 works. As he values the dissemination and democratization of scientific productions of excellence and high scientific rigor, he participates on the editorial board, as an academic editor and reviewer, of several scientific journals of recognized international prestige.

Carmine Stolfi

Carmine Stolfi is an assistant professor at the University of Rome, "Tor Vergata". Dr. Stolfi's basic research has been mostly focused on the molecular mechanisms and immune/inflammatory signals that drive and sustain inflammatory bowel diseases (IBD) and colon carcinogenesis. During his PhD program, he focused his research on colorectal cancer (CRC) prevention, and his studies identified some of the basic mechanisms by which mesalazine, an anti-inflammatory compound largely used in the management of patients with IBD, interferes with CRC cell biology. During his postdoctoral career, his efforts aimed at unraveling the immune-inflammatory networks involved in the pathogenesis of inflammation-associated and sporadic CRCs. He found that the cytokine interleukin (IL)-21 is highly expressed during the course of both colitis-associated and sporadic CRC and plays a crucial role in the mechanisms that control the incidence and ultimate growth of colonic tumors driven by chronic inflammation. In 2011, he was the winner of a My First AIRC Grant from the Italian Association for Cancer Research. Studies supported by these funds contributed to characterizing the type of immune cell infiltrate in sporadic colon cancer tissue, thus providing a detailed analysis of immune cell-derived signals that stimulate CRC cell growth.

Preface

Inflammatory bowel disease (IBD) is the term used to describe a group of chronic and relapsing inflammatory diseases of the gastrointestinal tract. Crohn's disease (CD) and ulcerative colitis (UC) are the two main clinical forms. Although the specific etiopathogenesis of IBD is unknown, it is widely recognized that immunological, genetic, and environmental factors are involved. A greater understanding of the multiple signaling pathways involved in the pathophysiology of IBD has led to the development of different therapies in recent decades. Although these treatments have dramatically transformed the course of IBD, to date, there is still no permanent cure. Individuals treated with the available therapies do not always respond satisfactorily to treatment, and when they do, eventual adverse effects limit the use of such therapies. The present Special Issue of the journal *Pharmaceuticals*, "Drug Treatments for Inflammatory Bowel Diseases", features original research articles and review articles on management strategies and therapeutic alternatives for the treatment of IBD. The Special Issue published one editorial, eight original research articles, and three review articles, involving the contributions of nearly seventy authors. The objective was to provide possible new treatment alternatives to address needs not yet met by clinical practice. We appreciate the significant contributions of all authors to this Special Issue and hope that the readers enjoy the content.

Anderson Luiz-Ferreira and Carmine Stolfi
Editors

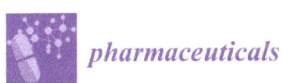

Editorial

Special Issue "Drug Treatments for Inflammatory Bowel Diseases"

Anderson Luiz-Ferreira [1,*] and Carmine Stolfi [2]

1 Inflammatory Bowel Disease Research Laboratory, Department of Biological Sciences, Institute of Biotechnology, Federal University of Catalão (UFCAT), Catalão 75704-020, GO, Brazil
2 Department of Systems Medicine, University of Rome "Tor Vergata", 00133 Rome, Italy; carmine.stolfi@uniroma2.it
* Correspondence: luiz_ferreira@ufcat.edu.br

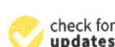

Citation: Luiz-Ferreira, A.; Stolfi, C. Special Issue "Drug Treatments for Inflammatory Bowel Diseases". *Pharmaceuticals* **2024**, *17*, 59. https://doi.org/10.3390/ph17010059

Received: 1 December 2023
Accepted: 8 December 2023
Published: 29 December 2023

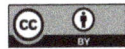

Copyright: © 2023 by the authors. Licensee MDPI, Basel, Switzerland. This article is an open access article distributed under the terms and conditions of the Creative Commons Attribution (CC BY) license (https://creativecommons.org/licenses/by/4.0/).

Inflammatory bowel diseases (IBD), including Crohn's disease (CD) and ulcerative colitis (UC), are chronic idiopathic, relapsing and remitting inflammatory diseases that affect the gastrointestinal tract, causing significant morbidity and loss of quality of life in affected individuals [1]. In UC, inflammation is mainly restricted to the mucosa and involves only the colon, although the extent of colic involvement may vary among patients and over time [2]. In CD, the inflammatory process is transmural and affects any portion of the gastrointestinal tract, from the mouth to the anus, and may be associated with penetrating phenomena such as intraperitoneal abscesses or fistulas [3]. Although the etiology is unknown, it is believed that the interaction between environmental factors and the gut microbiota of a genetically susceptible host leads to the abnormal immune response of the colic mucosa observed in these diseases [4].

Traditionally, the process of drug development for the treatment of IBD involves the discovery and selection of targets, followed by biological confirmation in cellular and animal models. When promising results are found at this stage, phase I, II and III clinical studies are carried out to investigate the safety, pharmacokinetics, clinical efficacy, and dosage of the drug [5].

Conventional therapies such as aminosalicylic acid, corticosteroids, immunomodulators and anti-tumor necrosis factor agents continue to demonstrate therapeutic efficacy, particularly when used in combination. However, despite the variety of therapeutic compounds available and the improved management strategies, a portion of IBD patients with moderate to severe degrees of the disease do not benefit from the existing treatments or experience side effects caused by the drugs used [6,7]. This has been a driving force for the intensive search for new drugs aimed at IBD therapy as well as the evaluation of potential IBD-related adverse effects [7].

In fact, aiming to increase the range of therapeutic options, new strategies with other biological agents and, more recently, with small-molecule drugs have been explored. Based on more accurate and targeted management of the disease, treatments with fewer adverse effects have been sought. In recent efforts, new inhibitors, whose targets include cytokines (such as IL-12/23 inhibitors, PDE4 inhibitors) [8,9], integrins (such as integrin inhibitors) [10], cytokine signaling pathways (such as Janus Kinases—JAK inhibitors) [11], and cell signaling receptors (such as Sphingosine 1-Phosphate Receptor—S1p modulators) [12], have become potentially promising therapeutic choices for many IBD patients.

Computational methods have also been employed in the development of drugs for the treatment of IBD, aiming to discover drugs in a more sustainable and economical way. These methods, together with the traditional drug development process, have contributed not only to the identification of more specific therapeutic targets, but also to novel applications of existing drugs [13].

This Special Issue included eight current research articles and three review articles with contributions to therapeutic decision-making and propositions of new therapeutic targets for IBD. We emphasize that it is not the objective of this Editorial to make a detailed description of each of the works, but rather to encourage the reader to explore them.

Two research studies published in this Special Issue aimed to investigate how two antidiabetic drugs of the thiazolidinedione class of agonists of the nuclear hormone receptor 'peroxisome proliferator-activated receptor gamma' (PPARγ), rosiglitazone and pioglitazone, can affect the risk of IBD.

In the first of these studies, Tseng (contribution 1) demonstrated that the use of rosiglitazone does not affect IBD risk, based on information from the reimbursement database of Taiwan's National Health Insurance. However, as this was an observational study with a small number of cases of UC, it was not possible to exclude the benefit of rosiglitazone for patients affected specifically by this pathology. In the second study, using the same database, Tseng further observed that pioglitazone had no effect on IBD at the doses used for the Taiwanese population (contribution 2).

With the objective of improving disease management strategies, two articles published in this Special Issue addressed strategies that can, in some way, assist in therapeutic decision-making: one related to the gene expression of mediators in the colic mucosa and the other related to changes in the form of drug administration.

Alafarj et al. (contribution 3) investigated changes in gene expression in the colic mucosa of IBD patients treated with 5-amino salicylic acid or biological therapy (anti-TNF drugs), IBD patients receiving no medication, and individuals without IBD. The study showed the importance of molecular analysis of biomarkers in the evaluation of inflammation, contributing to therapeutic decision-making.

Oršić Frič et al. (contribution 4) compared the vedolizumab serum trough concentration, efficacy and safety before and six months after changing the route of administration from intravenous to subcutaneous, but in a low number of patients. The authors demonstrated that the mean trough serum concentration of subcutaneous vedolizumab was significantly higher than that of intravenous vedolizumab, with the efficacy and safety previously established for patients on maintenance therapy with intravenous vedolizumab.

Four articles addressed the search for therapeutic alternatives for the treatment of IBD (contributions 5 to 8).

Lebish et al. (contribution 5) used inhibitors of the MAPK-activated protein kinase 2 (MK2) pathway, an important pathway in the regulation of cytokines in IBD and highly expressed and activated in tissues of patients affected by CD, to study a new therapeutic alternative. It was identified that MK2 regulates the expression of specific matrix metalloproteinases, and its inhibition decreases not only T-cell activity, but also the production of inflammatory cytokines. In view of previously published data on the safety of MK2 inhibitors in humans and the results presented in this study, Lebish et al. suggested that MK2 could be a new therapeutic target for CD.

Saber et al. (contribution 6) introduced a new therapeutic approach in order to improve the treatment of chronic UC. In this study, (R,R)-BD-AcAc2, a type of ketone ester (KE), improved the macroscopic and microscopic characteristics of the colon, exhibiting anti-inflammatory properties by reducing the production of pro-inflammatory cytokines. Although the use of an animal model cannot fully capture the intricate complexities of human pathophysiology, the authors concluded that this preclinical study indicated a potential therapeutic benefit of ketosis and ketone production in the treatment of IBD.

Assuming that the transforming growth factor-β/Smad (TGF-β/Smad) signaling pathway is inactivated in CD patients by Smad 7 overexpression and that clinical studies using oral Smad 7 antisense oligonucleotides were discontinued, Tsujimura et al. (contribution 7) tested the complex formed by microRNA (miR-497a-5p) and apatite super carbonate nanoparticle (sCA-miR-497a-5p) in the DSS-induced colitis model. Through the regulation of multiple genes rather than a single molecule, sCA-miR-497a-5p exerted a potent anti-inflammatory effect through the activation of the TGF-β/Smad signaling pathway and the inhibition of secretion inflammatory cytokines. Therefore, the authors suggested that this complex may have a therapeutic ability against IBD.

Jin et al. (contribution 8) investigated the activity of Ren-Shen-Bai-Du powder (RSBDP), which is already currently used for the treatment of IBD in China. RSBDP protected the colic mucosa of DSS-challenged animals by reducing the concentration of pro-inflammatory cytokines and promoting apoptosis of intestinal epithelial cells. The authors attributed the pharmacological effects shown by RSBDP to the main specialized metabolites (quercetin, kaempferol, luteolin, naringenin, and sitosterol) present in its constitution and provided contributions regarding the anti-inflammatory mechanisms of the currently used RSBDP in IBD therapy.

In addition to research articles, three interesting review articles were published in this Special Issue.

In the first, Blagov et al. (contribution 9) conducted a review of studies published with experimental models and clinical studies and described in detail the involvement of oxidative stress, with the accumulation of reactive oxygen species (ROS), in the chronic inflammation observed in IBD. The effects and mechanism of action of several natural antioxidants, as well as other antioxidants that have not yet been tested in the treatment of IBD, were also considered in this work.

The second review article (contribution 10) assembled the major targets and agents currently directed at the production of pro-inflammatory cytokines and lymphatic trafficking in order to contribute to the development of new drugs for IBD.

Finally, Imbrizi et al. (contribution 11) carried out a narrative review that elegantly presented the therapeutic advances in the treatment of IBD, the mechanisms of action, and the challenges facing the therapeutic goals in the treatment of IBD. Interestingly, the authors showed that despite the different mechanisms of action of the different classes of drugs, the general rates of effectiveness are similar, including the latest therapeutic classes approved for the treatment of IBD, JAK inhibitors and S1p modulators.

In conclusion, conventional therapies are still widely used, especially in the treatment of mild and moderate levels of IBD. However, the variable responses of IBD patients can lead to relapses, and this highlights the need to explore new treatment alternatives capable of addressing unmet needs and reducing adverse effects. The development of new therapeutic classes, as well as the combination of biological agents and small molecules, can bring substantial benefits for the therapeutic management of IBD. Finally, computational approaches have been used to identify metabolite–target interactions, providing several new drug targets for potential immune therapies.

We hope that the articles and reviews in this Special Issue meet the expectations of readers in the field and further promote investigations on the treatment of IBD by the scientific community.

Author Contributions: A.L.-F.: conceptualization, literature search, writing—review and editing. C.S.: conceptualization, literature search, writing—review and editing. All authors have read and agreed to the published version of the manuscript.

Funding: This research received no external funding.

Institutional Review Board Statement: Not applicable.

Informed Consent Statement: Not applicable.

Data Availability Statement: Data is contained within the article.

Acknowledgments: The Guest Editors wish to thank of all the authors for their valuable contributions to this Special Issue. We also thank of all the reviewers for their work in evaluating the submitted.

Conflicts of Interest: The authors declare no conflicts of interest.

List of Contributions:

1. Tseng, C.-H. Rosiglitazone Does Not Affect the Risk of Inflammatory Bowel Disease: A Retrospective Cohort Study in Taiwanese Type 2 Diabetes Patients. *Pharmaceuticals* 2023, 16, 679. https://doi.org/10.3390/ph16050679.

2. Tseng, C.-H. Pioglitazone Has a Null Association with Inflammatory Bowel Disease in Patients with Type 2 Diabetes Mellitus. *Pharmaceuticals* **2022**, *15*, 1538. https://doi.org/10.3390/ph15121538.
3. Alarfaj, S.J.; Mostafa, S.A.; Negm, W.A.; El-Masry, T.A.; Kamal, M.; Elsaeed, M.; El Nakib, A.M. Mucosal Genes Expression in Inflammatory Bowel Disease Patients: New Insights. *Pharmaceuticals* **2023**, *16*, 324. https://doi.org/10.3390/ph16020324.
4. Oršić Frič, V.; Borzan, V.; Šahinović, I.; Borzan, A.; Kurbel, S. Real-World Study on Vedolizumab Serum Concentration, Efficacy, and Safety after the Transition from Intravenous to Subcutaneous Vedolizumab in Inflammatory Bowel Disease Patients: Single-Center Experience. *Pharmaceuticals* **2023**, *16*, 239. https://doi.org/10.3390/ph16020239.
5. Lebish, E.J.; Morgan, N.J.; Valentine, J.F.; Beswick, E.J. MK2 Inhibitors as a Potential Crohn's Disease Treatment Approach for Regulating MMP Expression, Cleavage of Checkpoint Molecules and T Cell Activity. *Pharmaceuticals* **2022**, *15*, 1508. https://doi.org/10.3390/ph15121508.
6. Saber, S.; Alamri, M.M.S.; Alfaifi, J.; Saleh, L.A.; Abdel-Ghany, S.; Aboregela, A.M.; Farrag, A.A.; Almaeen, A.H.; Adam, M.I.E.; AlQahtani, A.A.J.; et al. (R,R)-BD-AcAc2 Mitigates Chronic Colitis in Rats: A Promising Multi-Pronged Approach Modulating Inflammasome Activity, Autophagy, and Pyroptosis. *Pharmaceuticals* **2023**, *16*, 953. https://doi.org/10.3390/ph16070953.
7. Tsujimura, N.; Ogino, T.; Hiraki, M.; Kai, T.; Yamamoto, H.; Hirose, H.; Yokoyama, Y.; Sekido, Y.; Hata, T.; Miyoshi, N.; et al. Super Carbonate Apatite-miR-497a-5p Complex Is a Promising Therapeutic Option against Inflammatory Bowel Disease. *Pharmaceuticals* **2023**, *16*, 618. https://doi.org/10.3390/ph16040618.
8. Jin, N.; Liu, Y.; Xiong, P.; Zhang, Y.; Mo, J.; Huang, X.; Zhou, Y. Exploring the Underlying Mechanism of Ren-Shen-Bai-Du Powder for Treating Inflammatory Bowel Disease Based on Network Pharmacology and Molecular Docking. *Pharmaceuticals* **2022**, *15*, 1038. https://doi.org/10.3390/ph15091038.
9. Blagov, A.V.; Orekhova, V.A.; Sukhorukov, V.N.; Melnichenko, A.A.; Orekhov, A.N. Potential Use of Antioxidant Compounds for the Treatment of Inflammatory Bowel Disease. *Pharmaceuticals* **2023**, *16*, 1150. https://doi.org/10.3390/ph16081150.
10. Song, Y.; Yuan, M.; Xu, Y.; Xu, H. Tackling Inflammatory Bowel Diseases: Targeting Proinflammatory Cytokines and Lymphocyte Homing. *Pharmaceuticals* **2022**, *15*, 1080. https://doi.org/10.3390/ph15091080.
11. Imbrizi, M.; Magro, F.; Coy, C.S.R. Pharmacological Therapy in Inflammatory Bowel Diseases: A Narrative Review of the Past 90 Years. *Pharmaceuticals* **2023**, *16*, 1272. https://doi.org/10.3390/ph16091272.

References

1. Alves de Almeida, A.C.; de-Faria, F.M.; Dunder, R.J.; Manzo, L.P.B.; Souza-Brito, A.R.M.; Luiz-Ferreira, A. Recent Trends in Pharmacological Activity of Alkaloids in Animal Colitis: Potential Use for Inflammatory Bowel Disease. *Evid.-Based Complement. Altern. Med.* **2017**, *2017*, 8528210. [CrossRef] [PubMed]
2. Biamonte, P.; D'Amico, F.; Fasulo, E.; Barà, R.; Bernardi, F.; Allocca, M.; Zilli, A.; Danese, S.; Furfaro, F. New Technologies in Digestive Endoscopy for Ulcerative Colitis Patients. *Biomedicines* **2023**, *11*, 2139. [CrossRef] [PubMed]
3. Pasternak, G.; Chrzanowski, G.; Aebisher, D.; Myśliwiec, A.; Dynarowicz, K.; Bartusik-Aebisher, D.; Sosna, B.; Cieślar, G.; Kawczyk-Krupka, A.; Filip, R. Crohn's Disease: Basic Characteristics of the Disease, Diagnostic Methods, the Role of Biomarkers, and Analysis of Metalloproteinases: A Review. *Life* **2023**, *13*, 2062. [CrossRef] [PubMed]
4. Agrawal, M.; Allin, K.H.; Petralia, F.; Colombel, J.-F.; Jess, T. Multiomics to Elucidate Inflammatory Bowel Disease Risk Factors and Pathways. *Nat. Rev. Gastroenterol. Hepatol.* **2022**, *19*, 399–409. [CrossRef]
5. Danese, S.; Fiocchi, C.; Panés, J. Drug Development in IBD: From Novel Target Identification to Early Clinical Trials. *Gut* **2016**, *65*, 1233–1239. [CrossRef] [PubMed]
6. Sobczak, M.; Fabisiak, A.; Murawska, N.; Wesołowska, E.; Wierzbicka, P.; Wlazłowski, M.; Wójcikowska, M.; Zatorski, H.; Zwolińska, M.; Fichna, J. Current Overview of Extrinsic and Intrinsic Factors in Etiology and Progression of Inflammatory Bowel Diseases. *Pharmacol. Rep.* **2014**, *66*, 766–775. [CrossRef] [PubMed]
7. Salvatori, S.; Neri, B.; Marafini, I.; Brigida, M.; Monteleone, G. Emerging Oral Drug Options for Ulcerative Colitis. *Expert Opin. Emerg. Drugs* **2023**, *28*, 191–201. [CrossRef] [PubMed]
8. Ma, C.; Panaccione, R.; Khanna, R.; Feagan, B.G.; Jairath, V. IL12/23 or Selective IL23 Inhibition for the Management of Moderate-to-Severe Crohn's Disease? *Best Pract. Res. Clin. Gastroenterol.* **2019**, *38–39*, 101604. [CrossRef] [PubMed]
9. Picchianti-Diamanti, A.; Spinelli, F.R.; Rosado, M.M.; Conti, F.; Laganà, B. Inhibition of Phosphodiesterase-4 in Psoriatic Arthritis and Inflammatory Bowel Diseases. *Int. J. Mol. Sci.* **2021**, *22*, 2638. [CrossRef] [PubMed]

10. Sandborn, W.J.; Vermeire, S.; Tyrrell, H.; Hassanali, A.; Lacey, S.; Tole, S.; Tatro, A.R. The Etrolizumab Global Steering Committee Etrolizumab for the Treatment of Ulcerative Colitis and Crohn's Disease: An Overview of the Phase 3 Clinical Program. *Adv. Ther.* **2020**, *37*, 3417–3431. [CrossRef] [PubMed]
11. Parigi, T.L.; D'Amico, F.; Danese, S. Upadacitinib for Crohn's Disease and Ulcerative Colitis Treatment: Hitting the Selective JAKpot. *Gastroenterology* **2021**, *160*, 1472–1474. [CrossRef] [PubMed]
12. Verstockt, B.; Vetrano, S.; Salas, A.; Nayeri, S.; Duijvestein, M.; Vande Casteele, N.; Alimentiv Translational Research Consortium (ATRC); Danese, S.; D'Haens, G.; Eckmann, L.; et al. Sphingosine 1-Phosphate Modulation and Immune Cell Trafficking in Inflammatory Bowel Disease. *Nat. Rev. Gastroenterol. Hepatol.* **2022**, *19*, 351–366. [CrossRef] [PubMed]
13. Johnson, T.O.; Akinsanmi, A.O.; Ejembi, S.A.; Adeyemi, O.E.; Oche, J.-R.; Johnson, G.I.; Adegboyega, A.E. Modern Drug Discovery for Inflammatory Bowel Disease: The Role of Computational Methods. *World J. Gastroenterol.* **2023**, *29*, 310–331. [CrossRef] [PubMed]

Disclaimer/Publisher's Note: The statements, opinions and data contained in all publications are solely those of the individual author(s) and contributor(s) and not of MDPI and/or the editor(s). MDPI and/or the editor(s) disclaim responsibility for any injury to people or property resulting from any ideas, methods, instructions or products referred to in the content.

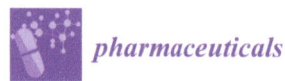

Article

Rosiglitazone Does Not Affect the Risk of Inflammatory Bowel Disease: A Retrospective Cohort Study in Taiwanese Type 2 Diabetes Patients

Chin-Hsiao Tseng [1,2,3]

1 Department of Internal Medicine, National Taiwan University College of Medicine, Taipei 10051, Taiwan; ccktsh@ms6.hinet.net
2 Division of Endocrinology and Metabolism, Department of Internal Medicine, National Taiwan University Hospital, Taipei 10002, Taiwan
3 National Institute of Environmental Health Sciences of the National Health Research Institutes, Zhunan 35053, Taiwan

Abstract: Human studies on the effect of rosiglitazone on inflammatory bowel disease (IBD) are still lacking. We investigated whether rosiglitazone might affect IBD risk by using the reimbursement database of Taiwan's National Health Insurance to enroll a propensity-score-matched cohort of ever users and never users of rosiglitazone. The patients should have been newly diagnosed with diabetes mellitus between 1999 and 2006 and should have been alive on 1 January 2007. We then started to follow the patients from 1 January 2007 until 31 December 2011 for a new diagnosis of IBD. Propensity-score-weighted hazard ratios were estimated with regards to rosiglitazone exposure in terms of ever users versus never users and in terms of cumulative duration and cumulative dose of rosiglitazone therapy for dose–response analyses. The joint effects and interactions between rosiglitazone and risk factors of psoriasis/arthropathies, dorsopathies, and chronic obstructive pulmonary disease/tobacco abuse and the use of metformin were estimated by Cox regression after adjustment for all covariates. A total of 6226 ever users and 6226 never users were identified and the respective numbers of incident IBD were 95 and 111. When we compared the risk of IBD in ever users to that of the never users, the estimated hazard ratio (0.870, 95% confidence interval: 0.661–1.144) was not statistically significant. When cumulative duration and cumulative dose of rosiglitazone therapy were categorized by tertiles and hazard ratios were estimated by comparing the tertiles of rosiglitazone exposure to the never users, none of the hazard ratios reached statistical significance. In secondary analyses, rosiglitazone has a null association with Crohn's disease, but a potential benefit on ulcerative colitis (UC) could not be excluded. However, because of the low incidence of UC, we were not able to perform detailed dose–response analyses for UC. In the joint effect analyses, only the subgroup of psoriasis/arthropathies (-)/rosiglitazone (-) showed a significantly lower risk in comparison to the subgroup of psoriasis/arthropathies (+)/rosiglitazone (-). No interactions between rosiglitazone and the major risk factors or metformin use were observed. We concluded that rosiglitazone has a null effect on the risk of IBD, but the potential benefit on UC awaits further investigation.

Keywords: Crohn's disease; inflammatory bowel disease; pharmacoepidemiology; rosiglitazone; Taiwan; type 2 diabetes mellitus; ulcerative colitis

Citation: Tseng, C.-H. Rosiglitazone Does Not Affect the Risk of Inflammatory Bowel Disease: A Retrospective Cohort Study in Taiwanese Type 2 Diabetes Patients. *Pharmaceuticals* 2023, 16, 679. https://doi.org/10.3390/ph16050679

Academic Editors: Anderson Luiz-Ferreira and Carmine Stolfi

Received: 14 March 2023
Revised: 27 April 2023
Accepted: 29 April 2023
Published: 1 May 2023

Copyright: © 2023 by the author. Licensee MDPI, Basel, Switzerland. This article is an open access article distributed under the terms and conditions of the Creative Commons Attribution (CC BY) license (https://creativecommons.org/licenses/by/4.0/).

1. Introduction

Inflammatory bowel disease (IBD) is a chronic relapsing inflammatory disease of the intestinal tract mediated by immunity. It may have varying courses and complications, and both the innate immune system and the adaptive immune system can be involved [1–3]. Proinflammatory immune mediators such as interleukin 17, interleukin 23, interferon gamma, and tumor necrosis factor alpha are always excessively expressed [4–6].

IBD is generally classified as Crohn's disease (CD) and ulcerative colitis (UC) [7] and the clinical manifestations may include watery diarrhea, fatigue, weight loss, abdominal pain, and bleeding [4]. Diarrhea may be insidious and episodic and can occur intermittently for many years before IBD is diagnosed, and patients may have suffered from significant body weight loss and malnutrition at the time of its diagnosis [4]. Intestinal fistulas to adjacent structures such as bowel, vagina, bladder, or skin can happen in 20–40% of the patients with CD [4]. Perianal fistula is associated with a more aggressive phenotype of the disease [4]. Chronic inflammation may lead to the development of strictures and intestinal obstruction [4]. Fever is usually low grade but higher fever may indicate more severe inflammation or is a sign of abscess formation or perforation [4]. Sometimes IBD can be life-threatening because of severe bleeding in 1–2% of the patients [4,8].

Extraintestinal involvement of skin, joints, eyes, liver, bile ducts, kidney, bone, and cardiovascular system can be seen in up to half of the patients [4,9–11]. Furthermore, IBD may increase the risk of colorectal cancer [12,13] and patients with IBD may have a higher incidence of atherosclerotic cardiovascular diseases, heart failure, atrial fibrillation [14], psoriasis [15], Alzheimer's disease [16,17], depression, and anxiety [18–20].

Because biomarkers, such as C-reactive protein, fecal calprotectin, interleukins, tumor necrosis factor alpha, antibodies, etc., are nonspecific and clinical presentations always have difficulty differentiating between the two disease entities of CD and UC, laboratory examinations such as colonoscopy, ultrasonography, computed tomography enterography, or magnetic resonance enterography are necessary for aiding in the diagnosis of IBD [4,21,22].

Some type of colitis may occur in approximately 10–15% of the population [8]. The highest prevalence rates of IBD (approximately 0.3%) are reported in Europe and North America, but its incidence seems to be stable or decreasing in these countries [23]. The incidence and prevalence of IBD in Asia, South America, and Africa are usually lower than those observed in Western countries [2,23–26]. However, the incidence of IBD has been increasing in these newly industrialized countries since 1990s [2,23–26]. In South Korea, IBD prevalence and incidence in 2015 were approximately 108.4 per 100,000 population and 9 per 100,000 population, respectively [27]. IBD increased by approximately 2.3% from 2010 to 2019 in South Korea [28]. In Taiwan, the respective prevalence and incidence rates were 16.7 and 1.4 per 100,000 population in 2015 [27], and the annual percentage change in the increasing incidence of IBD from 1998 to 2008 has been estimated to be 4% to 5% [23]. In China, it was reported that the age-standardized incidence and prevalence both increased by approximately 2.5-fold within a period of 30 years from 1990 to 2019 [29]. Asian immigrants to Western countries also experience an increasing incidence of IBD [30].

Though not fully elucidated, the etiology of IBD involves the interplay among host, microbiota, and environmental factors [1,2,8,31–36]. Researchers have identified more than 230 genetic loci associated with IBD. These genes are primarily involved in major histocompatibility complex, pattern recognition, inflammation, and apoptosis [4,37–39]. Environmental risk factors relating to industrialization and excessive sanitation and hygiene have been reported. More specifically, risk factors may include metabolic syndrome, lack of exercise, work shift, psychological stress, vitamin D deficiency, and dietary patterns (more consumption of calorically dense diet, animal protein, high-fat diet and high-sugar diet and less intake of fiber-containing vegetables, fruits, cereals, and nuts) [2,37,40–43]. In addition, milk formula feeding, history of childhood infection and vaccination, and medications such as antibiotics, nonsteroidal anti-inflammatory drugs, and oral contraceptives have also been reported [2,37,40–43]. On the other hand, breastfeeding is protective against IBD [2]. Studies also suggested that cigarette smoking and appendectomy both aggravate CD but may alleviate UC [2]. Gut microbiota are pivotal in the development of IBD because they may produce metabolites that affect the hosts' immune response and control the release of inflammatory cytokines [44].

The peroxisome proliferator–activator receptors (PPARs) belong to the nuclear hormone receptors' superfamily which contains three isoforms, i.e., PPARα, PPARβ/δ, and PPARγ [1,8]. They act as transcription factors that activate the expression of various genes [1]. PPARγ is abundantly expressed in colonic epithelial cells and exerts antiproliferative, anti-inflammatory, and immune modulating effects [1,8,45,46]. The usefulness of PPARγ in the treatment of IBD has long been investigated in preclinical studies [1,8,47–52]. Emodin is a Chinese herb drug that has been used to treat IBD. Its potential mode of action is through the activation of PPARγ-related signaling [53].

A class of oral antidiabetic drugs known as thiazolidinedione (TZD) improves insulin resistance by targeting PPARγ. In Taiwan, only two drugs in the class, i.e., rosiglitazone and pioglitazone, have been marketed [54]. However, rosiglitazone has been withdrawn from the market in many countries, including Taiwan, following the publication of a meta-analysis in 2007 that suggested a significantly higher risk of cardiovascular disease [55]. Pioglitazone survived the market even though a signal of increased risk of bladder cancer was raised in 2011 [56].

To our knowledge, there are scanty population-based studies investigating the potential role of antidiabetic drugs in the class of TZD in the prevention of IBD in humans. In our recent study, we found a null association between pioglitazone (the only TZD currently available in Taiwan) exposure and IBD risk in Taiwanese patients with type 2 diabetes mellitus [57]. Although rosiglitazone is not currently used in clinical practice in Taiwan, it remains a clinically important issue to look into the potential usefulness of rosiglitazone in the prevention of an intractable disease of IBD. In the present study, we investigated IBD risk with regard to rosiglitazone exposure in a cohort of patients with type 2 diabetes mellitus matched on propensity score by using the reimbursement database derived from the nationwide National Health Insurance (NHI) in Taiwan.

2. Results

As shown in Table 1, ever users and never users of rosiglitazone derived from the NHI database and matched on propensity score (PS) are well balanced in all characteristics because none of the variables showed a value of standardized difference between ever users and never users of rosiglitazone > 10%.

Table 1. Characteristics of enrolled subjects with regard to rosiglitazone exposure in a propensity-score-matched cohort.

Variable	Never Users of Rosiglitazone (n = 6226)		Ever Users of Rosiglitazone (n = 6226)		p Value	Standardized Difference
	n	%	n	%		
Basic information						
Age * (years)	63.83	12.13	63.85	11.92	0.9488	−0.03
Sex (men)	3392	54.48	3330	53.49	0.2649	−2.10
Diabetes duration * (years)	5.69	2.18	5.69	2.07	0.9845	0.15
Occupation					0.9402	
I	2638	42.37	2643	42.45		
II	1276	20.49	1250	20.08		−1.01
III	1123	18.04	1127	18.10		0.32
IV	1189	19.10	1206	19.37		0.64
Living region					0.5279	
Taipei	2531	40.65	2472	39.70		
Northern	575	9.24	593	9.52		0.97
Central	1671	26.84	1734	27.85		2.42
Southern	644	10.34	659	10.58		0.87
Kao-Ping and Eastern	805	12.93	768	12.34		−1.85

Table 1. *Cont.*

Variable	Never Users of Rosiglitazone (*n* = 6226)		Ever Users of Rosiglitazone (*n* = 6226)		*p* Value	Standardized Difference
	n	%	n	%		
Major comorbidities associated with diabetes mellitus						
Hypertension	5295	85.05	5290	84.97	0.9001	−0.25
Dyslipidemia	5168	83.01	5150	82.72	0.6686	−0.76
Obesity	319	5.12	340	5.46	0.4006	1.48
Diabetes-related complications						
Ischemic heart disease	3209	51.54	3153	50.64	0.3154	−1.87
Stroke	2185	35.09	2167	34.81	0.7351	−0.70
Peripheral arterial disease	1785	28.67	1785	28.67	0.6492	0.74
Diabetic polyneuropathy	2042	32.80	2093	33.62	0.3318	1.67
Eye disease	2480	39.83	2498	40.12	0.7419	0.61
Nephropathy	1942	31.19	1959	31.46	0.7426	0.48
Factors that might affect exposure/outcome						
Gingival and periodontal diseases	5393	86.62	5396	86.67	0.9370	0.22
Pulmonary tuberculosis	262	4.21	293	4.71	0.1782	2.26
Pneumonia	1106	17.76	1187	19.07	0.0611	3.27
Head injury	242	3.89	236	3.79	0.7796	−0.47
Dementia	502	8.06	521	8.37	0.5352	0.99
Parkinson's disease	204	3.28	207	3.32	0.8804	0.32
Hypoglycemia	446	7.16	470	7.55	0.4100	1.40
Osteoporosis	1295	20.80	1338	21.49	0.3453	1.67
Human immunodeficiency virus infection	6	0.10	5	0.08	0.7629	−0.63
Cancer	1091	17.52	1093	17.56	0.9624	−0.01
Alcohol-related diagnoses	344	5.53	346	5.56	0.9376	0.22
Tobacco abuse	183	2.94	189	3.04	0.7521	0.47
Chronic obstructive pulmonary disease	3070	49.31	3111	49.97	0.4624	1.08
Heart failure	1379	22.15	1386	22.26	0.8800	0.18
Valvular heart disease	704	11.31	745	11.97	0.2519	2.03
Dorsopathies	4789	76.92	4790	76.94	0.9830	−0.02
Arthropathies and related disorders	4949	79.49	4913	78.91	0.4267	−1.50
Psoriasis and similar disorders	173	2.78	176	2.83	0.8706	0.26
Organ transplantation	44	0.71	43	0.69	0.9143	−0.15
Hepatitis B virus infection	250	4.02	234	3.76	0.4582	−1.27
Hepatitis C virus infection	294	4.72	268	4.30	0.2617	−1.89
Liver cirrhosis	247	3.97	212	3.41	0.0960	−2.86
Other chronic nonalcoholic liver diseases	553	8.88	583	9.36	0.3505	1.72
Antidiabetic drugs						
Insulin	259	4.16	260	4.18	0.9642	0.33
Sulfonylureas	4495	72.20	4432	71.19	0.2101	−2.43
Metformin	4111	66.03	4068	65.34	0.4170	−1.28
Meglitinide	419	6.73	432	6.94	0.6443	0.76
Acarbose	708	11.37	748	12.01	0.2646	2.15
Other commonly used medications						
Angiotensin converting enzyme inhibitors/Angiotensin receptor blockers	4932	79.22	4878	78.35	0.2366	−2.17
Calcium channel blockers	3863	62.05	3828	61.48	0.5187	−1.21
Statins	4672	75.04	4635	74.45	0.4454	−1.38
Fibrates	2676	42.98	2717	43.64	0.4584	1.29
Aspirin	4183	67.19	4201	67.48	0.7309	0.59
Corticosteroids	251	4.03	241	3.87	0.6455	−0.67

* Age and diabetes duration are expressed as continuous variables in mean and standard deviation.

Table 2 shows the incident case numbers, incidence rates, and hazard ratios of IBD in never users of rosiglitazone and in different subgroups of ever users in the primary analyses. All results suggested a nonsignificant association between rosiglitazone and

IBD. In secondary analyses, when IBD was analyzed separately for CD and UC, we found that most of the IBD cases were diagnosed as CD (97 cases in never users and 92 cases in ever users) and only 18 cases were diagnosed as UC (15 cases in never users and 3 in ever users). The estimated hazard ratios for CD and UC were 0.964 (95% confidence interval: 0.725–1.282, p = 0.8016) and 0.203 (95% confidence interval: 0.059–0.700, p = 0.0116), respectively. For the dose–response analyses for cumulative duration and cumulative dose, none of the tertiles reached statistical significance for the CD analyses. Because there were only three cases of UC among ever users, we actually did not have sufficient case numbers for the dose–response analyses for UC in terms of cumulative duration and cumulative dose.

Table 2. Incident case numbers, incidence rates, and hazard ratios of inflammatory bowel disease in never users and in different subgroups of ever users of rosiglitazone.

Rosiglitazone Use	Number of Incident Case	Number of Cases Followed	Person-Years	Incidence Rate (per 100,000 Person-Years)	Hazard Ratio	95% Confidence Interval	p Value
Never users	111	6226	27,597.94	402.20	1.000		
Ever users	95	6226	27,235.66	348.81	0.870	(0.661–1.144)	0.3174
Tertiles of cumulative duration of rosiglitazone therapy (months)							
Never users	111	6226	27,597.94	402.20	1.000		
<12.4	29	2056	8782.12	330.22	0.826	(0.549–1.244)	0.3605
12.4–25.3	28	2054	8999.12	311.14	0.776	(0.513–1.174)	0.2301
>25.3	38	2116	9454.43	401.93	0.996	(0.689–1.440)	0.9843
Tertiles of cumulative dose of rosiglitazone therapy (mg)							
Never users	111	6226	27,597.94	402.20	1.000		
<1624	30	2044	8875.26	338.02	0.844	(0.564–1.263)	0.4090
1624–3596	32	2065	9179.81	348.59	0.866	(0.584–1.283)	0.4723
>3596	33	2117	9180.59	359.45	0.897	(0.608–1.323)	0.5844

Table 3 shows the results that investigated the joint effects of and interactions between rosiglitazone use and major risk factors of IBD/metformin after adjustment for all covariates listed in Table 1. In the analyses of joint effects, except for the subgroup of psoriasis/arthropathies (-)/rosiglitazone (-) that showed a significantly lower risk in comparison to the subgroup of psoriasis/arthropathies (+)/rosiglitazone (-), none of the other hazard ratios was statistically significant. There was a lack of significant interaction between rosiglitazone and the risk factors/metformin use in any of the models.

Table 3. Joint effects of and interactions between rosiglitazone and risk factors/metformin use.

Risk Factor/Rosiglitazone Use	Incident Case Number	Cases Followed	Person-Years	Incidence Rate (per 100,000 Person-Years)	Hazard Ratio	95% Confidence Interval	p Value
Psoriasis/Arthropathies (+)/Rosiglitazone (-)	98	4979	22,081.13	443.82	1.000		
Psoriasis/Arthropathies (+)/Rosiglitazone (+)	81	4948	21,709.31	373.11	0.828	(0.616–1.112)	0.2097
Psoriasis/Arthropathies (-)/Rosiglitazone (-)	13	1247	5516.81	235.64	0.523	(0.287–0.954)	0.0345
Psoriasis/Arthropathies (-)/Rosiglitazone (+)	14	1278	5526.35	253.33	0.571	(0.319–1.023)	0.0595
P-interaction							0.3103
Dorsopathies (+)/Rosiglitazone (-)	92	4789	21,291.34	432.10	1.000		
Dorsopathies (+)/Rosiglitazone (+)	73	4790	21,003.45	347.56	0.796	(0.584–1.083)	0.1463
Dorsopathies (-)/Rosiglitazone (-)	19	1437	6306.60	301.27	0.846	(0.508–1.410)	0.5214
Dorsopathies (-)/Rosiglitazone (+)	22	1436	6232.21	353.00	0.986	(0.608–1.597)	0.9533
P-interaction							0.2777
COPD/Tobacco abuse (+)/Rosiglitazone (-)	62	3143	13,853.61	447.54	1.000		
COPD/Tobacco abuse (+)/Rosiglitazone (+)	46	3181	13,834.35	332.51	0.733	(0.500–1.076)	0.1125

Table 3. Cont.

Risk Factor/Rosiglitazone Use	Incident Case Number	Cases Followed	Person-Years	Incidence Rate (per 100,000 Person-Years)	Hazard Ratio	95% Confidence Interval	p Value
COPD/Tobacco abuse (-)/Rosiglitazone (-)	49	3083	13,744.33	356.51	0.788	(0.534–1.163)	0.2304
COPD/Tobacco abuse (-)/Rosiglitazone (+)	49	3045	13,401.32	365.64	0.802	(0.544–1.182)	0.2647
P-interaction							0.7492
Metformin (-)/Rosiglitazone (-)	40	2115	9177.49	435.85	1.000		
Metformin (-)/Rosiglitazone (+)	34	2158	9383.34	362.34	0.789	(0.495–1.258)	0.3201
Metformin (+)/Rosiglitazone (-)	71	4111	18,420.45	385.44	0.798	(0.535–1.191)	0.2694
Metformin (+)/Rosiglitazone (+)	61	4068	17,852.32	341.69	0.718	(0.477–1.081)	0.1128
P-interaction							0.6761

COPD: chronic obstructive pulmonary disease.

3. Discussion

3.1. Main Findings

The findings of this study did not support any effect of rosiglitazone use on the risk of IBD (Table 2). Furthermore, no interaction was observed between rosiglitazone and any of the risk factors and between rosiglitazone and metformin (Table 3).

3.2. Explanations for the Discrepant Findings in Preclinical Studies

In in vitro and in vivo studies, PPARγ may have a potential benefit on IBD through the crosstalk with metabolism and inflammation [1,8,47–53]. However, there is a lack of evidence to support such a benefit in humans. Our previous study on pioglitazone [57] and the present study on rosiglitazone do not support such a benefit of either TZD on the occurrence of IBD in humans. There are some possible explanations for such discrepancies between preclinical studies and the observational studies conducted in humans.

First, it should be mentioned that colitis in animal models of IBD in preclinical studies is induced mainly by chemicals. Commonly used chemicals include oxazolone, dextran sodium sulphate, dinitrobenzene sulfonic acid, trinitrobenzene sulfonic acid, and intracolonic instillation of acetic acid [8]. Because the pathogenesis of the colitis induced by these chemicals might not be the same as that seen in human IBD, findings derived from in vitro and animal studies should not be directly applied to humans. Colitis induced by chemicals might lead to inflammation following the toxic damages to the colon, which is different from what we know about human IBD that is characterized by inflammation mainly induced by the induction of autoantibodies and the destruction by cytokines.

Second, the doses of rosiglitazone used in in vitro and in vivo studies and the concentrations of rosiglitazone in the medium or in the animals' blood derived from such administered doses might not be corresponding to the clinically used doses and the blood concentrations that might have been derived in patients with type 2 diabetes mellitus. In clinical trials, rosiglitazone is generally used in a daily dose of 2 to 12 mg [58]. In Taiwan, the generally prescribed daily dose of rosiglitazone is either 4 mg or 8 mg. Whether these clinically used doses of rosiglitazone can be translated to the concentrations used in in vitro or in animal studies [59–61] remains to be investigated.

Third, the blood concentration of rosiglitazone derived from oral administration while used for the treatment of hyperglycemia in humans does not guarantee a delivery of sufficient rosiglitazone to the colon for the activation of PPARγ locally. Recent drug development by using nanotechnology [59] or topical administration of rosiglitazone [61] may provide more specific delivery of rosiglitazone to the target organ and tissue and is worthy of more in-depth investigation. Novel PPARγ activators are also being investigated for the treatment of colitis in animals [46].

Fourth, the effects of rosiglitazone and pioglitazone may differ among different species, and the activation of PPARγ by rosiglitazone and pioglitazone in different cells may result in different biological functions, some even counteracting each other, resulting in a variety of different clinical effects. These may explain the different clinical effects of rosiglitazone and pioglitazone observed in different cancer and noncancer diseases in humans. For example, rosiglitazone may adversely affect lipid profile [62] and we did observe a lack of association between rosiglitazone and bladder cancer [63] and dementia [64] but a significantly lower risk of thyroid cancer [65]. On the other hand, pioglitazone improves lipid profiles [62], is associated with a significant risk reduction of dementia [66], and shows a null association with thyroid cancer [67]. Though controversial, a potentially higher risk of bladder cancer associated with pioglitazone use [56] should be cautiously attended. Therefore, rosiglitazone and pioglitazone should be viewed as different entities and they should be investigated separately and not together.

Fifth, though not statistically significant, the overall hazard ratio of 0.870 (95% confidence interval: 0.661–1.144) in Table 2 favored a risk reduction of approximately 13% associated with rosiglitazone use. We could not exclude the possibility of a lack of statistical power and a lack of adjustment for some unmeasured confounders such as microbiota and nutritional and dietary factors in the primary analyses. In secondary analyses, when CD and UC were separately analyzed, although the risk for CD associated with rosiglitazone use was not significant, we did observe a significantly lower risk of UC associated with rosiglitazone. Because there were only three cases of UC among ever users, we did not have sufficient incident case numbers for dose–response analyses for UC. We recognize that the currently available database is not competent to answer whether the effects of rosiglitazone might not be the same for CD and UC, and we cannot completely exclude a possible benefit of rosiglitazone on UC. Future analyses based on an additional request for a larger database from the NHI should be considered to answer these questions.

3.3. Potential Explanations for the Discrepant Findings between Metformin and TZDs

The discrepant findings between metformin [68], which shows a significantly reduced risk of IBD, and TZDs including pioglitazone [57] and rosiglitazone (the findings of the present study), which show a null association with IBD, implied some clues to the pathogenesis of IBD in patients with type 2 diabetes mellitus and deserved discussion.

PPARγ is abundantly expressed in the intestinal epithelium, where it plays important roles in maintaining a healthy intestinal tract by inhibiting the expression of inflammatory cytokines activated via either the innate or adaptive immune system [1–3]. However, environmental factors such as obesity [42] and compositional changes of the gut microbiota by diet or medications [1] are crucial in the development of IBD. The emergence of these environmental risk factors following the industrialization of our societies and Westernization of our lifestyle may contribute to the increasing trends of IBD in recent years in developing countries, including Taiwan [2,23–30], because genetic mutations may not be responsible for the rapid evolving change of the disease.

Downregulation of PPARγ expression may be triggered by these environmental risk factors, resulting in the activation of the immune-mediated inflammatory processes seen in IBD [1]. Although TZDs used in patients with type 2 diabetes mellitus may theoretically alleviate inflammation via the activation of PPARγ [69], such a benefit has not been well demonstrated in humans. TZDs may significantly increase body weight when used for glycemic control [70] and they do not significantly change the composition of gut microbiota either by rosiglitazone [71,72] or by pioglitazone [73]. Therefore, the anti-inflammatory effect of TZDs might have been offset by the body weight gain following their use.

On the other hand, metformin has some pleiotropic effects that TZDs do not possess. First, metformin does not increase body weight and it may even have a mild weight reduction effect [74]. Second, patients with IBD show a reduced relative abundance of *Akkermansia muciniphila*, and administration of this bacterial species has shown some promising results in the treatment of IBD [75–77]. A recent study suggests that metformin significantly increases the relative abundance of *Akkermansia* but pioglitazone fails to do so [78]. Another study shows that rosiglitazone treatment cannot restore the microbiota composition in mice fed with a high-fat diet [72]. *Akkermansia muciniphila* may produce metabolites including propionate and butyrate [76,79–81], which are important in amplifying the PPARγ transcriptional activities involving in the alleviation of the inflammatory processes of IBD [1].

In addition, metformin has an additional benefit of inhibiting the mammalian target of rapamycin (mTOR) [74], which is activated in patients with IBD and may be responsible for triggering the inflammatory process in IBD [82]. An early study showed that rosiglitazone might activate the mTOR signaling pathway, which mediates its adipogenic effect [83]. Another recent study confirmed the involvement of mTOR in rosiglitazone's regulation of adiponectin production and secretion and the oxidative metabolism of branched-chain amino acids [84]. Therefore, the anti-inflammatory benefits following the use of TZDs might have further been mitigated by their activation of the mTOR pathway which is actually inhibited by the use of metformin.

Our recent study suggested that metformin plays an important role in the inhibition of immune-mediated skin diseases including urticaria, allergic contact dermatitis, and psoriasis [85]. This observation provides a clue that metformin might also be able to modulate the autoimmune processes of IBD.

Because metformin [74] and TZDs [86] share similar effects on the improvement of insulin resistance and reduction of blood glucose, these metabolic actions may not satisfactorily explain the discrepant findings between these two classes of drugs.

Taken together, it seems reasonable to suggest that rectifying the PPARγ signaling pathways by TZDs, even if they really work, would not actually prevent the development of IBD clinically. On the other hand, the use of metformin may affect the development of IBD, probably through its exceptional ability to change the gut microbiota, to maintain or reduce body weight, to modulate autoimmunity, and to inhibit the mTOR pathway. All of these pleiotropic effects of metformin may collectively contribute to a significant and sustained alleviation of the inflammatory processes of IBD. The improvement in insulin resistance and glycemic control associated with the use of either metformin or TZDs may not be responsible for the discrepant findings observed in the development of IBD between these two classes of antidiabetic drugs.

3.4. Implications

There are several clinical implications from the present study. First, the potential benefits of rosiglitazone on IBD derived from preclinical studies should not be immediately interpreted as a potential usefulness in the treatment of human IBD; at least, our present study did not favor such a benefit of rosiglitazone. Together with the finding of a null association with pioglitazone [57], the usefulness of TZDs in the prevention or treatment of IBD in humans is not very optimistic, at least in their current formulations.

Second, because we found a potential benefit of rosiglitazone on UC but not on CD in the secondary analyses when IBD was analyzed for UC and CD separately, we were interested to know whether similar findings could be seen in patients treated with pioglitazone. We additionally analyzed the data in association with pioglitazone use (this was not conducted in our previously published paper [57]) and found that pioglitazone had a null effect on either UC or CD (data not shown). Therefore, future research should focus on more detailed analyses on the potential benefit of rosiglitazone on UC by enrolling enough case numbers of UC and with more adequate consideration of potential confounders.

Third, although rosiglitazone does not cause hypoglycemia and may have some potential benefits in the risk reduction of some cancers [65], it potentially increases the risk of heart failure [87] and cardiovascular disease [55]. Therefore, the reuse of rosiglitazone as an antidiabetic drug for treating hyperglycemia in patients with type 2 diabetes mellitus needs additional research to balance the potential risk and benefit.

3.5. Strengths

The use of a nationwide database that covers >99% of Taiwan's population may have some inherent merits. First, because of a lower risk of selection bias, we believe that the generalization of the findings to the whole population might be more confident. Second, the risk of information bias resulting from self-reporting was minimal because of the use of the objective medical records documented in the database. Third, it is less likely to have detection bias as a result of different socioeconomic status in the study because the healthcare services provided in the NHI system require very low drug cost-sharing and the copayment can even be waived when the patients receive prescription refills for chronic disease or when the patients have a low-income household or when the patients are veterans. Finally, we considered the timeframes of enrollment of patients and follow-up period by taking into account the potential psychological impacts of the attending physicians leading to their behavioral changes in the prescription of the drug and the possible nonadherence to the drug by the patients even when it had been prescribed when the issue of a potential risk of cardiovascular disease might be induced by rosiglitazone was brought up [55].

3.6. Limitations

The following study limitations must be considered. First, most confounders in the database were not collected primarily and we did not have measurement data such as family history, genetic parameters, lifestyle, smoking, alcohol drinking, anthropometric factors, dietary pattern, and nutritional status.

Second, biochemical data of levels of inflammatory cytokines, C-reactive protein, fecal calprotectin, glucose, and insulin were not available for analyses in the database.

Third, it should be mentioned that unmeasured confounders can never be statistically adjusted for. Therefore, we could not exclude the possible existence of some important confounders that might have influenced the results.

Fourth, because the average follow-up time was approximately 4.4 years in either the never users or the ever users (Table 2), we did not know whether such a relatively short period of time would be sufficient to capture the long-term effects of rosiglitazone on the risk of IBD.

Fifth, we did not have clinical information and laboratory data to investigate the severity of IBD in the patients.

Sixth, because of the lack of colonoscopic examination for the diagnosis of the outcome, misdiagnosis in some patients was possible. However, if the misclassification was not differential, we would expect a bias toward the null in the estimated hazard ratios [88,89].

Seventh, as mentioned earlier, we could not exclude the possibility of a lack of statistical power and the potential benefit of rosiglitazone on UC in secondary analysis. We think that future investigation with a request of a larger database of the NHI is warranted.

Finally, because this is a retrospective matched cohort study, the interpretation of the results in terms of causal inference should be cautious and future prospective cohort studies or clinical trials are needed to confirm our findings.

Because of these potential limitations, the conclusions of the present work may not be directly extrapolated to clinical situations.

4. Materials and Methods

4.1. Taiwan's National Health Insurance

Taiwan has implemented a nationwide and compulsory healthcare insurance since 1 March 1995. This healthcare insurance is called the NHI and it covers more than 99.6% of Taiwan's population. To provide comprehensive and equal medical care to the insurants, the Bureau of the NHI has contracted with all hospitals and more than 93% of all medical settings in Taiwan. All medical records and reimbursement information, including disease diagnoses, medication prescriptions, and performed procedures, are stored in computerized files before submitting for reimbursement. Researchers can apply for academic use of the database after ethics review and approval. This study was approved by the Research Ethics Committee of the National Health Research Institutes with an approval number NHIRD-102-175.

Throughout the research period, the disease coding system used in the database was the International Classification of Diseases, Ninth Revision, Clinical Modification (ICD-9-CM). We used the codes of 250.XX as a diagnosis of diabetes mellitus. The codes of 555 (regional enteritis or CD) and/or 556 (ulcerative enterocolitis or UC) were used for IBD diagnosis, as previously used in our study investigating the effect of pioglitazone [57].

4.2. Enrollment of Study Subjects

This was a retrospective cohort study. We enrolled from the NHI database a cohort of 1:1 matched pairs of ever users and never users of rosiglitazone based on PS. The flowchart in Figure 1 shows the procedures that we followed in the enrollment of the subjects used for analyses. At first, we identified 444,984 new-onset diabetes patients within the period from 1999 to 2006. We did not include patients who had a diagnosis of diabetes mellitus between 1996 and 1998 to ensure that the patients' diagnosis of diabetes mellitus was made after 1999. To confirm a correct diagnosis of diabetes mellitus, the enrolled patients should have received prescriptions of antidiabetic drugs for at least two times at the outpatient clinics. We tried to maximize from the available database as many eligible patients as possible for follow-up and therefore we restricted the exclusion criteria to a minimum without unnecessary exclusions of eligible patients according to the steps shown in Figure 1. As a result, we identified an unmatched cohort consisting of 6226 ever users and 284,300 never users of rosiglitazone. Logistic regression that included all characteristics listed in Table 1 as independent variables was then used to create PS. The Greedy 8 → 1 digit match algorithm proposed by Parson [90] was then used to create a matched cohort consisting of 6226 ever users and 6226 never users.

In Taiwan, we have had only two drugs, namely, rosiglitazone and pioglitazone, marketed in the class of TZD. Following the challenge of a potential risk of cardiovascular disease associated with the use of rosiglitazone in a meta-analysis published in 2007 [55], rosiglitazone has been withdrawn from the markets of many countries, including Taiwan. To avoid the potential impact of some unknown factors following the publication of this meta-analysis, we restricted our analyses by enrolling patients of ever users of rosiglitazone based on the prescription of the drug before 2007 and excluding those who had a prescription of rosiglitazone after 2007 (Figure 1).

Users of pioglitazone were deliberately excluded for analyses (Figure 1) because of the following reasons:

Besides the glucose lowering effect, very different safety profiles in terms of cardiovascular disease, cancer, and dementia have been shown between rosiglitazone and pioglitazone. For example, rosiglitazone may have a potential risk of myocardial infarction and cardiovascular death [55]. On the other hand, pioglitazone may significantly improve lipid profiles [62], reduce cardiovascular events in patients with type 2 diabetes mellitus [91], and prevent secondary stroke in patients with insulin resistance and a previous ischemic stroke [92]. With regard to cancer, a potential risk of bladder cancer has been reported in patients who had been treated with pioglitazone, as shown in the interim analysis of the Kaiser Permanente Northern California study published in 2011 [56]. Furthermore, rosiglitazone significantly reduces the risk of thyroid cancer [65], but pioglitazone shows a null association with thyroid cancer [67]. Pioglitazone and rosiglitazone also show different effects on their association with dementia. As shown in our previous observational studies, a significantly lower risk of dementia was associated with pioglitazone [66] but not with rosiglitazone [64]. Therefore, rosiglitazone and pioglitazone should be viewed as two different entities when we intend to analyze the safety profile or the risk associated with cancer or noncancer diseases.

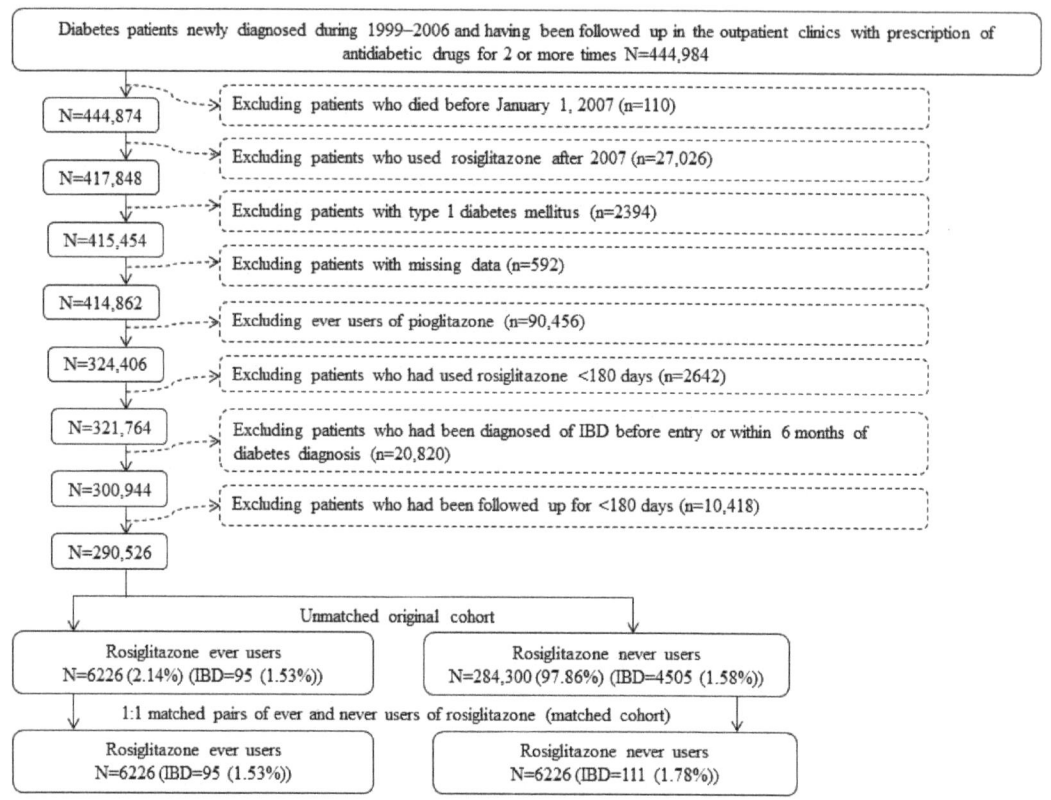

Figure 1. The procedures followed in the enrollment of study subjects. IBD: inflammatory bowel disease.

4.3. Potential Confounders and Statistical Analyses

Potential confounders are shown in Table 1. The ICD-9-CM codes for the related diagnoses have been reported previously [57].

The matched cohort was used for statistical analyses with the aid of the SAS statistical software, version 9.4 (SAS Institute, Cary, NC, USA). A $p < 0.05$ was used as a cutoff for indicating statistical significance.

Standardized difference was calculated for each covariate listed in Table 1 to examine the potential risk of confounding by indication. We used a cutoff value of >10% to indicate the potential existence of such a confounding from the variable. This is the generally recommended cutoff value by most investigators [93].

We calculated the cumulative duration in months and cumulative dose in mg of rosiglitazone therapy and categorized ever users according to the tertiles of these parameters for the assessment of a dose–response relationship. We calculated incidence density of IBD with regard to rosiglitazone exposure in never users, ever users, and subgroups of ever users categorized by the tertiles of cumulative duration and cumulative dose. We identified newly diagnosed cases of IBD during follow-up with regard to the different subgroups of rosiglitazone exposure. The numerators of the incidence density were the case numbers of newly diagnosed IBD in the respective subgroups. The denominators of the incidence density were the person-years of follow-up in the respective subgroups. We set the date of start of follow-up as 1 January 2007 and the patients were then followed up until 31 December 2011 when a new diagnosis of IBD was made, or the last reimbursement record, or the date of death, whichever occurred first.

For primary analyses, we estimated hazard ratios and their 95% confidence intervals for IBD by Cox proportional hazards regression model incorporated with the inverse probability of treatment weighting using the PS. In comparison to the never users, hazard ratios were estimated for ever users and for each tertile of cumulative duration and cumulative dose. In consideration that CD and UC may have different characteristics and clinical patterns, we also estimated the hazard ratios for CD and UC separately as secondary analyses.

We also evaluated the joint effects of rosiglitazone and some major risk factors of IBD by using the traditional Cox regression after adjustment for all covariates listed in Table 1. These major risk factors included psoriasis/arthropathies, dorsopathies (ankylosing spondylitis is associated with IBD [94]), and chronic obstructive pulmonary disease/tobacco abuse (as a surrogate marker for smoking that can affect IBD [2,95]). The joint effects were evaluated by estimating hazard ratios with regard to the presence and absence of risk factors and rosiglitazone use in the following subgroups: (1) risk factor (+)/rosiglitazone (-) as the referent group; (2) risk factor (+)/rosiglitazone (+); (3) risk factor (-)/rosiglitazone (-); and (4) risk factor (-)/rosiglitazone (+). We also estimated the value of P-interaction for each model.

Because we previously showed that metformin may reduce the risk of IBD [68], we additionally investigated the joint effect of and interaction between metformin and rosiglitazone.

5. Conclusions

The findings of the present study suggest that rosiglitazone does not affect the risk of IBD and that rosiglitazone does not interact with major risk factors or metformin in the development of IBD in patients with type 2 diabetes mellitus. However, we cannot exclude the possible benefit of rosiglitazone on UC in secondary analyses. Because this is an observational study that may have potential limitations including a lack of sufficient power (especially the small case numbers of UC) and an inability to consider all confounders, we acknowledge that further confirmation of the null effect of rosiglitazone on IBD observed in the present study is recommended. Personalized medicine [27] and application of nanotechnology [59,96,97] and artificial intelligence [98] may help to identify patients at a high risk of developing IBD and its related complications, and to identify subgroups of patients who can benefit from rosiglitazone treatment. These novel technologies should be incorporated in future research.

Funding: This research was funded by the Ministry of Science and Technology (MOST 103-2314-B-002-187-MY3) of Taiwan.

Institutional Review Board Statement: The study was conducted in accordance with the Declaration of Helsinki, and approved by the Ethics Committee of the National Health Research Institutes (approval number NHIRD-102-175).

Informed Consent Statement: Patient consent was waived because the personal information had been deidentified and the patient could not be contacted according to local regulations.

Data Availability Statement: The datasets in this article are not readily available because local regulations restrict public availability of the dataset to protect privacy. Requests to access the datasets should be directed to C.T., ccktsh@ms6.hinet.net.

Acknowledgments: The author thanks Ting-Ting Chan for her excellent performance in the statistical analyses for the study.

Conflicts of Interest: The author declares no conflict of interest.

References

1. Caioni, G.; Viscido, A.; d'Angelo, M.; Panella, G.; Castelli, V.; Merola, C.; Frieri, G.; Latella, G.; Cimini, A.; Benedetti, E. Inflammatory bowel disease: New insights into the interplay between environmental factors and PPARγ. *Int. J. Mol. Sci.* **2021**, *22*, 985. [CrossRef] [PubMed]
2. Baumgart, D.C.; Carding, S.R. Inflammatory bowel disease: Cause and immunobiology. *Lancet* **2007**, *369*, 1627–1640. [CrossRef] [PubMed]
3. Saez, A.; Herrero-Fernandez, B.; Gomez-Bris, R.; Sánchez-Martinez, H.; Gonzalez-Granado, J.M. Pathophysiology of inflammatory bowel disease: Innate immune system. *Int. J. Mol. Sci.* **2023**, *24*, 1526. [CrossRef]
4. Flynn, S.; Eisenstein, S. Inflammatory bowel disease presentation and diagnosis. *Surg. Clin. N. Am.* **2019**, *99*, 1051–1062. [CrossRef] [PubMed]
5. Parigi, T.L.; Iacucci, M.; Ghosh, S. Blockade of IL-23: What is in the pipeline? *J. Crohn's Colitis* **2022**, *16* (Suppl. S2), ii64–ii72. [CrossRef]
6. Noviello, D.; Mager, R.; Roda, G.; Borroni, R.G.; Fiorino, G.; Vetrano, S. The IL23-IL17 immune axis in the treatment of ulcerative colitis: Successes, defeats, and ongoing challenges. *Front. Immunol.* **2021**, *12*, 611256. [CrossRef]
7. Verstockt, B.; Bressler, B.; Martinez-Lozano, H.; McGovern, D.; Silverberg, M.S. Time to revisit disease classification in inflammatory bowel disease: Is the current classification of inflammatory bowel disease good enough for optimal clinical management? *Gastroenterology* **2022**, *162*, 1370–1382. [CrossRef]
8. Decara, J.; Rivera, P.; López-Gambero, A.J.; Serrano, A.; Pavón, F.J.; Baixeras, E.; Rodríguez de Fonseca, F.; Suárez, J. Peroxisome proliferator-activated receptors: Experimental targeting for the treatment of inflammatory bowel diseases. *Front. Pharmacol.* **2020**, *11*, 730. [CrossRef]
9. Pagani, K.; Lukac, D.; Bhukhan, A.; McGee, J.S. Cutaneous manifestations of inflammatory bowel disease: A basic overview. *Am. J. Clin. Dermatol.* **2022**, *23*, 481–497. [CrossRef]
10. Van Hoeve, K.; Hoffman, I. Renal manifestations in inflammatory bowel disease: A systematic review. *J. Gastroenterol.* **2022**, *57*, 619–629. [CrossRef]
11. Masood, F.; Ehrenpreis, E.D.; Rubin, G.; Russell, J.; Guru, S.; Luzzi, P. State of the art review: Coronary artery disease in patients with inflammatory bowel disease: Mechanisms, prevalence, and outcomes. *Acta. Cardiol.* **2022**, *77*, 297–306. [CrossRef] [PubMed]
12. Shah, S.C.; Itzkowitz, S.H. Colorectal cancer in inflammatory bowel disease: Mechanisms and management. *Gastroenterology* **2022**, *162*, 715–730.e3. [CrossRef]
13. Nagao-Kitamoto, H.; Kitamoto, S.; Kamada, N. Inflammatory bowel disease and carcinogenesis. *Cancer Metastasis Rev.* **2022**, *41*, 301–316. [CrossRef] [PubMed]
14. Chen, B.; Collen, L.V.; Mowat, C.; Isaacs, K.L.; Singh, S.; Kane, S.V.; Farraye, F.A.; Snapper, S.; Jneid, H.; Lavie, C.J.; et al. Inflammatory bowel disease and cardiovascular diseases. *Am. J. Med.* **2022**, *135*, 1453–1460. [CrossRef] [PubMed]
15. Li, Y.; Guo, J.; Cao, Z.; Wu, J. Causal association between inflammatory bowel disease and psoriasis: A two-sample bidirectional mendelian randomization study. *Front. Immunol.* **2022**, *13*, 916645. [CrossRef] [PubMed]
16. Wang, D.; Zhang, X.; Du, H. Inflammatory bowel disease: A potential pathogenic factor of Alzheimer's disease. *Prog. Neuropsychopharmacol. Biol. Psychiatry* **2022**, *119*, 110610. [CrossRef] [PubMed]
17. Zhang, M.N.; Shi, Y.D.; Jiang, H.Y. The risk of dementia in patients with inflammatory bowel disease: A systematic review and meta-analysis. *Int. J. Colorectal. Dis.* **2022**, *37*, 769–775. [CrossRef]
18. Luo, J.; Xu, Z.; Noordam, R.; van Heemst, D.; Li-Gao, R. Depression and inflammatory bowel disease: A didirectional two-sample mendelian randomization study. *J. Crohn's Colitis* **2022**, *16*, 633–642. [CrossRef]
19. Bisgaard, T.H.; Allin, K.H.; Keefer, L.; Ananthakrishnan, A.N.; Jess, T. Depression and anxiety in inflammatory bowel disease: Epidemiology, mechanisms and treatment. *Nat. Rev. Gastroenterol. Hepatol.* **2022**, *19*, 717–726. [CrossRef]
20. Masanetz, R.K.; Winkler, J.; Winner, B.; Günther, C.; Süß, P. The gut-immune-brain axis: An important route for neuropsychiatric morbidity in inflammatory bowel disease. *Int. J. Mol. Sci.* **2022**, *23*, 11111. [CrossRef]
21. Nardone, O.M.; Cannatelli, R.; Ghosh, S.; Iacucci, M. New endoscopic tools in inflammatory bowel disease. *United Eur. Gastroenterol. J.* **2022**, *10*, 1103–1112. [CrossRef] [PubMed]
22. Christian, M.; Giovanni, M.; Torsten, K.; Mariangela, A. Ultrasonography in inflammatory bowel disease—So far we are? *United Eur. Gastroenterol. J.* **2022**, *10*, 225–232. [CrossRef]
23. Ng, S.C.; Shi, H.Y.; Hamidi, N.; Underwood, F.E.; Tang, W.; Benchimol, E.I.; Panaccione, R.; Ghosh, S.; Wu, J.C.Y.; Chan, F.K.L.; et al. Worldwide incidence and prevalence of inflammatory bowel disease in the 21st century: A systematic review of population-based studies. *Lancet* **2018**, *390*, 2769–2778. [CrossRef] [PubMed]
24. Park, J.; Cheon, J.H. Incidence and prevalence of inflammatory bowel disease across Asia. *Yonsei Med. J.* **2021**, *62*, 99–108. [CrossRef] [PubMed]
25. Watermeyer, G.; Katsidzira, L.; Setshedi, M.; Devani, S.; Mudombi, W.; Kassianides, C.; Gastroenterology and Hepatology Association of sub-Saharan Africa (GHASSA). Inflammatory bowel disease in sub-Saharan Africa: Epidemiology, risk factors, and challenges in diagnosis. *Lancet Gastroenterol. Hepatol.* **2022**, *7*, 952–961. [CrossRef]
26. Agrawal, M.; Jess, T. Implications of the changing epidemiology of inflammatory bowel disease in a changing world. *United Eur. Gastroenterol. J.* **2022**, *10*, 1113–1120. [CrossRef]

27. Park, S.H.; Park, S.H. Personalized medicine in inflammatory bowel disease: Perspectives on Asia. *J. Gastroenterol. Hepatol.* **2022**, *37*, 1434–1445. [CrossRef]
28. Lee, J.W.; Eun, C.S. Inflammatory bowel disease in Korea: Epidemiology and pathophysiology. *Korean J. Intern. Med.* **2022**, *37*, 885–894. [CrossRef]
29. Zhang, Y.; Liu, J.; Han, X.; Jiang, H.; Zhang, L.; Hu, J.; Shi, L.; Li, J. Long-term trends in the burden of inflammatory bowel disease in China over three decades: A joinpoint regression and age-period-cohort analysis based on GBD 2019. *Front. Public Health* **2022**, *10*, 994619. [CrossRef]
30. Aniwan, S.; Santiago, P.; Loftus, E.V., Jr.; Park, S.H. The epidemiology of inflammatory bowel disease in Asia and Asian immigrants to Western countries. *United Eur. Gastroenterol. J.* **2022**, *10*, 1063–1076. [CrossRef]
31. Dipasquale, V.; Romano, C. Genes vs environment in inflammatory bowel disease: An update. *Expert Rev. Clin. Immunol.* **2022**, *18*, 1005–1013. [CrossRef] [PubMed]
32. Verdugo-Meza, A.; Ye, J.; Dadlani, H.; Ghosh, S.; Gibson, D.L. Connecting the dots between inflammatory bowel disease and metabolic syndrome: A focus on gut-derived metabolites. *Nutrients* **2020**, *12*, 1434. [CrossRef] [PubMed]
33. Singh, N.; Bernstein, C.N. Environmental risk factors for inflammatory bowel disease. *United Eur. Gastroenterol. J.* **2022**, *10*, 1047–1053. [CrossRef]
34. Upadhyay, K.G.; Desai, D.C.; Ashavaid, T.F.; Dherai, A.J. Microbiome and metabolome in inflammatory bowel disease. *J. Gastroenterol. Hepatol.* **2023**, *38*, 34–43. [CrossRef]
35. Yan, J.; Wang, L.; Gu, Y.; Hou, H.; Liu, T.; Ding, Y.; Cao, H. Dietary patterns and gut microbiota changes in inflammatory bowel disease: Current insights and future challenges. *Nutrients* **2022**, *14*, 4003. [CrossRef]
36. Andoh, A.; Nishida, A. Alteration of the gut microbiome in inflammatory bowel disease. *Digestion* **2023**, *104*, 16–23. [CrossRef]
37. Actis, G.C.; Pellicano, R.; Fagoonee, S.; Ribaldone, D.G. History of inflammatory bowel diseases. *J. Clin. Med.* **2019**, *8*, 1970. [CrossRef] [PubMed]
38. Nambu, R.; Warner, N.; Mulder, D.J.; Kotlarz, D.; McGovern, D.P.B.; Cho, J.; Klein, C.; Snapper, S.B.; Griffiths, A.M.; Iwama, I.; et al. A systematic review of monogenic inflammatory bowel disease. *Clin. Gastroenterol. Hepatol.* **2022**, *20*, e653–e663. [CrossRef]
39. Jarmakiewicz-Czaja, S.; Zielińska, M.; Sokal, A.; Filip, R. Genetic and epigenetic etiology of inflammatory bowel disease: An update. *Genes* **2022**, *13*, 2388. [CrossRef]
40. Celiberto, L.S.; Graef, F.A.; Healey, G.R.; Bosman, E.S.; Jacobson, K.; Sly, L.M.; Vallance, B.A. Inflammatory bowel disease and immunonutrition: Novel therapeutic approaches through modulation of diet and the gut microbiome. *Immunology* **2018**, *155*, 36–52. [CrossRef]
41. Triantos, C.; Aggeletopoulou, I.; Mantzaris, G.J.; Mouzaki, A. Molecular basis of vitamin D action in inflammatory bowel disease. *Autoimmun. Rev.* **2022**, *21*, 103136. [CrossRef]
42. Ananthakrishnan, A.N.; Kaplan, G.G.; Bernstein, C.N.; Burke, K.E.; Lochhead, P.J.; Sasson, A.N.; Agrawal, M.; Tiong, J.H.T.; Steinberg, J.; Kruis, W.; et al. International Organization for Study of Inflammatory Bowel Diseases. Lifestyle, behaviour, and environmental modification for the management of patients with inflammatory bowel diseases: An International Organization for Study of Inflammatory Bowel Diseases consensus. *Lancet Gastroenterol. Hepatol.* **2022**, *7*, 666–678. [PubMed]
43. Infantino, C.; Francavilla, R.; Vella, A.; Cenni, S.; Principi, N.; Strisciuglio, C.; Esposito, S. Role of vitamin D in celiac disease and inflammatory bowel diseases. *Nutrient* **2022**, *14*, 5154. [CrossRef]
44. Lavelle, A.; Sokol, H. Gut microbiota-derived metabolites as key actors in inflammatory bowel disease. *Nat. Rev. Gastroenterol. Hepatol.* **2020**, *17*, 223–237. [CrossRef] [PubMed]
45. Matthiessen, M.W.; Pedersen, G.; Albrektsen, T.; Adamsen, S.; Fleckner, J.; Brynskov, J. Peroxisome proliferator-activated receptor expression and activation in normal human colonic epithelial cells and tubular adenomas. *Scand. J. Gastroenterol.* **2005**, *40*, 198–205. [CrossRef] [PubMed]
46. Choo, J.; Lee, Y.; Yan, X.J.; Noh, T.H.; Kim, S.J.; Son, S.; Pothoulakis, C.; Moon, H.R.; Jung, J.H.; Im, E. A novel peroxisome proliferator-activated receptor (PPAR)γ agonist 2-hydroxyethyl 5-chloro-4,5-didehydrojasmonate exerts anti-inflammatory effects in colitis. *J. Biol. Chem.* **2015**, *290*, 25609–25619. [CrossRef]
47. Dubuquoy, L.; Rousseaux, C.; Thuru, X.; Peyrin-Biroulet, L.; Romano, O.; Chavatte, P.; Chamaillard, M.; Desreumaux, P. PPARgamma as a new therapeutic target in inflammatory bowel diseases. *Gut* **2006**, *55*, 1341–1349. [CrossRef]
48. Vetuschi, A.; Pompili, S.; Gaudio, E.; Latella, G.; Sferra, R. PPAR-γ with its anti-inflammatory and anti-fibrotic action could be an effective therapeutic target in IBD. *Eur. Rev. Med. Pharmacol. Sci.* **2018**, *22*, 8839–8848.
49. Venkataraman, B.; Ojha, S.; Belur, P.D.; Bhongade, B.; Raj, V.; Collin, P.D.; Adrian, T.E.; Subramanya, S.B. Phytochemical drug candidates for the modulation of peroxisome proliferator-activated receptor γ in inflammatory bowel diseases. *Phytother. Res.* **2020**, *34*, 1530–1549. [CrossRef]
50. Korolczuk, A.; Madro, A.; Slomka, M. Comparison of the anti-inflammatory and therapeutic actions of PPAR-gamma agonists rosiglitazone and troglitazone in experimental colitis. *J. Physiol. Pharmacol.* **2012**, *63*, 631–640.
51. Celinski, K.; Dworzanski, T.; Fornal, R.; Korolczuk, A.; Madro, A.; Brzozowski, T.; Slomka, M. Comparison of anti-inflammatory properties of peroxisome proliferator-activated receptor gamma agonists rosiglitazone and troglitazone in prophylactic treatment of experimental colitis. *J. Physiol. Pharmacol.* **2013**, *64*, 587–595. [PubMed]
52. Fang, J.; Wang, H.; Xue, Z.; Cheng, Y.; Zhang, X. PPARγ: The central mucus barrier coordinator in ulcerative colitis. *Inflamm. Bowel Dis.* **2021**, *27*, 732–741. [CrossRef]

53. Luo, S.; He, J.; Huang, S.; Wang, X.; Su, Y.; Li, Y.; Chen, Y.; Yang, G.; Huang, B.; Guo, S.; et al. Emodin targeting the colonic metabolism via PPARγ alleviates UC by inhibiting facultative anaerobe. *Phytomedicine* **2022**, *104*, 154106. [CrossRef]
54. Tseng, C.H. A review on thiazolidinediones and bladder cancer in human studies. *J. Environ. Sci. Health C Environ. Carcinog. Ecotoxicol. Rev.* **2014**, *32*, 1–45. [CrossRef]
55. Nissen, S.E.; Wolski, K. Effect of rosiglitazone on the risk of myocardial infarction and death from cardiovascular causes. *N. Engl. J. Med.* **2007**, *356*, 2457–2471. [CrossRef] [PubMed]
56. Lewis, J.D.; Ferrara, A.; Peng, T.; Hedderson, M.; Bilker, W.B.; Quesenberry, C.P., Jr.; Vaughn, D.J.; Nessel, L.; Selby, J.; Strom, B.L. Risk of bladder cancer among diabetic patients treated with pioglitazone: Interim report of a longitudinal cohort study. *Diabetes Care* **2011**, *34*, 916–922. [CrossRef]
57. Tseng, C.H. Pioglitazone has a null association with inflammatory bowel disease in patients with type 2 diabetes mellitus. *Pharmaceuticals* **2022**, *15*, 1538. [CrossRef] [PubMed]
58. Balfour, J.A.; Plosker, G.L. Rosiglitazone. *Drugs* **1999**, *57*, 921–930. [CrossRef]
59. Sun, T.; Kwong, C.H.T.; Gao, C.; Wei, J.; Yue, L.; Zhang, J.; Ye, R.D.; Wang, R. Amelioration of ulcerative colitis via inflammatory regulation by macrophage-biomimetic nanomedicine. *Theranostics* **2020**, *10*, 10106–10119. [CrossRef]
60. Da Silva, S.; Keita, Å.V.; Mohlin, S.; Påhlman, S.; Theodorou, V.; Påhlman, I.; Mattson, J.P.; Söderholm, J.D. A novel topical PPARγ agonist induces PPARγ activity in ulcerative colitis mucosa and prevents and reverses inflammation in induced colitis models. *Inflamm. Bowel Dis.* **2018**, *24*, 792–805. [CrossRef]
61. Pedersen, G.; Brynskov, J. Topical rosiglitazone treatment improves ulcerative colitis by restoring peroxisome proliferator-activated receptor-gamma activity. *Am. J. Gastroenterol.* **2010**, *105*, 1595–1603. [CrossRef] [PubMed]
62. Goldberg, R.B.; Kendall, D.M.; Deeg, M.A.; Buse, J.B.; Zagar, A.J.; Pinaire, J.A.; Tan, M.H.; Khan, M.A.; Perez, A.T.; Jacober, S.J.; et al. A comparison of lipid and glycemic effects of pioglitazone and rosiglitazone in patients with type 2 diabetes and dyslipidemia. *Diabetes Care* **2005**, *28*, 1547–1554. [CrossRef] [PubMed]
63. Tseng, C.H. Rosiglitazone is not associated with an increased risk of bladder cancer. *Cancer Epidemiol.* **2013**, *37*, 385–389. [CrossRef] [PubMed]
64. Tseng, C.H. Rosiglitazone has a neutral effect on the risk of dementia in type 2 diabetes patients. *Aging* **2019**, *11*, 2724–2734. [CrossRef] [PubMed]
65. Tseng, C.H. Rosiglitazone may reduce thyroid cancer risk in patients with type 2 diabetes. *Ann. Med.* **2013**, *45*, 539–544. [CrossRef]
66. Tseng, C.H. Pioglitazone reduces dementia risk in patients with type 2 diabetes mellitus: A retrospective cohort analysis. *J. Clin. Med.* **2018**, *7*, 306. [CrossRef]
67. Tseng, C.H. Pioglitazone and thyroid cancer risk in Taiwanese patients with type 2 diabetes. *J. Diabetes* **2014**, *6*, 448–450. [CrossRef]
68. Tseng, C.H. Metformin use is associated with a lower risk of inflammatory bowel disease in patients with type 2 diabetes mellitus. *J. Crohn's Colitis* **2021**, *15*, 64–73. [CrossRef]
69. Tseng, C.H.; Tseng, F.H. Peroxisome proliferator-activated receptor agonists and bladder cancer: Lessons from animal studies. *J. Environ. Sci. Health C Environ. Carcinog. Ecotoxicol. Rev.* **2012**, *30*, 368–402. [CrossRef]
70. Tseng, C.H.; Huang, T.S. Pioglitazone with sulfonylurea: Glycemic and lipid effects in Taiwanese diabetic patients. *Diabetes Res. Clin. Pract.* **2005**, *70*, 193–194. [CrossRef]
71. Madsen, M.S.A.; Grønlund, R.V.; Eid, J.; Christensen-Dalsgaard, M.; Sommer, M.; Rigbolt, K.; Madsen, M.R.; Jelsing, J.; Vrang, N.; Hansen, H.H.; et al. Characterization of local gut microbiome and intestinal transcriptome responses to rosiglitazone treatment in diabetic db/db mice. *Biomed. Pharmacother.* **2021**, *133*, 110966. [CrossRef] [PubMed]
72. Tomas, J.; Mulet, C.; Saffarian, A.; Cavin, J.B.; Ducroc, R.; Regnault, B.; Kun Tan, C.; Duszka, K.; Burcelin, R.; Wahli, W.; et al. High-fat diet modifies the PPAR-γ pathway leading to disruption of microbial and physiological ecosystem in murine small intestine. *Proc. Natl. Acad. Sci. USA* **2016**, *113*, E5934–E5943. [CrossRef] [PubMed]
73. Bai, J.; Zhu, Y.; Dong, Y. Response of gut microbiota and inflammatory status to bitter melon (*Momordica charantia* L.) in high fat diet induced obese rats. *J. Ethnopharmacol.* **2016**, *194*, 717–726. [CrossRef] [PubMed]
74. Amin, S.; Lux, A.; O'Callaghan, F. The journey of metformin from glycaemic control to mTOR inhibition and the suppression of tumour growth. *Br. J. Clin. Pharmacol.* **2019**, *85*, 37–46. [CrossRef]
75. Zhang, T.; Ji, X.; Lu, G.; Zhang, F. The potential of *Akkermansia muciniphila* in inflammatory bowel disease. *Appl. Microbiol. Biotechnol.* **2021**, *105*, 5785–5794. [CrossRef] [PubMed]
76. Rodrigues, V.F.; Elias-Oliveira, J.; Pereira, Í.S.; Pereira, J.A.; Barbosa, S.C.; Machado, M.S.G.; Carlos, D. *Akkermansia muciniphila* and gut immune system: A good friendship that attenuates inflammatory bowel disease, obesity, and diabetes. *Front. Immunol.* **2022**, *13*, 934695. [CrossRef]
77. Zheng, M.; Han, R.; Yuan, Y.; Xing, Y.; Zhang, W.; Sun, Z.; Liu, Y.; Li, J.; Mao, T. The role of *Akkermansia muciniphila* in inflammatory bowel disease: Current knowledge and perspectives. *Front. Immunol.* **2023**, *13*, 1089600. [CrossRef] [PubMed]
78. Wang, D.; Liu, J.; Zhong, L.; Ding, L.; Zhang, Q.; Yu, M.; Li, M.; Xiao, X. Potential benefits of metformin and pioglitazone combination therapy via gut microbiota and metabolites in high-fat diet-fed mice. *Front. Pharmacol.* **2022**, *13*, 1004617. [CrossRef]
79. Liu, M.J.; Yang, J.Y.; Yan, Z.H.; Hu, S.; Li, J.Q.; Xu, Z.X.; Jian, Y.P. Recent findings in Akkermansia muciniphila-regulated metabolism and its role in intestinal diseases. *Clin. Nutr.* **2022**, *41*, 2333–2344. [CrossRef]
80. Vallianou, N.G.; Stratigou, T.; Tsagarakis, S. Metformin and gut microbiota: Their interactions and their impact on diabetes. *Hormones* **2019**, *18*, 141–144. [CrossRef] [PubMed]

81. Ojo, O.; Wang, X.; Ojo, O.O.; Brooke, J.; Jiang, Y.; Dong, Q.; Thompson, T. The effect of prebiotics and oral anti-diabetic agents on gut microbiome in patients with type 2 diabetes: A systematic review and network meta-analysis of randomised controlled trials. *Nutrients* **2022**, *14*, 5139. [CrossRef] [PubMed]
82. Lashgari, N.A.; Roudsari, N.M.; Momtaz, S.; Abdolghaffari, A.H. Mammalian target of rapamycin-novel insight for management of inflammatory bowel diseases. *World J. Pharmacol.* **2022**, *11*, 1–5. [CrossRef]
83. Blanchard, P.G.; Festuccia, W.T.; Houde, V.P.; St-Pierre, P.; Brûlé, S.; Turcotte, V.; Côté, M.; Bellmann, K.; Marette, A.; Deshaies, Y. Major involvement of mTOR in the PPARγ-induced stimulation of adipose tissue lipid uptake and fat accretion. *J. Lipid Res.* **2012**, *53*, 1117–1125. [CrossRef]
84. Andrade, M.L.; Gilio, G.R.; Perandini, L.A.; Peixoto, A.S.; Moreno, M.F.; Castro, É.; Oliveira, T.E.; Vieira, T.S.; Ortiz-Silva, M.; Thomazelli, C.A.; et al. PPARγ-induced upregulation of subcutaneous fat adiponectin secretion, glyceroneogenesis and BCAA oxidation requires mTORC1 activity. *Biochim. Biophys. Acta Mol. Cell Biol. Lipids* **2021**, *1866*, 158967. [CrossRef] [PubMed]
85. Tseng, C.H. Differential effects of metformin on immune-mediated and androgen-mediated non-cancer skin diseases in diabetes patients: A retrospective cohort study. *Dermatology*, 2023; *Online ahead of print*. [CrossRef]
86. Wang, S.; Dougherty, E.J.; Danner, R.L. PPARγ signaling and emerging opportunities for improved therapeutics. *Pharmacol. Res.* **2016**, *111*, 76–85. [CrossRef] [PubMed]
87. Xu, B.; Xing, A.; Li, S. The forgotten type 2 diabetes mellitus medicine: Rosiglitazone. *Diabetol. Int.* **2021**, *13*, 49–65. [CrossRef] [PubMed]
88. Pearce, N.; Checkoway, H.; Kriebel, D. Bias in occupational epidemiology studies. *Occup. Environ. Med.* **2007**, *64*, 562–568. [CrossRef]
89. Kesmodel, U.S. Information bias in epidemiological studies with a special focus on obstetrics and gynecology. *Acta Obstet. Gynecol. Scand.* **2018**, *97*, 417–423. [CrossRef]
90. Parsons, L.S. Performing a 1:N Case-Control Match on Propensity Score. Available online: http://www2.sas.com/proceedings/sugi29/165-29.pdf (accessed on 1 April 2023).
91. Dormandy, J.A.; Charbonnel, B.; Eckland, D.J.; Erdmann, E.; Massi-Benedetti, M.; Moules, I.K.; Skene, A.M.; Tan, M.H.; Lefèbvre, P.J.; Murray, G.D.; et al. PROactive investigators. Secondary prevention of macrovascular events in patients with type 2 diabetes in the PROactive Study (PROspective pioglitAzone Clinical Trial In macroVascular Events): A randomised controlled trial. *Lancet* **2005**, *366*, 1279–1289. [CrossRef]
92. Kernan, W.N.; Viscoli, C.M.; Furie, K.L.; Young, L.H.; Inzucchi, S.E.; Gorman, M.; Guarino, P.D.; Lovejoy, A.M.; Peduzzi, P.N.; Conwit, R.; et al. IRIS Trial Investigators. Pioglitazone after ischemic stroke or transient ischemic attack. *N. Engl. J. Med.* **2016**, *374*, 1321–1331. [CrossRef]
93. Austin, P.C.; Stuart, E.A. Moving towards best practice when using inverse probability of treatment weighting (IPTW) using the propensity score to estimate causal treatment effects in observational studies. *Stat. Med.* **2015**, *34*, 3661–3679. [CrossRef] [PubMed]
94. Lin, A.; Inman, R.D.; Streutker, C.J.; Zhang, Z.; Pritzker, K.P.H.; Tsui, H.W.; Tsui, F.W.L. Lipocalin 2 links inflammation and ankylosis in the clinical overlap of inflammatory bowel disease (IBD) and ankylosing spondylitis (AS). *Arthritis Res. Ther.* **2020**, *22*, 51. [CrossRef] [PubMed]
95. Liu, T.C.; Kern, J.T.; VanDussen, K.L.; Xiong, S.; Kaiko, G.E.; Wilen, C.B.; Rajala, M.W.; Caruso, R.; Holtzman, M.J.; Gao, F.; et al. Interaction between smoking and ATG16L1T300A triggers Paneth cell defects in Crohn's disease. *J. Clin. Investig.* **2018**, *128*, 5110–5122. [CrossRef]
96. Viscido, A.; Capannolo, A.; Latella, G.; Caprilli, R.; Frieri, G. Nanotechnology in the treatment of inflammatory bowel diseases. *J. Crohn's Colitis* **2014**, *8*, 903–918. [CrossRef]
97. Yasmin, F.; Najeeb, H.; Shaikh, S.; Hasanain, M.; Naeem, U.; Moeed, A.; Koritala, T.; Hasan, S.; Surani, S. Novel drug delivery systems for inflammatory bowel disease. *World J. Gastroenterol.* **2022**, *28*, 1922–1933. [CrossRef]
98. Stidham, R.W.; Takenaka, K. Artificial intelligence for disease assessment in inflammatory bowel disease: How will it change our practice? *Gastroenterology* **2022**, *162*, 1493–1506. [CrossRef] [PubMed]

Disclaimer/Publisher's Note: The statements, opinions and data contained in all publications are solely those of the individual author(s) and contributor(s) and not of MDPI and/or the editor(s). MDPI and/or the editor(s) disclaim responsibility for any injury to people or property resulting from any ideas, methods, instructions or products referred to in the content.

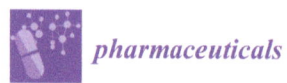

Article

Pioglitazone Has a Null Association with Inflammatory Bowel Disease in Patients with Type 2 Diabetes Mellitus

Chin-Hsiao Tseng [1,2,3]

1 Department of Internal Medicine, National Taiwan University College of Medicine, Taipei 10051, Taiwan; ccktsh@ms6.hinet.net
2 Division of Endocrinology and Metabolism, Department of Internal Medicine, National Taiwan University Hospital, Taipei 10002, Taiwan
3 National Institute of Environmental Health Sciences, Zhunan 35053, Taiwan

Abstract: Pioglitazone shows potential benefits in inflammatory bowel disease (IBD) in preclinical studies, but its effect in humans has not been researched. We used a nationwide database of Taiwan's National Health Insurance to investigate whether pioglitazone might affect IBD risk. We enrolled 12,763 ever users and 12,763 never users matched on a propensity score from patients who had a new diagnosis of type 2 diabetes mellitus between 1999 and 2008. The patients were alive on 1 January 2009, and they were followed up for a new diagnosis of IBD until 31 December 2011. Propensity score-weighted hazard ratios were estimated, and the interactions between pioglitazone and major risk factors of IBD (i.e., psoriasis, arthropathies, dorsopathies, chronic obstructive pulmonary disease/tobacco abuse, and any of the above) and metformin were investigated. At the end of the follow-up, 113 ever users and 139 never users were diagnosed with IBD. When compared to never users, the hazard ratio for ever users was 0.809 (95% confidence interval: 0.631–1.037); and none of the hazard ratios for ever users categorized by tertiles of cumulative duration and cumulative dose reached statistical significance. No interactions with major risk factors or metformin were observed. Our findings suggested a null effect of pioglitazone on IBD.

Keywords: diabetes mellitus; inflammatory bowel disease; pharmacoepidemiology; pioglitazone; Taiwan

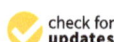

Citation: Tseng, C.-H. Pioglitazone Has a Null Association with Inflammatory Bowel Disease in Patients with Type 2 Diabetes Mellitus. *Pharmaceuticals* 2022, 15, 1538. https://doi.org/10.3390/ph15121538

Academic Editors: Anderson Luiz-Ferreira and Carmine Stolfi

Received: 2 November 2022
Accepted: 9 December 2022
Published: 11 December 2022

Publisher's Note: MDPI stays neutral with regard to jurisdictional claims in published maps and institutional affiliations.

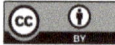

Copyright: © 2022 by the author. Licensee MDPI, Basel, Switzerland. This article is an open access article distributed under the terms and conditions of the Creative Commons Attribution (CC BY) license (https://creativecommons.org/licenses/by/4.0/).

1. Introduction

Inflammatory bowel disease (IBD), generally classified as Crohn's disease (CD) and ulcerative colitis (UC) in clinical practice, is characterized by chronic and relapsing colitis due to excessive expression of various inflammatory mediators. Clinical manifestations include watery diarrhea, fatigue, weight loss, abdominal pain, and bleeding, and sometimes it can be life-threatening [1,2]. It is difficult to differentiate between CD and UC from clinical presentations, and laboratory examinations, including colofibroscope, are necessary for more accurate diagnosis [1]. It has been estimated that 10–15% of the population may have some type of colitis [2]. The prevalence of IBD is approximately 0.3% in North America, Oceania, and Europe, and its incidence is either stable or decreasing in these countries. However, since the 1990s, an increased incidence has been observed in newly industrialized countries in Asia, South America, and Africa [3,4]. In Taiwan, the incidence is increasing, and the annual percentage change has been estimated to be 4% to 5% [3].

The etiology of IBD remains to be investigated, but the interplay among the host, microbiota, and environmental factors is important [2,5,6]. More than 230 genetic loci relating to major histocompatibility complex, pattern recognition, inflammation, and apoptosis have been identified [1,7]. However, environmental risk factors relating to industrialization, sanitation, and hygiene are important, and specific risk factors may include metabolic syndrome, lack of exercise, work shift, dietary patterns (less intake of fiber-containing vegetables, fruit, cereal, and nuts, and more intake of calorically dense diet, elaborate meat, high-fat diet, and high-sugar diet), animal protein, milk formula feeding, vitamin D deficiency, excessive sanitation, psychological stress, history of childhood infection and vaccination and use of oral contraceptives, non-steroidal anti-inflammatory drugs and antibiotics [4,7,8]. On the other hand, breastfeeding may provide protection against IBD [4]. Cigarette smoking and appendectomy both seemed to aggravate CD but might alleviate UC [4]. Metabolites derived from gut microbiota play important roles in mediating the hosts' immune response and release of inflammatory cytokines and, thus, are pivotal in the development of IBD [9].

Thiazolidinedione (TZD) activates the peroxisome proliferator-activator receptor gamma (PPARγ) and improves insulin resistance and has been used for lowering blood glucose in patients with type 2 diabetes mellitus. In in vitro and in vivo preclinical studies, PPARγ activation has been shown to play a role in the regulation of inflammation and immune response in the colon [10], and the role of PPARγ in the treatment of IBD has long been under investigation [2,5,11–15]. Emodin, a Chinese herb-drug used to treat IBD, may act through its activation of PPARγ-related signaling [16]. A recent study showed that the attenuation of IBD by pioglitazone in cellular and animal studies might act through the prevention of cleaving of annexin A1 in macrophages, leading to reduced secretion of inflammatory cytokines [17]. However, evidence of the use of PPARγ agonists in the treatment of human IBD remains to be explored.

To our knowledge, a population-based study investigating the potential role of PPARγ agonists in the development of IBD in humans is still lacking. In the present study, we aimed to investigate the effect of pioglitazone, a PPARγ agonist in the class of TZD, on the risk of IBD in patients with type 2 diabetes mellitus in Taiwan.

2. Results

Table 1 shows the characteristics of never users and ever users in the matched cohort. The two groups were balanced in the distributions of all variables because none of the values of standardized difference was >10%.

Table 1. Characteristics of pioglitazone never users and ever users.

Characteristics	Never Users (n = 12,763)		Ever Users (n = 12,763)		Standardized Difference
	n	%	n	%	
Basic data					
Age * (years)	61.01	12.17	60.95	11.50	−0.68
Diabetes duration * (years)	6.51	2.74	6.50	2.59	−0.40
Sex (men)	7219	56.56	7218	56.55	−0.03
Occupation					
I	4966	38.91	4920	38.55	
II	2814	22.05	2800	21.94	−0.25
III	2505	19.63	2533	19.85	0.50
IV	2478	19.42	2510	19.67	0.68
Living region					
Taipei	5068	39.71	5097	39.94	
Northern	1326	10.39	1327	10.40	0.10
Central	2044	16.02		15.69	−0.84
Southern	1574	12.33	1609	12.61	0.78
Kao-Ping and Eastern	2751	21.55	2727	21.37	−0.48
Major comorbidities associated with diabetes mellitus					
Hypertension	10,370	81.25	10,422	81.66	0.97
Dyslipidemia	10,915	85.52	10,907	85.46	−0.17
Obesity	715	5.60	785	6.15	2.32

Table 1. *Cont.*

Characteristics	Never Users (n = 12,763)		Ever Users (n = 12,763)		Standardized Difference
	n	%	n	%	
Diabetes-related complications					
Nephropathy	3290	25.78	3245	25.43	−0.91
Eye disease	4302	33.71	4352	34.10	0.85
Diabetic polyneuropathy	3610	28.28	3617	28.34	0.08
Stroke	3113	24.39	3175	24.88	1.02
Ischemic heart disease	5419	42.46	5479	42.93	0.84
Peripheral arterial disease	3116	24.41	3090	24.21	−0.49
Factors that might affect exposure/outcome					
Head injury	436	3.42	440	3.45	0.12
Parkinson's disease	286	2.24	272	2.13	−0.81
Hypoglycemia	473	3.71	496	3.89	0.85
Chronic obstructive pulmonary disease	5759	45.12	5812	45.54	0.76
Tobacco abuse	486	3.81	504	3.95	0.65
Alcohol-related diagnoses	702	5.50	698	5.47	0.02
Heart failure	1932	15.14	1948	15.26	0.25
Gingival and periodontal diseases	11,232	88.00	11,181	87.60	−1.16
Pneumonia	1576	12.35	1595	12.50	0.29
Pulmonary tuberculosis	388	3.04	444	3.48	2.40
Osteoporosis	2108	16.52	2195	17.20	1.74
Human immunodeficiency virus infection	12	0.09	8	0.06	−1.31
Cancer	1579	12.37	1657	12.98	1.80
Dementia	677	5.30	653	5.12	−0.99
Valvular heart disease	1025	8.03	1043	8.17	0.51
Arthropathies	9628	75.44	9685	75.88	1.02
Psoriasis	419	3.28	374	2.93	−2.19
Dorsopathies	9777	76.60	9792	76.72	0.25
Liver cirrhosis	360	2.82	352	2.76	−0.45
Other chronic non-alcoholic liver diseases	1171	9.17	1210	9.48	0.99
Hepatitis B virus infection	452	3.54	465	3.64	0.52
Hepatitis C virus infection	419	3.28	451	3.53	1.32
Organ transplantation	33	0.26	24	0.19	−1.57
Antidiabetic drugs and drugs that are commonly prescribed to diabetes patients or drugs that might affect exposure/outcome					
Insulin	380	2.98	388	3.04	0.43
Sulfonylureas	8849	69.33	8894	69.69	0.58
Metformin	9381	73.50	9389	73.56	0.15
Meglitinide	905	7.09	879	6.89	−1.00
Acarbose	1702	13.34	1742	13.65	0.89
Angiotensin converting enzyme inhibitors/Angiotensin receptor blockers	9404	73.68	9487	74.33	1.38
Calcium channel blockers	7273	56.99	7358	57.65	1.27
Statins	9457	74.10	9505	74.47	0.91
Fibrates	5736	44.94	5728	44.88	−0.15
Aspirin	7594	59.50	7587	59.45	−0.21
Corticosteroids	359	2.81	331	2.59	−1.48

* Age and diabetes duration are shown as mean and standard deviation.

Table 2 shows the incidence rates of IBD and the hazard ratios comparing pioglitazone-exposed patients to unexposed patients. The overall hazard ratios and the hazard ratios estimated for each tertile of pioglitazone exposure all favored a null association between pioglitazone use and IBD risk.

Table 2. Incidence rates of inflammatory bowel disease and hazard ratios comparing pioglitazone exposed groups to the unexposed group.

Pioglitazone Use	Incident Case Number	Cases Followed	Person-Years	Incidence Rate (per 100,000 Person-Years)	Hazard Ratio	95% Confidence Interval	p Value
Never users	139	12,763	33,988.31	408.96	1.000		
Ever users	113	12,763	34,154.60	330.85	0.809	(0.631–1.037)	0.0937
Tertiles of cumulative duration of pioglitazone therapy (months)							
Never users	139	12,763	33,988.31	408.96	1.000		
<11.0	32	4147	10,833.86	295.37	0.727	(0.495–1.068)	0.1044
11.0–19.7	35	4282	11,466.87	305.23	0.745	(0.514–1.079)	0.1191
>19.7	46	4334	11,853.86	388.06	0.942	(0.675–1.315)	0.7253
Tertiles of cumulative dose of pioglitazone therapy (mg)							
Never users	139	12,763	33,988.31	408.96	1.000		
<7980	31	4155	10,897.90	284.46	0.700	(0.474–1.033)	0.0726
7980–14,940	37	4266	11,435.47	323.55	0.790	(0.550–1.135)	0.2018
>14,940	45	4342	11,821.23	380.67	0.925	(0.661–1.294)	0.6478

The joint effects of and the interactions between pioglitazone and the major risk factors of IBD are shown in Table 3. The joint effect of and the interaction between pioglitazone and metformin are shown in Table 4. All models suggested a null association without any interaction.

Table 3. Joint effects and interactions between pioglitazone and major risk factors of inflammatory bowel disease.

Risk Factor/Pioglitazone Use	Incident Case Number	Cases Followed	Person-Years	Incidence Rate (per 100,000 Person-Years)	Hazard Ratio	95% Confidence Interval	p Value
Psoriasis (+)/Pioglitazone (−)	3	419	1124.62	266.76	1.000		
Psoriasis (+)/Pioglitazone (+)	6	374	994.22	603.49	2.329	(0.581–9.332)	0.2325
Psoriasis (−)/Pioglitazone (−)	136	12,344	32,863.69	413.83	1.602	(0.509–5.043)	0.4206
Psoriasis (−)/Pioglitazone (+)	107	12,389	33,160.38	322.67	1.250	(0.396–3.947)	0.7042
P-interaction							0.1286
Arthropathies (+)/Pioglitazone (−)	117	9628	25,741.21	454.52	1.000		
Arthropathies (+)/Pioglitazone (+)	90	9685	25,978.83	346.44	0.763	(0.580–1.005)	0.0546
Arthropathies (−)/Pioglitazone (−)	22	3135	8247.10	266.76	0.687	(0.427–1.107)	0.1228
Arthropathies (−)/Pioglitazone (+)	23	3078	8175.77	281.32	0.731	(0.457–1.169)	0.1906
P-interaction							0.3149
Dorsopathies (+)/Pioglitazone (−)	113	9777	26,118.94	432.64	1.000		
Dorsopathies (+)/Pioglitazone (+)	93	9792	26,258.73	354.17	0.820	(0.623–1.079)	0.1558
Dorsopathies (−)/Pioglitazone (−)	26	2986	7869.37	330.39	0.942	(0.603–1.471)	0.7920
Dorsopathies (−)/Pioglitazone (+)	20	2971	7895.87	253.30	0.726	(0.444–1.188)	0.2026
P-interaction							0.8522
COPD/Tobacco abuse (+)/Pioglitazone (−)	72	5960	15,908.15	452.60	1.000		

Table 3. Cont.

Risk Factor/Pioglitazone Use	Incident Case Number	Cases Followed	Person-Years	Incidence Rate (per 100,000 Person-Years)	Hazard Ratio	95% Confidence Interval	p Value
COPD/Tobacco abuse (+)/Pioglitazone (+)	56	6038	16,163.84	346.45	0.760	(0.536–1.079)	0.1252
COPD/Tobacco abuse (−)/Pioglitazone (−)	67	6803	18,080.16	370.57	0.860	(0.609–1.215)	0.3932
COPD/Tobacco abuse (−)/Pioglitazone (+)	57	6725	17,990.76	316.83	0.744	(0.520–1.066)	0.1074
P-interaction							0.9709
Any of the four (+)/Pioglitazone (−)	130	11,333	30,243.27	429.85	1.000		
Any of the four (+)/Pioglitazone (+)	104	11,370	30,483.71	341.17	0.797	(0.615–1.031)	0.0843
All of the four (−)/Pioglitazone (−)	9	1430	3745.04	240.32	0.660	(0.332–1.310)	0.2347
All of the four (−)/Pioglitazone (+)	9	1393	3670.88	245.17	0.668	(0.336–1.327)	0.2492
P-interaction							0.6240

COPD: chronic obstructive pulmonary disease.

Table 4. Joint effect and interaction between metformin and pioglitazone on inflammatory bowel disease.

Metformin/Pioglitazone Use	Incident Case Number	Cases Followed	Person-Years	Incidence Rate (per 100,000 Person-Years)	Hazard Ratio	95% Confidence Interval	p Value
Metformin (−)/Pioglitazone (−)	33	3382	8911.51	370.31	1.000		
Metformin (−)/Pioglitazone (+)	27	3374	8986.75	300.44	0.840	(0.503–1.402)	0.5043
Metformin (+)/Pioglitazone (−)	106	9381	25,076.80	422.70	1.186	(0.793–1.771)	0.4061
Metformin (+)/Pioglitazone (+)	86	9389	25,167.85	341.71	0.950	(0.630–1.433)	0.8074
P-interaction							0.6002

3. Discussion

Main Findings

There was a lack of any association between pioglitazone use and IBD (Table 2), and no interaction was observed between pioglitazone and any of the risk factors (Table 3) or pioglitazone and metformin use (Table 4).

a. *Discrepancies with preclinical studies*

Although PPARγ can play a role in the treatment of IBD through the crosstalk between metabolism and inflammation [5] and preclinical studies favor a potential usefulness of pioglitazone in the treatment of IBD [2,5], such a benefit of pioglitazone could not be observed in humans in this observational study. The discrepancies between preclinical in vitro and in vivo studies and this human observational study require some discussion.

First, animal models of colitis are mainly induced by chemicals such as dextran sodium sulfate, trinitrobenzene sulfonic acid, dinitrobenzene sulfonic acid, oxazolone, and intracolonic instillation of acetic acid [2]. It remains to be explored whether colitis induced by these chemicals can completely mimic human IBD. Furthermore, the administered doses of pioglitazone in in vitro and in vivo studies might be much higher than the available concentrations of pioglitazone derived from the clinical doses used for the treatment of hyperglycemia. In Taiwan, the generally accepted maximum dose of pioglitazone is 30 mg, and we rarely use a dosage of up to 45 mg as has been used in Caucasians [18].

Second, the blood concentration of pioglitazone derived from oral administration does not guarantee a sufficient level of pioglitazone to be delivered to the colon for local activation of PPARγ. Recent drug development for the treatment of IBD focuses on more specific delivery of the drugs by using nanotechnology [19] or topically applied PPARγ agonists [20]. Whether these may improve the efficacy of pioglitazone on IBD prevention or treatment are interesting research topics worthy of investigation.

Third, pioglitazone can target multiple organs and tissues, and activation of PPARγ that acts jointly with retinoid X receptor in different types of cells may result in different biological functions, some even counteracting each other. These may explain the various clinical effects observed for different types of cancer and non-cancer diseases in patients treated with pioglitazone. For example, we did observe an improvement in lipid profiles after pioglitazone treatment in a small clinical trial [21] and a significant risk reduction in dementia [22] and chronic obstructive pulmonary disease [23] in observational studies. However, a potentially higher risk of bladder cancer [24] should be attended to in clinical practice.

However, though not statistically significant, the overall hazard ratio of 0.809 (Table 2) favored an approximately 20% risk reduction in association with pioglitazone use. We could not exclude the possibility of lack of power and the confounding by some unmeasured variables such as microbiota and nutrients.

b. *Implications*

At least two clinical implications can be derived from the present study. First, findings observed in preclinical studies suggesting potential usefulness in the treatment of IBD by pioglitazone should never be immediately extrapolated to a clinical implication. At least, our present study did not favor such a benefit of pioglitazone.

Second, pioglitazone does not cause hypoglycemia and shows benefits for cardiovascular diseases [18], especially ischemic stroke [25], and is minimally excreted by the kidney [26]. It should be a candidate drug for glucose lowering in patients who fail their treatment by the first-line drug of metformin, especially when the patients have renal insufficiency or are at a high risk of stroke, dementia, and/or chronic obstructive pulmonary disease. However, pioglitazone should better be avoided in patients with a previous diagnosis of bladder cancer or who are at a high risk of developing bladder cancer, such as a positive family history.

c. *Strengths*

The study has several merits. First, because of the use of a nationwide database of the National Health Insurance (NHI) that has high coverage of >99% of Taiwan's population, it is reasonable to generalize the findings to the whole population. Second, because we used objective medical records, potential recall bias relating to self-reporting could be avoided. Third, detection biases resulting from different socioeconomic statuses could be minimized because the drug cost-sharing in the NHI is low and can always be waived in veterans, in patients with low income, and in patients who receive prescription refills for chronic disease.

d. *Limitations*

This study also has some limitations. First, we did not have measurement data of some confounders such as anthropometric factors, lifestyle, physical activity, exposure history to some chemicals, history of childhood infection, stress in life, smoking, alcohol drinking, dietary pattern, nutritional status, micronutrient supplementation, family history, and genetic parameters. Second, we did not have biochemical data such as levels of inflammatory cytokines, glucose, insulin, and lipid profiles. Neither did we have indicators of insulin resistance or β-cell function and gut microbiota information for analyses. Third, the outcome of IBD was defined by the International Classification of Diseases, Ninth Revision, Clinical Modification (ICD-9-CM) codes and not by colofibroscopic examinations. Therefore, we could not exclude the potential risk of misdiagnosis in some patients. Because the misclassification was expected to be non-differential, the estimated hazard ratios were supposed to bias toward the null [27,28]. Finally, because the daily dose of pioglitazone used in the Taiwanese and probably also in other Asian populations rarely exceeds 30 mg, whether the clinical use of 45 mg in the Caucasian people [18] would exert a different effect on IBD is an interesting issue that requires additional studies.

4. Materials and Methods

4.1. The National Health Insurance in Taiwan

Taiwan started to implement the so-called NHI on 1 March 1995. The NHI is compulsory and covers >99.6% of Taiwan's population. The Bureau of NHI signs contracts with all in-hospitals and more than 93% of all medical settings in Taiwan to provide medical care to the insurants. For reimbursement purposes, computerized medical records, including disease diagnoses, medication prescriptions, and performed procedures, have to be submitted to the Bureau of the NHI. The database can be used for academic research after ethics review and approval. The present study was approved (approval number NHIRD-102-175) by the Research Ethics Committee of the National Health Research Institutes. The readers may refer to our previously published paper for a more detailed description of the database [29].

4.2. Enrollment of Study Subjects

Throughout the research period, the ICD-9-CM was used as the disease coding system. Accordingly, diabetes mellitus was coded 250.XX and IBD were coded 555 (regional enteritis) and/or 556 (ulcerative enterocolitis).

We created a cohort consisting of propensity score (PS)-matched pairs of ever users and never users of pioglitazone from the NHI database. Figure 1 shows the stepwise procedures. First, we excluded patients whose diagnosis of diabetes mellitus was made during 1995–1998 and then enrolled 477,207 patients who had a first diagnosis of diabetes mellitus made between 1999 and 2008 with a prescription of antidiabetic drugs for at least two times at outpatient clinics. We then excluded step-by-step the following ineligible patients: (1) patients who died before 1 January 2009 ($n = 188$), (2) patients who used pioglitazone for the first time after 2009 ($n = 58,835$), (3) patients who were diagnosed of type 1 diabetes mellitus ($n = 2534$), (4) patients who had ever been treated with rosiglitazone ($n = 51,017$), (5) patients who had used pioglitazone for a short period of <180 days ($n = 6399$), (6) patients who had a diagnosis of IBD before entry or within 6 months of diabetes diagnosis ($n = 27,374$), and (7) patients who had a short follow-up duration of <180 days ($n = 13,692$). As a result, we identified an unmatched cohort consisting of 12,763 ever users and 304,405 never users. We then created PS-matched pairs consisting of 12,763 ever users and 12,763 never users (the matched cohort) based on the Greedy 8→1 digit match algorithm. The PS was created by logistic regression from independent variables that included all characteristics listed in Table 1, as described in more detail previously [29].

We deliberately excluded users of rosiglitazone in the analyses for the following reasons. In Taiwan, only rosiglitazone and pioglitazone in the class of TZD have ever been marketed. In addition to their glucose-lowering effects, these two drugs show different safety profiles in several clinical aspects. For example, the meta-analysis published in 2007 that suggested a potential link between rosiglitazone and myocardial infarction and cardiovascular death [30] has led to the withdrawal of rosiglitazone from the markets or the discontinuation of its use in many countries, including Taiwan. On the contrary, clinical trials suggest that pioglitazone significantly improves lipid profiles [21] and reduces cardiovascular diseases in patients with type 2 diabetes mellitus [18] or in patients with ischemic stroke and insulin resistance [25]. Therefore, in the analyses of the safety profile and the risk association with cancer or other non-cancer diseases, pioglitazone and rosiglitazone should be viewed as two different entities.

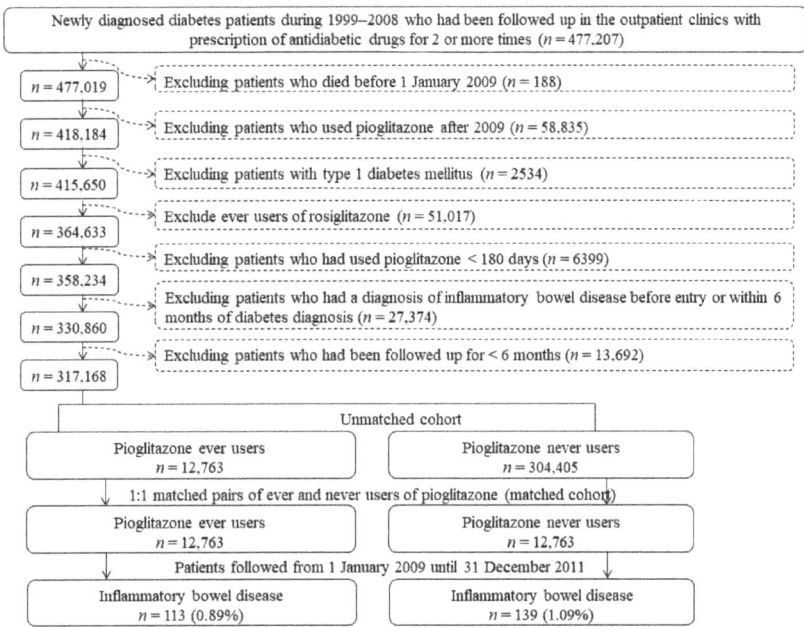

Figure 1. Flowchart showing the stepwise procedures followed in the enrollment of propensity score-matched pairs of pioglitazone ever users and never users.

4.3. Potential Confounders

Potential confounders included in the analyses are listed in Table 1. The occupation was classified as class I (civil servants, teachers, employees of governmental or private businesses, professionals and technicians), class II (people without a specific employer, self-employed people or seamen), class III (farmers or fishermen), and class IV (low-income families supported by social welfare, or veterans). We defined the use of corticosteroids as a consistent use of ≥ 90 days. The ICD-9-CM codes for the disease diagnoses have been reported previously [22].

4.4. Statistical Analyses

We used the SAS statistical software version 9.4 (SAS Institute, Cary, NC, USA), as a tool for analyses being conducted in the matched cohort. $p < 0.05$ was considered statistically significant.

We calculated the standardized difference for each covariate and defined a value > 10% as an indicator of potential confounding from the variable, which is generally adopted by many investigators [31].

We calculated two parameters for the assessment of a potential dose-response relationship, i.e., the cumulative duration of pioglitazone therapy (expressed in months) and the cumulative dose of pioglitazone therapy (expressed in mg). The incidence density of IBD was calculated with regard to pioglitazone exposure. The numerator of the incidence was the number of new cases of IBD identified during follow-up, and the denominator was the follow-up duration in person-years. We set the follow-up starting date on 1 January 2009 and ended the follow-up on a date no later than 31 December 2011 when whichever of the following events occurred first: a new diagnosis of IBD, death, or the last reimbursement record. We ended follow-up by the end of 2011 because the concern of a potential risk of bladder cancer associated with pioglitazone was raised in that year [24], which might have led to changes in prescription behavior in the attending physicians and nonadherence to the treatment on the side of the patients.

We estimated hazard ratios and their 95% confidence intervals that compared pioglitazone exposure to non-exposure by applying Cox proportional hazards regression incorporated with the inverse probability of treatment weighting using the PS.

Psoriasis, arthropathies, dorsopathies, and chronic obstructive pulmonary disease/tobacco abuse were viewed as potential risk factors for IBD. To evaluate the joint effects of and the interactions between pioglitazone and these risk factors, we estimated hazard ratios in subgroups categorized by the presence and absence of risk factors and pioglitazone, i.e., (1) risk factor (+)/pioglitazone (−) as the referent group; (2) risk factor (+)/pioglitazone (+); (3) risk factor (−)/pioglitazone (−); and (4) risk factor (−)/pioglitazone (+). The value of P-interaction was also estimated for each model.

Metformin use is associated with a reduced risk of IBD in our previous study [32]. Therefore, we also investigated the joint effect of and interaction between metformin and pioglitazone on the risk of IBD.

5. Conclusions

There is a lack of association between pioglitazone use and IBD risk in Taiwanese patients with type 2 diabetes mellitus, and there are no significant interactions between pioglitazone and major risk factors or metformin. Because of the observational design, the potential risk of lack of sufficient power, and the inability to include all potential confounders, further confirmation of our finding is warranted. The daily dose of pioglitazone in Taiwan is generally not more than 30 mg. Whether the use of a higher dose of 45 mg of pioglitazone in Caucasians may exert a clinical benefit on IBD requires further investigation.

Funding: This research was funded by the Ministry of Science and Technology (MOST 103-2314-B-002-187-MY3) of Taiwan.

Institutional Review Board Statement: The study was conducted in accordance with the Declaration of Helsinki and approved by the Ethics Committee of the National Health Research Institutes (approval number NHIRD-102-175).

Informed Consent Statement: Patient consent was waived because the personal information had been de-identified, and the patient could not be contacted according to local regulations.

Data Availability Statement: Data contained within the article are not readily available because local regulations restrict the public availability of the dataset to protect privacy. Requests to access the datasets should be directed to C.T., ccktsh@ms6.hinet.net.

Acknowledgments: The author wishes to thank Ting-Ting Chan for her excellent performance in the analyses of the data.

Conflicts of Interest: The author declares no conflict of interest.

References

1. Flynn, S.; Eisenstein, S. Inflammatory bowel disease presentation and diagnosis. *Surg. Clin. N. Am.* **2019**, *99*, 1051–1062. [CrossRef] [PubMed]
2. Decara, J.; Rivera, P.; López-Gambero, A.J.; Serrano, A.; Pavón, F.J.; Baixeras, E.; Rodríguez de Fonseca, F.; Suárez, J. Peroxisome proliferator-activated receptors: Experimental targeting for the treatment of inflammatory bowel diseases. *Front. Pharmacol.* **2020**, *11*, 730. [CrossRef] [PubMed]
3. Ng, S.C.; Shi, H.Y.; Hamidi, N.; Underwood, F.E.; Tang, W.; Benchimol, E.I.; Panaccione, R.; Ghosh, S.; Wu, J.C.Y.; Chan, F.K.L.; et al. Worldwide incidence and prevalence of inflammatory bowel disease in the 21st century: A systematic review of population-based studies. *Lancet* **2018**, *390*, 2769–2778. [CrossRef] [PubMed]
4. Baumgart, D.C.; Carding, S.R. Inflammatory bowel disease: Cause and immunobiology. *Lancet* **2007**, *369*, 1627–1640. [CrossRef] [PubMed]
5. Caioni, G.; Viscido, A.; d'Angelo, M.; Panella, G.; Castelli, V.; Merola, C.; Frieri, G.; Latella, G.; Cimini, A.; Benedetti, E. Inflammatory bowel disease: New insights into the interplay between environmental factors and PPARγ. *Int. J. Mol. Sci.* **2021**, *22*, 985. [CrossRef]
6. Verdugo-Meza, A.; Ye, J.; Dadlani, H.; Ghosh, S.; Gibson, D.L. Connecting the dots between inflammatory bowel disease and metabolic syndrome: A focus on gut-derived metabolites. *Nutrients* **2020**, *12*, 1434. [CrossRef]

7. Actis, G.C.; Pellicano, R.; Fagoonee, S.; Ribaldone, D.G. History of inflammatory bowel diseases. *J. Clin. Med.* **2019**, *8*, 1970. [CrossRef]
8. Celiberto, L.S.; Graef, F.A.; Healey, G.R.; Bosman, E.S.; Jacobson, K.; Sly, L.M.; Vallance, B.A. Inflammatory bowel disease and immunonutrition: Novel therapeutic approaches through modulation of diet and the gut microbiome. *Immunology* **2018**, *155*, 36–52. [CrossRef]
9. Lavelle, A.; Sokol, H. Gut microbiota-derived metabolites as key actors in inflammatory bowel disease. *Nat. Rev. Gastroenterol. Hepatol.* **2020**, *17*, 223–237. [CrossRef]
10. Speca, S.; Dubuquoy, L.; Desreumaux, P. Peroxisome proliferator-activated receptor gamma in the colon: Inflammation and innate antimicrobial immunity. *J. Clin. Gastroenterol.* **2014**, *48* (Suppl. 1), S23–S27. [CrossRef]
11. Dubuquoy, L.; Rousseaux, C.; Thuru, X.; Peyrin-Biroulet, L.; Romano, O.; Chavatte, P.; Chamaillard, M.; Desreumaux, P. PPARgamma as a new therapeutic target in inflammatory bowel diseases. *Gut* **2006**, *55*, 1341–1349. [CrossRef] [PubMed]
12. Vetuschi, A.; Pompili, S.; Gaudio, E.; Latella, G.; Sferra, R. PPAR-γ with its anti-inflammatory anti-fibrotic action could be an effective therapeutic target in IBD. *Eur. Rev. Med. Pharmacol. Sci.* **2018**, *22*, 8839–8848. [PubMed]
13. Venkataraman, B.; Ojha, S.; Belur, P.D.; Bhongade, B.; Raj, V.; Collin, P.D.; Adrian, T.E.; Subramanya, S.B. Phytochemical drug candidates for the modulation of peroxisome proliferator-activated receptor γ in inflammatory bowel diseases. *Phytother. Res.* **2020**, *34*, 1530–1549. [CrossRef] [PubMed]
14. Celinski, K.; Dworzanski, T.; Fornal, R.; Korolczuk, A.; Madro, A.; Brzozowski, T.; Slomka, M. Comparison of anti-inflammatory properties of peroxisome proliferator-activated receptor gamma agonists rosiglitazone and troglitazone in prophylactic treatment of experimental colitis. *J. Physiol. Pharmacol.* **2013**, *64*, 587–595.
15. Fang, J.; Wang, H.; Xue, Z.; Cheng, Y.; Zhang, X. PPARγ: The central mucus barrier coordinator in ulcerative colitis. *Inflamm. Bowel Dis.* **2021**, *27*, 732–741. [CrossRef]
16. Luo, S.; He, J.; Huang, S.; Wang, X.; Su, Y.; Li, Y.; Chen, Y.; Yang, G.; Huang, B.; Guo, S.; et al. Emodin targeting the colonic metabolism via PPARγ alleviates UC by inhibiting facultative anaerobe. *Phytomedicine* **2022**, *104*, 154106. [CrossRef]
17. da Rocha, G.H.O.; de Paula-Silva, M.; Broering, M.F.; Scharf, P.R.D.S.; Matsuyama, L.S.A.S.; Maria-Engler, S.S.; Farsky, S.H.P. Pioglitazone-mediated attenuation of experimental colitis relies on cleaving of annexin A1 released by macrophages. *Front. Pharmacol.* **2020**, *11*, 591561. [CrossRef]
18. Dormandy, J.A.; Charbonnel, B.; Eckland, D.J.; Erdmann, E.; Massi-Benedetti, M.; Moules, I.K.; Skene, A.M.; Tan, M.H.; Lefèbvre, P.J.; Murray, G.D.; et al. PROactive investigators. Secondary prevention of macrovascular events in patients with type 2 diabetes in the PROactive Study (PROspective pioglitAzone Clinical Trial In macroVascular Events): A randomised controlled trial. *Lancet* **2005**, *366*, 1279–1289. [CrossRef]
19. Sun, T.; Kwong, C.H.T.; Gao, C.; Wei, J.; Yue, L.; Zhang, J.; Ye, R.D.; Wang, R. Amelioration of ulcerative colitis via inflammatory regulation by macrophage-biomimetic nanomedicine. *Theranostics* **2020**, *10*, 10106–10119. [CrossRef]
20. Da Silva, S.; Keita, Å.V.; Mohlin, S.; Påhlman, S.; Theodorou, V.; Påhlman, I.; Mattson, J.P.; Söderholm, J.D. A novel topical PPARγ agonist induces PPARγ activity in ulcerative colitis mucosa and prevents and reverses inflammation in induced colitis models. *Inflamm. Bowel Dis.* **2018**, *24*, 792–805. [CrossRef]
21. Tseng, C.H.; Huang, T.S. Pioglitazone with sulfonylurea: Glycemic and lipid effects in Taiwanese diabetic patients. *Diabetes Res. Clin. Pract.* **2005**, *70*, 193–194. [CrossRef] [PubMed]
22. Tseng, C.H. Pioglitazone reduces dementia risk in patients with type 2 diabetes mellitus: A retrospective cohort analysis. *J. Clin. Med.* **2018**, *7*, 306. [CrossRef] [PubMed]
23. Tseng, C.H. Pioglitazone and risk of chronic obstructive pulmonary disease in patients with type 2 diabetes mellitus. *Int J COPD.* **2022**, *17*, 285–295. [CrossRef] [PubMed]
24. Lewis, J.D.; Ferrara, A.; Peng, T.; Hedderson, M.; Bilker, W.B.; Quesenberry, C.P., Jr.; Vaughn, D.J.; Nessel, L.; Selby, J.; Strom, B.L. Risk of bladder cancer among diabetic patients treated with pioglitazone: Interim report of a longitudinal cohort study. *Diabetes Care* **2011**, *34*, 916–922. [CrossRef]
25. Kernan, W.N.; Viscoli, C.M.; Furie, K.L.; Young, L.H.; Inzucchi, S.E.; Gorman, M.; Guarino, P.D.; Lovejoy, A.M.; Peduzzi, P.N.; Conwit, R.; et al. IRIS Trial Investigators. Pioglitazone after ischemic stroke or transient ischemic attack. *N. Engl. J. Med.* **2016**, *374*, 1321–1331. [CrossRef]
26. Al-Majed, A.; Bakheit, A.H.; Abdel Aziz, H.A.; Alharbi, H.; Al-Jenoobi, F.I. Pioglitazone. *Profiles Drug Subst. Excip. Relat. Methodol.* **2016**, *41*, 379–438.
27. Pearce, N.; Checkoway, H.; Kriebel, D. Bias in occupational epidemiology studies. *Occup. Environ. Med.* **2007**, *64*, 562–568. [CrossRef]
28. Kesmodel, U.S. Information bias in epidemiological studies with a special focus on obstetrics and gynecology. *Acta Obstet. Gynecol. Scand.* **2018**, *97*, 417–423. [CrossRef]
29. Tseng, C.H. Metformin is associated with a lower risk of colorectal cancer in Taiwanese patients with type 2 diabetes: A retrospective cohort analysis. *Diabetes Metab.* **2017**, *43*, 438–445. [CrossRef]
30. Nissen, S.E.; Wolski, K. Effect of rosiglitazone on the risk of myocardial infarction and death from cardiovascular causes. *N. Engl. J. Med.* **2007**, *356*, 2457–2471. [CrossRef]

31. Austin, P.C.; Stuart, E.A. Moving towards best practice when using inverse probability of treatment weighting (IPTW) using the propensity score to estimate causal treatment effects in observational studies. *Stat. Med.* **2015**, *34*, 3661–3679. [CrossRef] [PubMed]
32. Tseng, C.H. Metformin use is associated with a lower risk of inflammatory bowel disease in patients with type 2 diabetes mellitus. *J. Crohn's Colitis* **2021**, *15*, 64–73. [CrossRef] [PubMed]

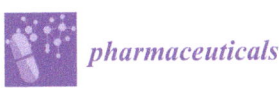

Article

Mucosal Genes Expression in Inflammatory Bowel Disease Patients: New Insights

Sumaiah J. Alarfaj [1,†], Sally Abdallah Mostafa [2,†], Walaa A. Negm [3,*], Thanaa A. El-Masry [4], Marwa Kamal [5], Mohamed Elsaeed [6,†] and Ahmed Mohamed El Nakib [7,†]

1. Department of Pharmacy Practice, College of Pharmacy, Princess Nourah Bint Abdulrahman University, P.O. Box 84428, Riyadh 11671, Saudi Arabia
2. Department of Medical Biochemistry and Molecular Biology, Faculty of Medicine, Mansoura University, Mansoura 35511, Egypt
3. Department of Pharmacognosy, Faculty of Pharmacy, Tanta University, Tanta 31527, Egypt
4. Department of Pharmacology and Toxicology, Faculty of Pharmacy, Tanta University, Tanta 31527, Egypt
5. Department of Clinical Pharmacy, Faculty of Pharmacy, Fayoum University, Fayoum 63514, Egypt
6. Department of General Surgery, Faculty of Medicine, Mansoura University, Mansoura 35511, Egypt
7. Department of Tropical Medicine, Faculty of Medicine, Mansoura University, Mansoura 35511, Egypt
* Correspondence: walaa.negm@pharm.tanta.edu.eg
† These authors contributed equally to this work.

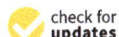

Abstract: Individual differences in IBD illness severity, behavior, progression, and therapy response are evident. Since a break in the intestinal epithelial barrier causes IBD to begin, mucosal gene expression in IBD is crucial. Due to its high sensitivity and dynamic nature, molecular analysis of biomarkers in intestinal biopsies is feasible and provides a reliable means of evaluating localized inflammation. The goal of this investigation was to discover alterations in gene expression in the inflamed mucosa of IBD patients undergoing treatment with 5-amino salicylic acid (5ASA) (N = 39) or anti-TNF drugs (N = 22). The mucosal expression of numerous IBD-related genes was evaluated using qPCR. We discovered that the levels of the proteins Lipocalin-2 (LCN2), Nitric Oxide Synthase 2 (NOS2), Mucin 2 (MUC2), Mucin 5AC (MUC5AC), and Trefoil factor 1 (TFF1), which are overexpressed in untreated IBD patients compared to non-IBD subjects, are decreased by both therapy regimens. On the other hand, anti-TNF medicine helped the levels of ABCB1 and E-cadherin return to normal in IBD patients who were not receiving treatment.

Keywords: 5-ASA; anti-TNF; gene expression; Crohn's disease; ulcerative colitis

1. Introduction

Inflammatory bowel disease is a long-term inflammatory condition of the gut that can present clinically as Crohn's disease (CD), ulcerative colitis (UC), or IBD undefined (IBD-U) [1–3].

The intensity, behavior, progression, and response to therapy for IBD disease show significant individual diversity [2,4–6]. Both clinical factors and molecular signatures have been linked to many elements of disease progression. Previous studies dealing with molecular investigations have been demonstrated and are used for clinical practice and therapeutic decision-making in IBD patients [7–9].

In the past 20 years, numerous innovative therapeutic agents targeting different immune pathways have also been developed, in addition to tumor necrosis factor (anti-TNF) inhibitors [10]. Taking these medications has improved the long-term results for both CD and UC, despite a significant increase in the expense burden on many health care systems [11].

The current therapy goals for IBD now include steroid-free remission, endoscopic remission, and lowering surgery rates [12]. Although the primary therapeutic purpose

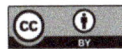

was to alleviate patient symptoms, in addition to the fact that over 30% of IBD patients do not respond to treatment, among those who do, the response vanishes in 23–46% of instances after a year of medication use [13]. In order to improve the overall IBD disease management, a treatment plan based on molecular perturbations and the detection of predictors of nonresponse can be chosen [14].

In IBD patients, mucosal gene expression is particularly significant because a breach in the intestinal epithelium barrier is thought to be the source of the disease's development. Due to their high sensitivity and dynamic nature, various molecular biomarkers in intestinal biopsies are feasible and offer a reliable approach to evaluating localized inflammation.

Mucosal genes play an essential role in mucosal integrity and play an important role in the pathogenesis of IBD. Genes within several IBD-associated loci indicate a position for barrier integrity in disease predisposition [15].

Another difficulty in controlling IBD disease is monitoring the pathophysiological mechanisms behind the chronic inflammatory process and the effects of treatment. Studies on molecular mucosal profiling are scarce in this area [15].

This study aimed to find differences in the gene expression between the mucosa of IBD patients receiving 5-aminosalicylic acid (5ASA) or biological therapies in the form of anti-TNF treatment and IBD patients receiving no medication or control subjects without IBD.

2. Results

2.1. Histological Changes

At the time of enrolment, 22 patients (27.5%) were receiving anti-TNF (anti-TNF) therapy, 39 patients (48.75%) were receiving (5-ASA), and 19 patients (23.75%) were drug-free. Among the treated patients, 59 were still in the active phase, and 21 showed endoscopically as being in remission. Clinical response for all patients was performed using the A MAYO partial score and Crohn's Disease Activity Index (CDAI) score (Figures 1–4).

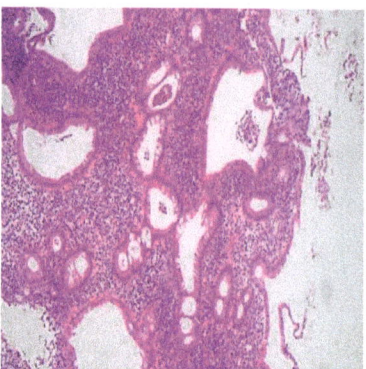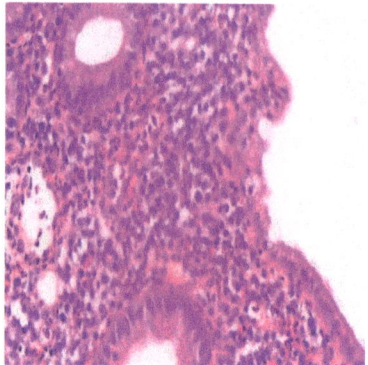

Figure 1. Moderate diffuse active colitis consistent with IBD (ulcerative colitis).

Multiple snips of colonic mucosa. Lamina was widened by dense mixed inflammatory cellular infiltrate involving muscularis mucosa. The infiltrate was mainly lymphoplasmacytic with mixed neutrophils and eosinophils. There was crypt irregularity with branching and a reduction in mucin production. There was detected cryptitis and crypt abscesses (Left: 200×/Right: 400×, H&E staining).

Multiple snips of colonic mucosa with focal ulceration. Lamina was widened by dense mixed inflammatory cellular infiltrate involving muscularis mucosa. The infiltrate was mainly lymphoplasmacytic with mixed neutrophils and eosinophils. There was crypt irregularity with branching and a reduction in mucin production. Cryptitis and crypt abscesses were detected (Left: 200×/Right: 400×, H&E staining).

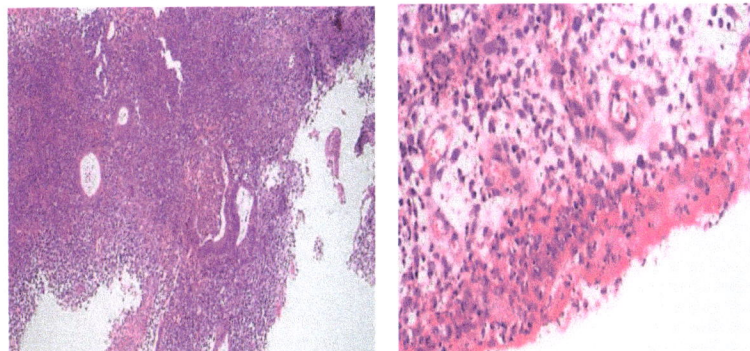

Figure 2. Severe diffuse active colitis consistent with IBD (ulcerative colitis).

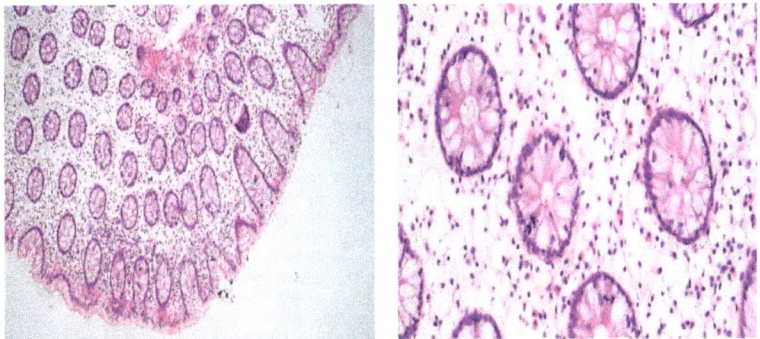

Figure 3. Mild focal colitis (quiescent stage of IBD)/(known case of ulcerative colitis).

Multiple snips of colonic mucosa with preserved mucin production and no significant crypt irregularity. Lamina propria was the seat of chronic inflammatory cellular infiltrate with some eosinophils about 15/HPF. No detected cryptitis or crypt abscesses (Left: 200×/Right: 400×).

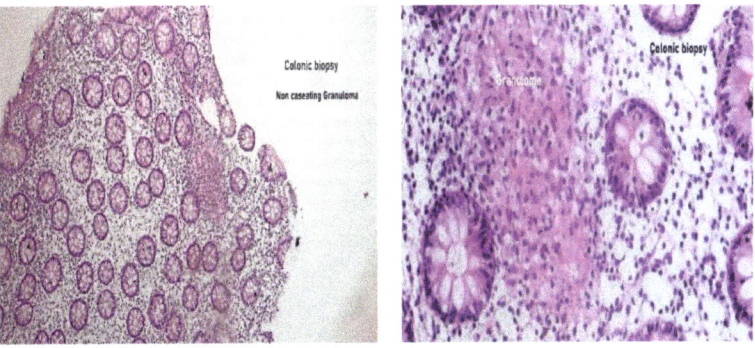

Figure 4. Moderate diffuse colitis with non-caseating epithelioid granulomatous inflammatory lesion highly suggestive of Crohn's disease.

Snips of colonic mucosa. Crypts were regular. The lamina propria was the seat of moderate inflammatory cellular infiltrate. The infiltrate was formed of lymphocytes and neutrophils with focal cryptitis. Multiple epithelioid granulomas were detected, which were non-caseating (Left: 200×/Right: 400×, H&E staining).

2.2. Patients' and Non-IBD Control Participants' Characteristics

The IBD patients' age, gender distribution, and smoking habits did not differ from those of the non-IBD control subjects. When patients were taken into account, there was no discernible difference in the length of the treatments for the 5-ASA and anti-TNF groups (Table 1).

Table 1. Characteristics of the IBD and control participants.

IBD Patients	N = 80
Age (mean ± SD)	46.75 ± 6.648
Sex (%M)	(N = 56) 70%
Sex (%F)	(N = 24) 30%
Smoking Behavior	
Non-smokers	(N = 62) 77.5%
Mild	(N = 12) 15%
Moderate	(N = 3) 3.75%
Severe	(N = 3) 3.75%
Type of Disease	
(%UC)	(N = 62) 77.5%
(%CD)	(N = 18) 22.5%
Disease Activity	
% Active	(N = 59) 73.75%
% Remission	(N = 21) 26.25%
Treatment Duration	
Drug-free	23.75% (19 patients)
5-ASA treatment	48.75% (3–24 months) (31 UC patients & 8 CD patients)
Anti-TNF treatment	27.5% (3–24 months) (12 UC patients & 10 CD patients)
Non-IBD subjects	N = 80
Age (mean ± SD)	49.78 ± 4.352
Sex (%M)	(N = 55) 68.75%
Sex (%F)	(N = 25) 31.25%
Smoking Behavior	
Non-smokers	(N = 70) 87.5%
Mild	(N = 5) 6.25%
Moderate	(N = 2) 2.5%
Severe	(N = 3) 3.75%

2.3. Gene Expression among Studied Groups

The results are displayed in Table S1 and Figure 5.

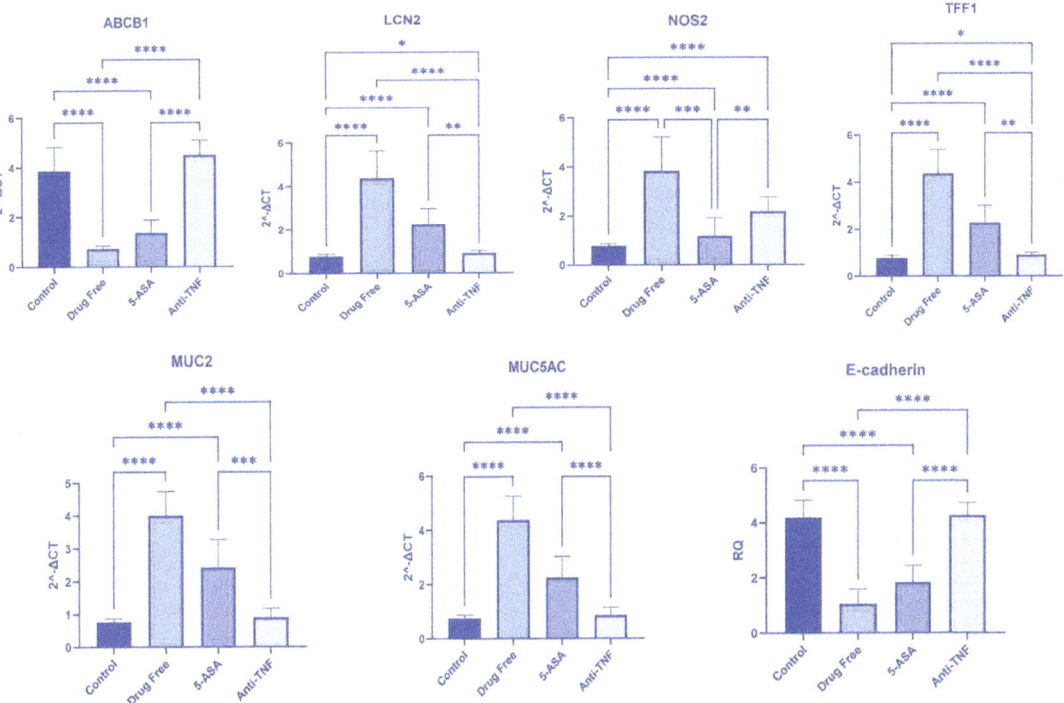

Figure 5. Gene expression in different groups. This shows the gene expression of various genes among the other studied groups (* significant at $p < 0.05$, ** at $p < 0.01$, *** at $p < 0.001$, **** at $p < 0.0001$).

2.3.1. ABCB1 Gene Expression

Regarding ABCB1 gene expression, there was a statistically substantial difference between patients receiving anti-TNF-α and those receiving 5-ASA ($p < 0.0001$). There was also a significant difference between participants receiving anti-TNF-α and those who received no treatment ($p < 0.0001$). There was no statistical difference between patients obtaining anti-TNF-α and the control group ($p = 0.4361$).

2.3.2. LCN2 Gene Expression

Regarding LCN2 gene expression, there was a statistically marked difference between participants receiving anti-TNF-α and those receiving 5-ASA ($p = 0.0012$). There was a statistically substantial difference between patients receiving anti-TNF-α and those who received no treatment ($p < 0.0001$). There was a statistically marked difference between patients obtaining anti-TNF-α and the control group ($p = 0.0139$).

2.3.3. NOS2 Gene Expression

There was a statistically significant difference between participants receiving anti-TNF-α and those receiving 5-ASA in NOS2 gene expression ($p = 0.0095$). There was no statistically significant difference between patients receiving anti-TNF-α and those receiving no treatment ($p > 0.9999$). There was a statistically significant difference between the anti-TNF-α treated patients and the control group ($p < 0.0001$).

2.3.4. TFF1 Gene Expression

Regarding TFF1 gene expression, patients receiving anti-TNF-α and those receiving 5-ASA differed statistically significantly ($p = 0.0016$). There was a statistically significant difference between the patients taking anti-TNF-α and those who received no treatment ($p < 0.0001$). There was a statistically marked difference between patients taking anti-TNF-α and the control group ($p = 0.0188$) [16].

2.3.5. MUC2 Gene Expression

Regarding MUC2 gene expression, there was a statistically substantial difference between patients receiving anti-TNF-α and those receiving 5-ASA ($p = 0.0003$). There was a statistically significant difference between patients receiving anti-TNF-α and those who received no treatment ($p < 0.0001$). There was no statistically significant difference between patients receiving anti-TNF-α and the control group ($p = 0.2564$).

2.3.6. MUC5AC Gene Expression

There was a statistically marked variation in MUC5AC gene expression between patients receiving anti-TNF-α and those receiving 5-ASA ($p < 0.0001$). There was a statistically marked difference between the patients receiving anti-TNF-α and those who received no treatment ($p < 0.0001$). There was no statistically significant difference between patients receiving anti-TNF-α and the control group ($p > 0.9999$).

2.3.7. E-Cadherin Gene Expression

Regarding E-cadherin gene expression, there was a statistically substantial variation between those receiving anti-TNF-α and 5-ASA ($p < 0.0001$). There was a statistically marked difference between patients obtaining anti-TNF-α and those who received no treatment ($p < 0.0001$). There was no statistically substantial difference between patients taking anti-TNF-α and the control group ($p > 0.9999$) [17].

2.4. ROC Curve Analysis for Different Gene Expression

The results are displayed in Figure 6.

For discrimination between the IBD patients and controls, ROC curve analysis was performed for different genes. The ABCB1 gene's cutoff value was <1.45, with a sensitivity of 100%, a specificity of 100%, and an AUC of 1. The AUC was 1, a sensitivity oof 100%, specificity was 100%, and >0.95 was the cutoff value for the LCN2 gene. The NOS2 gene's cutoff value was >0.85, with a sensitivity of 100%, a specificity of 76.3%, and an AUC of 0.981. The TFF1 gene's cutoff value was >1.45, with a sensitivity of 100%, a specificity of 100%, and an AUC of 1. The MUC2 gene's cutoff value was >1.45, with a sensitivity of 100%, a specificity of 100%, and an AUC of 1. The MUC5AC gene's cutoff value was >1.45, with a sensitivity of 100%, a specificity of 100%, and an AUC of 1. The E-cadherin gene's cutoff value was <2.5, with a sensitivity of 94.7%, a specificity of 100%, and an AUC of 0.0997.

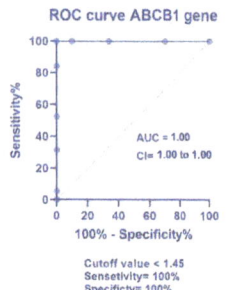
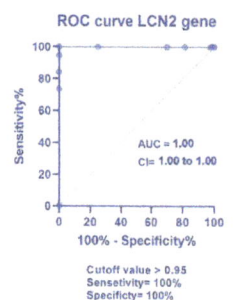
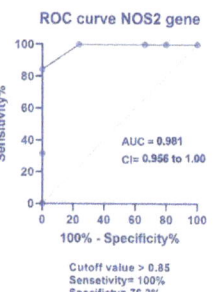
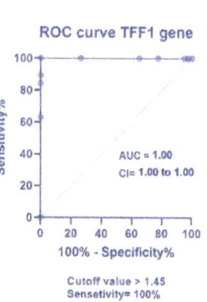

Figure 6. *Cont.*

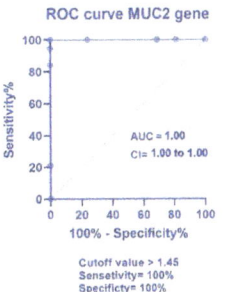 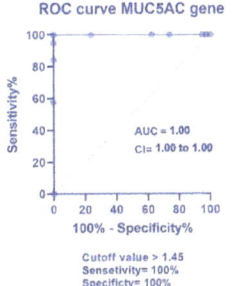 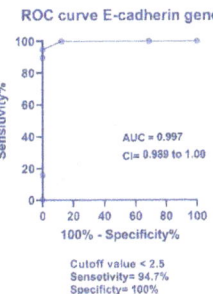

Figure 6. The ROC curve analysis of the different genes.

2.5. Correlation between Different Genes

The correlation between different genes is explained in Figure 7 and Table S2. There was a strong negative relationship between the ABCB1 gene and E-cadherin gene, LCN2 gene, MUC2 gene, MUC5AC gene, and TFF1 gene (r = −0.73, −0.77, −0.76, −0.77, and −078 respectively). There was a negligible relationship between the ABCB1 gene and the NOS2 gene (r = −0.14).

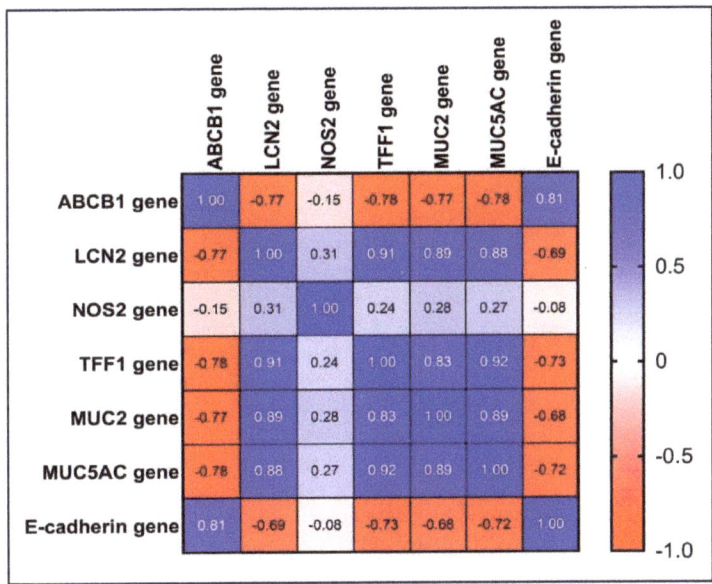

Figure 7. Correlation between different genes.

There was a strong positive relationship between the LCN2 gene and E-cadherin gene, MUC2 gene, MUC5AC, and TFF1 gene (r = 0.88, 0.88, 0.87, 0.91, respectively). On the other hand, there was a moderate positive relationship between the LCN2 gene and the NOS2 gene (r = 0.31). There was a strong positive relationship between the MUC2 gene and both the E-cadherin gene and the MUC5AC gene (r = 0.9 and 0.88, respectively).

There was a strong relationship between the MU5AC gene and E-cadherin (r = 0.88).

There was a weak positive relationship between the NOS2 gene, MUC2 gene, MUC5AC gene, and TFF1 gene (r = 0.28, 0.26, and 0.23, respectively). On the other hand, there was a moderate positive relationship between the NOS2 gene and E-cadherin (r = 0.3).

There was a strong positive relationship between the TFF1 gene and the E-cadherin gene, MUC2 gene, and MUC5AC gene (r = 0.88, 0.83 and 0.91, respectively).

3. Discussion

In order to assess changes in the colonic mucosa of IBD patients under various therapy modalities, we used a bull's eye gene expression approach to look at genes implicated in inflammation, apoptosis, immunological response, cellular adhesion, and tissue remodeling. Previous studies comparing the molecular signature of patients undergoing various medications remain underrepresented, despite the extensive use of the transcriptional analysis of intestinal tissues comparing IBD patients and non-IBD controls to uncover new biomarkers.

Following anti-TNF medication, ABCB1 was increased after being downregulated in drug-free patients. P-Glycoprotein 1, an ATP-dependent transmembrane pump that transfers drugs from the intracellular to the extracellular area, is encoded by the ABCB1 gene, commonly known as the MDR1 gene. It has been proposed that reduced gut expression levels and ABCB1's lack of function are factors in the genesis of IBD. The typical gastrointestinal system expresses ABCB1 extensively [18].

Additionally, inconsistent results have been found in several genetic studies examining the connection between IBD susceptibility and the three SNPs (G2677T/A, C3435T, and C1236T) regarded to be the most clinically significant [19]. Numerous research has evaluated ABCB1's role in the responsiveness to anti-TNF medications. There was no significant correlation between the ABCB1 gene alternates and infliximab response in Italian and Hungarian patients with IBD [11,20,21]. In this study, we found that the low levels of ABCB1 in patients were markedly increased by anti-TNF medication, bringing them to levels that were equivalent to the non-IBD controls. One in vitro study using Caco-2 cell lines displayed that in vitro TNF reduced the MDR1 mRNA levels. However, the possible alteration of ABCB1 in the mucosa of IBD patients by anti-TNF therapy has not been studied [22].

Additionally, we found that ABCB1 expression was significantly increased by anti-TNF medication, reaching levels comparable to those seen in the control subjects free of IBD. These results were consistent with the earlier research by Milanesi et al. (2019) [14].

Our findings demonstrate that 5-ASA and anti-TNF medications can lower the mucosal expression levels of NOS2, TFF1, and LCN2, which were excessive in untreated cases relative to the controls. Interestingly, anti-TNF medicine had a more significant effect on TFF1 and LCN2; nonetheless, treatment returned their levels to normal for individuals who were not affected. The impacts of 5-ASA on NOS2 expression also seem more favorable, despite the differences from the non-IBD controls being noticeably different. These results were in line with those of an earlier investigation by Milanesi et al. (2019) [14]. The NOS2 and LCN2 genes encode two antimicrobial peptides (AMPs): nitric oxide synthase 2 and the neutrophil gelatinase-associated lipocalin (NGAL) system.

LCN2/NGAL prevents bacterial development by securing iron-containing siderophores, while NOS2 produces nitric oxide, a reactive free radical that is a biological moderator in antibacterial, neurotransmission, and anti-tumor effects.

Numerous studies have demonstrated that the mucosa of IBD patients has both highly elevated LCN2/NGAL and NOS2 levels [23,24]. Notably, the NGAL protein has been proposed as a potential biomarker in IBD patients since, if present in high concentrations, it is positively connected with the severity and activity of the disease. The LCN2/NGAL levels were shown to be higher in patients with active UC, and infliximab treatment resulted in a decrease in these levels [24].

A single high infliximab dosage effectively lowered the elevated LCN protein concentration in the urine of CD patients. This intriguing result was also shown in our research, where the treated group's LCN2 expression was lower [25].

Nitric oxide (NO) is produced by the enzyme NOS2, activated through a concoction of lipopolysaccharide and specific inflammatory mediators. Nitric oxide controls bowel epithelial cells, preserves the barrier's integrity, and supports tight junctions. Additionally, it starts the oxidation of proteins and lipids through a free radical process that causes a redox imbalance. It has been demonstrated that the colon mucosa of both UC and CD patients exhibit enhanced nitric oxide synthase activity [26,27].

Higher gene expression levels were found by Senhaji et al. in 2017 in the colonic mucosa of CD patients compared to the controls and in patients with active UC compared to patients with passive UC [28]. Numerous populations have demonstrated a relationship between NOS2 gene variations and IBD risk [28,29]. Luther and colleagues discovered that the colonic expression of NOS2 was higher in non-responders than responders in individuals who lost response to the TNF-antagonist [30].

TFF1 is another increased gene in untreated individuals, and 5-ASA and anti-TNF treatments impact it. It is related to the same family as the trefoils TFF1, TFF2, and TFF3 [31]. It has been demonstrated that these persistent secretory proteins contribute to the upkeep and restoration of epithelial surfaces because they are highly expressed in the gastrointestinal mucosa [32].

While chronic inflammation encourages TFF expression to limit the course of the disease, acute mucosal damage stimulates TFFs to expedite cell migration to seal the wounded zone from luminal contents. TFF1 was expressed in individuals with severe UC in immunohistochemical studies on colon biopsy specimens but not in normal tissue [33].

Shaoul et al. (2004) found that this trefoil protein was also expressed in the colons of patients with IBD [34]. The serum levels of the trefoil factors have also been investigated, and those with IBD had higher concentrations of TFF1 and TFF3 [35].

Additionally, in UC patients, the serum TFF3 concentration was associated with the clinical and biochemical indicators of disease activity [36].

In the inflamed IBD colon, E-cadherin gene expression was dramatically reduced. The loss and destruction of epithelial cells in the colon affected by IBD are likely to blame for the reduced expression.

Additionally, IBD responders to anti-TNF medication showed normalized expression of this gene, and these results were consistent with those of an earlier study conducted by Arijs et al. in 2011 [37].

Both the MUC2 and MUC5AC genes were found to be significantly expressed in the current study's untreated IBD patients, and their expression returned to normal after receiving anti-TNF medication.

MUC2 is the prominent colonic mucin in IBD, although it is not just found in healthy goblet cells. Clamp et al. [38] discovered that granular MUC2 is expressed by not phenotypical goblet cells in IBD and other inflammatory conditions of the colon. Contrary to the goblet cells of healthy people and IBD patients, who keep mature granular mucin and do not express immature mucin outside the Golgi, these cells express weakly glycosylated mucin present in secretory granules. This mucin is likely secreted as a juvenile, sparsely glycosylated product. This abnormal pattern of mucin glycosylation in IBD patients has also been proposed by others [38,39].

To make up for the loss of barrier and repair function caused by MUC2 and perhaps ITF expression alterations during inflammation, MUC5AC and TFF1 expression may be upregulated. It has been hypothesized that TFF1 aids in healing and regeneration [40].

Goblet cells that express MUC5ACTFF1 are frequently found in inflammatory conditions, indicating that this is a generic response to inflammation and may not always signify dysplastic alterations [34]. The cross-sectional nature of this study could be a possible drawback. Furthermore, the small size of our study prevented us from conducting additional subgroup analysis (UC and CD separately).

4. Materials and Methods

4.1. Patients

Eighty IBD patients and 80 healthy control participants from the Tropical Medicine Department at the Mansoura Faculty of Medicine were recruited for this study out of 1974 patients who underwent colonoscopy over three years (Figure 8).

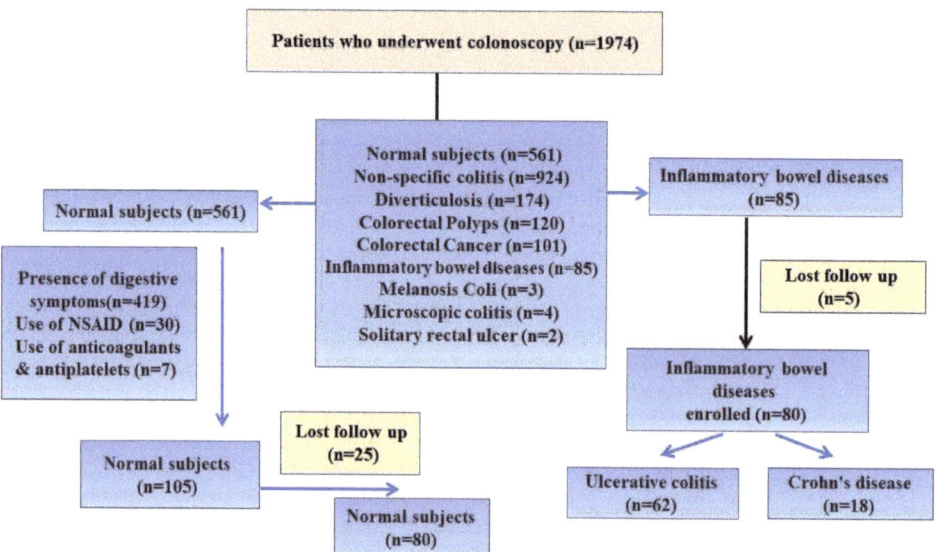

Figure 8. Flowchart of the study.

Multiple colonoscopic biopsies were taken from the inflamed mucosa in patients with active IBD, those IBD patients who were in remission, and from the healthy colonic mucosa from healthy control individuals. Before biopsy sampling, all individuals provided written informed consent. The Mansoura Faculty of Medicine's Institutional Review Board (MFM-IRB) authorized the study (Code number R.22.08.1786).

Crohn's disease (CD) and ulcerative colitis (UC) were identified in accordance with suggestions made by the European Crohn's and Colitis Organization (ECCO), which preclude that the diagnosis of CD or UC is based on a combination of clinical, biochemical, stool, endoscopic, cross-sectional imaging, and histological investigations [3]. According to Dobre et al. (2018) [14], the following exclusion criteria were applied to the non-IBD control subjects: the presence of gastrointestinal symptoms, current or previous use of non-steroidal anti-inflammatory drugs (within the last three months), and current or prior use of anticoagulants/antiplatelet drugs (within the last three months).

Monoclonal antibodies directed against TNF-α are fast-acting and potent anti-inflammatory agents. Anti-TNF therapies approved for treating IBD include infliximab, adalimumab, and certolizumab [3].

4.2. Total RNA Isolation and qPCR

For qPCR, a 7500 Fast Real-Time PCR system was used. The total RNA was extracted from fresh-frozen tissues using the RNeasy Mini Kit (Qiagen, Venlo, Germany), and the RNA quantity and quality were assessed using a spectrophotometric approach (NanoDrop 2000, Thermo Scientific™ ND2000USCAN, Waltham, MA, USA). The total RNA was then converted to complementary DNA (cDNA) using the SensiFAST™ cDNA Kit (Bioline, London, UK). As an internal control gene, glyceraldehyde 3-phosphate dehydrogenase (GAPDH) was employed along with the SensiFAST™ SYBR Green PCR Master Mix from

Bioline. We applied the 2CT approach to determine the fold change in gene expression. Table S3 shows the primer sequences of different genes, and the GAPDH gene was used as the control gene.

4.3. Statistical Analysis

Continuous variables were tested using the t-test, while categorical variables were tested using the Chi-square test. The gene expression data are displayed as the mean ± standard deviation (SD). To ascertain each gene's appropriate cutoff value and diagnostic accuracy, receiver operating characteristic (ROC) curves were built.

The differences in gene expression were estimated using Kruskal–Wallis and Dunn's multiple comparisons tests. The statistical analysis of each gene's expression was verified for normality using the Shapiro–Wilk normality test. The Spearman correlation test was used to examine the relationship among genes. GraphPad Prism was used for statistical analysis (version 9.3.1). At $p < 0.05$, significance was accepted.

5. Conclusions

Considering the potential drawbacks of our investigation, we identified a configuration of genes whose ectopic expression in IBD mucosa appears to be better controlled by biological therapy (anti-TNF therapy) than by 5-ASA medications. Lipocalin-2 (LCN2), Nitric Oxide Synthase 2 (NOS2), Mucin 2 (MUC2), Mucin 5AC (MUC5AC), and Trefoil factor 1 (TFF1) were overexpressed in the untreated IBD patients compared to the non-IBD patients and that 5ASA and anti-TNF-a treatment reduced these expressions. Anti-TNF therapy helped the levels of ABCB1 and E-cadherin in the untreated IBD patients return to normal. To find the gene expression profiles useful for assisting therapeutic decision-making, more extensive studies of treatment naive IBD with standardized sampling and the prospective follow-up of clinical outcomes are pertinent.

Supplementary Materials: The following supporting information can be downloaded at: https://www.mdpi.com/article/10.3390/ph16020324/s1, Table S1. Gene expression analysis among different groups, Table S2. Explanation of correlation between different genes, Table S3. Primer sequences of different genes.

Author Contributions: Conceptualization, A.M.E.N. and W.A.N.; Data curation, M.E.; Formal analysis, S.J.A.; Funding acquisition, T.A.E.-M.; Investigation, S.A.M., M.E., and A.M.E.N.; Methodology, S.A.M., M.K., and A.M.E.N.; Project administration, S.J.A.; Resources, S.J.A., and M.K.; Software, W.A.N., and M.K.; Supervision, T.A.E.-M. and W.A.N.; Writing—original draft, S.A.M., M.E., and A.M.E.N.; Writing—review & editing, W.A.N., M.K., S.J.A., and A.M.E.N. All authors have read and agreed to the published version of the manuscript.

Funding: This project was funded by Princess Nourah bint Abdulrahman University Researchers Supporting Project Number (PNURSP2023R167), Princess Nourah bint Abdulrahman University, Riyadh, Saudi Arabia.

Institutional Review Board Statement: The present study was permitted and approved by Mansoura Faculty of Medicine's Institutional Review Board (MFM-IRB) (Code number R.22.08.1786).

Informed Consent Statement: Written informed consent was obtained from all 160 participants in this study, and the study was approved by the ethical committee of the Mansoura Faculty of Medicine (Code number R.22.08.1786).

Data Availability Statement: The data presented in this study are available on request.

Acknowledgments: We greatly appreciate the support of Princess Nourah bint Abdulrahman University in funding this research through Princess Nourah bint Abdulrahman University Researchers Supporting Project Number (PNURSP2023R167), Princess Nourah bint Abdulrahman University, Riyadh, Saudi Arabia.

Conflicts of Interest: The authors declare no conflict of interest.

References

1. Gomollón, F.; Dignass, A.; Annese, V.; Tilg, H.; Van Assche, G.; Lindsay, J.O.; Peyrin-Biroulet, L.; Cullen, G.J.; Daperno, M.; Kucharzik, T., 3rd European evidence-based consensus on the diagnosis and management of Crohn's disease 2016: Part 1: Diagnosis and medical management. *J. Crohns Colitis* **2017**, *11*, 3–25. [CrossRef] [PubMed]
2. Thia, K.T.; Sandborn, W.J.; Harmsen, W.S.; Zinsmeister, A.R.; Loftus Jr, E.V. Risk factors associated with progression to intestinal complications of Crohn's disease in a population-based cohort. *Gastroenterology* **2010**, *139*, 1147–1155. [CrossRef] [PubMed]
3. Magro, F.; Gionchetti, P.; Eliakim, R.; Ardizzone, S.; Armuzzi, A.; Barreiro-de Acosta, M.; Burisch, J.; Gecse, K.B.; Hart, A.L.; Hindryckx, P. Third European evidence-based consensus on diagnosis and management of ulcerative colitis. Part 1: Definitions, diagnosis, extra-intestinal manifestations, pregnancy, cancer surveillance, surgery, and ileo-anal pouch disorders. *J. Crohns Colitis* **2017**, *11*, 649–670. [CrossRef] [PubMed]
4. Beaugerie, L.; Seksik, P.; Nion–Larmurier, I.; Gendre, J.P.; Cosnes, J. Predictors of Crohn's disease. *Gastroenterology* **2006**, *130*, 650–656. [CrossRef]
5. Monstad, I.; Hovde, Ø.; Solberg, I.C.; Moum, B.A. Clinical course and prognosis in ulcerative colitis: Results from population-based and observational studies. *Ann. Gastroenterol. Q. Publ. Hell. Soc. Gastroenterol.* **2014**, *27*, 95.
6. Alarfaj, S.J.; Mostafa, S.A.; Abdelsalam, R.A.; Negm, W.A.; El-Masry, T.A.; Hussein, I.A.; El Nakib, A.M. Helicobacter pylori Infection in Cirrhotic Patients with Portal Hypertensive Gastropathy: A New Enigma? *Front. Med.* **2022**, *9*, 902255. [CrossRef]
7. Martin, J.C.; Chang, C.; Boschetti, G.; Ungaro, R.; Giri, M.; Grout, J.A.; Gettler, K.; Chuang, L.-s.; Nayar, S.; Greenstein, A.J. Single-cell analysis of Crohn's disease lesions identifies a pathogenic cellular module associated with resistance to anti-TNF therapy. *Cell* **2019**, *178*, 1493–1508.e1420. [CrossRef]
8. Marigorta, U.M.; Denson, L.A.; Hyams, J.S.; Mondal, K.; Prince, J.; Walters, T.D.; Griffiths, A.; Noe, J.D.; Crandall, W.V.; Rosh, J.R. Transcriptional risk scores link GWAS to eQTLs and predict complications in Crohn's disease. *Nat. Genet.* **2017**, *49*, 1517–1521. [CrossRef]
9. Lee, J.C.; Lyons, P.A.; McKinney, E.F.; Sowerby, J.M.; Carr, E.J.; Bredin, F.; Rickman, H.M.; Ratlamwala, H.; Hatton, A.; Rayner, T.F. Gene expression profiling of CD8+ T cells predicts prognosis in patients with Crohn disease and ulcerative colitis. *J. Clin. Investig.* **2011**, *121*, 4170–4179. [CrossRef]
10. Reinisch, W.; Sandborn, W.J.; Rutgeerts, P.; Feagan, B.G.; Rachmilewitz, D.; Hanauer, S.B.; Lichtenstein, G.R.; De Villiers, W.J.; Blank, M.; Lang, Y. Long-term infliximab maintenance therapy for ulcerative colitis: The ACT-1 and-2 extension studies. *Inflamm. Bowel Dis.* **2012**, *18*, 201–211. [CrossRef]
11. Reinglas, J.; Gonczi, L.; Kurt, Z.; Bessissow, T.; Lakatos, P.L. Positioning of old and new biologicals and small molecules in the treatment of inflammatory bowel diseases. *World J. Gastroenterol.* **2018**, *24*, 3567. [CrossRef]
12. Atreya, R.; Neurath, M.F. Current and future targets for mucosal healing in inflammatory bowel disease. *Visc. Med.* **2017**, *33*, 82–88. [CrossRef]
13. Ben-Horin, S.; Chowers, Y. loss of response to anti-TNF treatments in Crohn's disease. *Aliment. Pharmacol. Ther.* **2011**, *33*, 987–995. [CrossRef]
14. Milanesi, E.; Dobre, M.; Manuc, T.E.; Becheanu, G.; Tieranu, C.G.; Ionescu, E.M.; Manuc, M. Mucosal gene expression changes induced by anti-TNF treatment in inflammatory bowel disease patients. *Drug Dev. Res.* **2019**, *80*, 831–836. [CrossRef]
15. D'Amico, F.; Netter, P.; Baumann, C.; Veltin, M.; Zallot, C.; Aimone-Gastin, I.; Danese, S.; Peyrin-Biroulet, L. Setting up a virtual calprotectin clinic in inflammatory bowel diseases: Literature review and nancy experience. *J. Clin. Med.* **2020**, *9*, 2697. [CrossRef]
16. Mostafa, S.A.; Mohammad, M.H.; Negm, W.A.; Batiha, G.E.S.; Alotaibi, S.S.; Albogami, S.M.; De Waard, M.; Tawfik, N.Z.; Abdallah, H.Y. Circulating microRNA203 and its target genes' role in psoriasis pathogenesis. *Front. Med.* **2022**, *9*, 988962. [CrossRef]
17. Muise, A.M.; Walters, T.D.; Glowacka, W.K.; Griffiths, A.M.; Ngan, B.; Lan, H.; Xu, W.; Silverberg, M.; Rotin, D. Polymorphisms in E-cadherin (CDH1) result in a mis-localised cytoplasmic protein that is associated with Crohn's disease. *Gut* **2009**, *58*, 1121–1127. [CrossRef]
18. Borg-Bartolo, S.P.; Boyapati, R.K.; Satsangi, J.; Kalla, R. Precision medicine in inflammatory bowel disease: Concept, progress and challenges. *F1000Research* **2020**, *9*, 54. [CrossRef]
19. Petryszyn, P.W.; Wiela-Hojeńska, A. The importance of the polymorphisms of the ABCB1 gene in disease susceptibility, behavior and response to treatment in inflammatory bowel disease: A literature review. *Adv. Clin. Exp. Med.* **2018**, *27*, 1459–1463. [CrossRef]
20. Palmieri, O.; Latiano, A.; Valvano, R.; D'inca, R.; Vecchi, M.; Sturniolo, G.; Saibeni, S.; Bossa, F.; Latiano, T.; Devoto, M. Multidrug resistance 1 gene polymorphisms are not associated with inflammatory bowel disease and response to therapy in Italian patients. *Aliment. Pharmacol. Ther.* **2005**, *22*, 1129–1138. [CrossRef]
21. Zintzaras, E. Is there evidence to claim or deny association between variants of the multidrug resistance gene (MDR1 or ABCB1) and inflammatory bowel disease? *Inflamm. Bowel Dis.* **2012**, *18*, 562–572. [CrossRef]
22. Belliard, A.M.; Lacour, B.; Farinotti, R.; Leroy, C. Effect of tumor necrosis factor-α and interferon-γ on intestinal P-glycoprotein expression, activity, and localization in Caco-2 cells. *J. Pharm. Sci.* **2004**, *93*, 1524–1536. [CrossRef] [PubMed]
23. Dobre, M.; Mănuc, T.E.; Milanesi, E.; Pleşea, I.E.; Ţieranu, E.N.; Popa, C.; Mănuc, M.; Preda, C.M.; Ţieranu, I.; Diculescu, M.M. Mucosal CCR1 gene expression as a marker of molecular activity in Crohn's disease: Preliminary data. *Rom. J. Morphol. Embryol* **2017**, *58*, 1263–1268. [PubMed]

24. Thorsvik, S.; Bakke, I.; van Beelen Granlund, A.; Røyset, E.S.; Damås, J.K.; Østvik, A.E.; Sandvik, A.K. Expression of neutrophil gelatinase-associated lipocalin (NGAL) in the gut in Crohn's disease. *Cell Tissue Res.* **2018**, *374*, 339–348. [CrossRef] [PubMed]
25. Bolignano, D.; Della Torre, A.; Lacquaniti, A.; Costantino, G.; Fries, W.; Buemi, M. Neutrophil gelatinase-associated lipocalin levels in patients with Crohn disease undergoing treatment with infliximab. *J. Investig. Med.* **2010**, *58*, 569–571. [CrossRef]
26. Guihot, G.; Guimbaud, R.; Bertrand, V.; Narcy-Lambare, B.; Couturier, D.; Duée, P.-H.; Chaussade, S.; Blachier, F. Inducible nitric oxide synthase activity in colon biopsies from inflammatory areas: Correlation with inflammation intensity in patients with ulcerative colitis but not with Crohn's disease. *Amino Acids* **2000**, *18*, 229–237. [CrossRef]
27. Alotaibi, B.; Mokhtar, F.A.; El-Masry, T.A.; Elekhnawy, E.; Mostafa, S.A.; Abdelkader, D.H.; Elharty, M.E.; Saleh, A.; Negm, W.A. Antimicrobial activity of brassica rapa L. Flowers extract on gastrointestinal tract infections and antiulcer potential against Indomethacin-Induced gastric ulcer in rats supported by metabolomics profiling. *J. Inflamm. Res.* **2021**, *14*, 7411. [CrossRef]
28. Senhaji, N.; Nadifi, S.; Zaid, Y.; Serrano, A.; Rodriguez, D.A.L.; Serbati, N.; Karkouri, M.; Badre, W.; Martín, J. Polymorphisms in oxidative pathway related genes and susceptibility to inflammatory bowel disease. *World J. Gastroenterol.* **2017**, *23*, 8300. [CrossRef]
29. Martín, M.C.; Martinez, A.; Mendoza, J.L.; Taxonera, C.; Díaz-Rubio, M.; Fernández-Arquero, M.; de la Concha, E.G.; Urcelay, E. Influence of the inducible nitric oxide synthase gene (NOS2A) on inflammatory bowel disease susceptibility. *Immunogenetics* **2007**, *59*, 833–837. [CrossRef]
30. Luther, J.; Gala, M.; Patel, S.J.; Dave, M.; Borren, N.; Xavier, R.J.; Ananthakrishnan, A.N. Loss of response to anti-tumor necrosis factor alpha therapy in Crohn's disease is not associated with emergence of novel inflammatory pathways. *Dig. Dis. Sci.* **2018**, *63*, 738–745. [CrossRef]
31. Kjellev, S. The trefoil factor family–small peptides with multiple functionalities. *Cell. Mol. Life Sci.* **2009**, *66*, 1350–1369. [CrossRef]
32. Aihara, E.; Engevik, K.A.; Montrose, M.H. Trefoil factor peptides and gastrointestinal function. *Annu. Rev. Physiol.* **2017**, *79*, 357. [CrossRef]
33. Longman, R.J.; Poulsom, R.; Corfield, A.P.; Warren, B.F.; Wright, N.A.; Thomas, M.G. Alterations in the composition of the supramucosal defense barrier in relation to disease severity of ulcerative colitis. *J. Histochem. Cytochem.* **2006**, *54*, 1335–1348. [CrossRef]
34. Shaoul, R.; Okada, Y.; Cutz, E.; Marcon, M.A. Colonic expression of MUC2, MUC5AC, and TFF1 in inflammatory bowel disease in children. *J. Pediatr. Gastroenterol. Nutr.* **2004**, *38*, 488–493. [CrossRef]
35. Vestergaard, E.; Brynskov, J.; Ejskjaer, K.; Clausen, P.; Thim, L.; Nexø, E.; Poulsen, S. Immunoassays of human trefoil factors 1 and 2: Measured on serum from patients with inflammatory bowel disease. *Scand. J. Clin. Lab. Investig.* **2004**, *64*, 146–156. [CrossRef]
36. Grønbæk, H.; Vestergaard, E.M.; Hey, H.; Nielsen, J.N.; Nexø, E. Serum trefoil factors in patients with inflammatory bowel disease. *Digestion* **2006**, *74*, 33–39. [CrossRef]
37. Arijs, I.; De Hertogh, G.; Machiels, K.; Van Steen, K.; Lemaire, K.; Schraenen, A.; Van Lommel, L.; Quintens, R.; Van Assche, G.; Vermeire, S. Mucosal gene expression of cell adhesion molecules, chemokines, and chemokine receptors in patients with inflammatory bowel disease before and after infliximab treatment. *Off. J. Am. Coll. Gastroenterol. ACG* **2011**, *106*, 748–761. [CrossRef]
38. Clamp, J.; Fraser, G.; Read, A. Study of the carbohydrate content of mucus glycoproteins from normal and diseased colons. *Clin. Sci.* **1981**, *61*, 229–234. [CrossRef]
39. Cui, M.; Zhang, M.; Liu, K. Colon-targeted drug delivery of polysaccharide-based nanocarriers for synergistic treatment of inflammatory bowel disease: A review. *Carbohydr. Polym.* **2021**, *272*, 118530. [CrossRef]
40. Khulusi, S.; Hanby, A.; Marrero, J.; Patel, P.; Mendall, M.; Badve, S.; Poulsom, R.; Elia, G.; Wright, N.; Northfield, T. Expression of trefoil peptides pS2 and human spasmolytic polypeptide in gastric metaplasia at the margin of duodenal ulcers. *Gut* **1995**, *37*, 205–209. [CrossRef]

Disclaimer/Publisher's Note: The statements, opinions and data contained in all publications are solely those of the individual author(s) and contributor(s) and not of MDPI and/or the editor(s). MDPI and/or the editor(s) disclaim responsibility for any injury to people or property resulting from any ideas, methods, instructions or products referred to in the content.

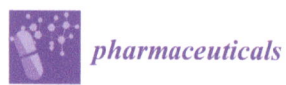

Article

Real-World Study on Vedolizumab Serum Concentration, Efficacy, and Safety after the Transition from Intravenous to Subcutaneous Vedolizumab in Inflammatory Bowel Disease Patients: Single-Center Experience

Vlasta Oršić Frič [1,2,*], Vladimir Borzan [1,2], Ines Šahinović [1,2], Andrej Borzan [1] and Sven Kurbel [1,3]

1. Faculty of Medicine, J. J. Strossmayer University of Osijek, 31000 Osijek, Croatia
2. Department of Clinical Laboratory Diagnostics, University Center Hospital Osijek, 31000 Osijek, Croatia
3. Poliklinika Aviva, 10000 Zagreb, Croatia
* Correspondence: vlasta.orsic@gmail.com

Abstract: Little is known about how the change from intravenous to subcutaneous vedolizumab in a real-life setting in inflammatory bowel disease patients on stable maintenance therapy affects clinical outcomes. We compared the data on vedolizumab serum trough concentration, efficacy, and safety prior to and six months after the switch from intravenous to subcutaneous vedolizumab. In total, 24 patients, 13 with ulcerative colitis (UC) and 11 with Crohn's disease (CD), were included. Mean serum trough concentration of intravenous vedolizumab was significantly lower than mean serum trough concentration of subcutaneous vedolizumab ($p = 0.002$). There was no significant difference between C-reactive protein levels, fecal calprotectin levels or clinical scores (Harvey–Bradshaw index or Partial Mayo score) prior to transition to subcutaneous vedolizumab and after 6 months. In four (16.7%) patients, two CD and two UC, therapy was discontinued during the follow-up period with a median of 5 months (minimum–maximum: 4–6). In all patients, therapy was discontinued due to loss of response. In total, 13 adverse events were reported by 11 patients, and the most common adverse event was COVID-19. No serious adverse events were reported. In conclusion, subcutaneous vedolizumab has shown to be effective and safe in patients on previously established maintenance therapy with intravenous vedolizumab.

Keywords: inflammatory bowel disease; vedolizumab; treatment outcome

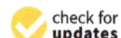

Citation: Oršić Frič, V.; Borzan, V.; Šahinović, I.; Borzan, A.; Kurbel, S. Real-World Study on Vedolizumab Serum Concentration, Efficacy, and Safety after the Transition from Intravenous to Subcutaneous Vedolizumab in Inflammatory Bowel Disease Patients: Single-Center Experience. *Pharmaceuticals* 2023, 16, 239. https://doi.org/10.3390/ph16020239

Academic Editors: Anderson Luiz-Ferreira and Carmine Stolfi

Received: 30 December 2022
Revised: 26 January 2023
Accepted: 2 February 2023
Published: 5 February 2023

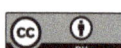

Copyright: © 2023 by the authors. Licensee MDPI, Basel, Switzerland. This article is an open access article distributed under the terms and conditions of the Creative Commons Attribution (CC BY) license (https:// creativecommons.org/licenses/by/ 4.0/).

1. Introduction

Crohn's disease (CD) and ulcerative colitis (UC) are chronic inflammatory diseases of the digestive tract, and anti-inflammatory drugs, whether conventional or biologics, have a central role in their treatment [1,2]. Vedolizumab is approved for the induction and maintenance of remission in patients with CD and UC. It is a humanized monoclonal antibody which binds to α4β7 protein on the surface of helper T lymphocytes and prevents its binding to mucosal vascular addressin cell adhesion molecule 1 (MadCAM1) on endothelial cells of blood vessels in the intestinal wall. This prevents lymphocyte migration and inflammatory response in the intestinal wall [3,4]. In Croatia, vedolizumab was approved in 2016 as a drug for intravenous application. From June 2021, a subcutaneous form of vedolizumab was approved as a maintenance therapy after the induction with at least two intravenous doses. In VISIBLE 1 and VISIBLE 2 studies, subcutaneous vedolizumab has proven to be more effective than placebo in the treatment of moderately to severely active UC and CD [5,6]. In both studies, subcutaneous vedolizumab was studied as a maintenance therapy in patients who responded to two intravenous doses of vedolizumab 300 mg at week 0 and 2. The primary endpoint was clinical remission in week 52. In VISIBLE 1, 46.2% of UC patients on subcutaneous vedolizumab achieved clinical remission vs. 14.3% of patients on placebo ($p < 0.001$). In VISIBLE 2, clinical remission at week 52 was achieved in 48.0% of CD patients receiving subcutaneous vedolizumab compared to 34.3% of patients on placebo ($p = 0.008$). Moreover, in the VISIBLE 1 study, the efficacy of the subcutaneous and intravenous forms of vedolizumab has proven to be comparable, as clinical remission at week 52 was achieved in 42.6% of patients receiving intravenous vedolizumab. In both studies, subcutaneous vedolizumab has proven to be safe and tolerable, with a safety profile comparable to that of intravenous vedolizumab (except for injection site reactions) [5,6].

Therapeutic drug monitoring (TDM) is used regularly in the treatment of patients with anti-tumor necrosis factor alpha (anti-TNF) drugs, but its role in treatment with newer biologics, including vedolizumab, is not completely clear [7]. Although pharmacokinetic data show that vedolizumab serum concentrations during induction and maintenance therapy correlate with clinical outcomes, it is probably not as evident as for anti-TNF drugs [7]. Moreover, there is no clear cut-off for vedolizumab serum concentration, neither for induction nor for maintenance therapy, with which positive clinical outcomes would be associated [8]. In the VISIBLE 1 clinical study, average steady state vedolizumab trough concentration in patients with UC treated with subcutaneous vedolizumab was 35.8 mg/L (SD ± 15.2), which is comparable to average vedolizumab through concentration for intravenous dosing every 4 weeks [9]. It has been shown, for both subcutaneous and intravenous vedolizumab, that with higher serum trough concentrations, more patients achieve clinical remission and endoscopic response [10].

Little is known about how the change from intravenous to subcutaneous vedolizumab in patients that are on stable maintenance therapy affects clinical outcomes. Recent real-world studies [11–14] showed that clinical outcomes did not significantly change in patients who changed to subcutaneous vedolizumab, but more data are still needed. In this study, we present data on vedolizumab serum concentration, efficacy, and safety in patients that transitioned from maintenance therapy with intravenous vedolizumab to the subcutaneous form of the drug.

2. Results

Thirty-two patients entered the study, but only patients that finished the 6-month visit were included in the further analysis. The study's algorithm is shown in Figure 1. In total, 24 patients, 13 with UC and 11 with CD, were included in the final analysis. Among CD patients, most patients had an inflammatory phenotype and ileocolonic localization, and among UC patients, most had left-sided colitis. A little over half of the patients were biologic-naïve prior to the beginning of the vedolizumab therapy (54.2%). Only one patient was taking corticosteroids (prednisone) at the time of transition to subcutaneous vedolizumab, but it was at a low dose and due to arthritis and not inflammatory bowel disease (IBD). Patients' baseline characteristics are presented in Table 1.

Mean steady-state serum trough concentration of intravenous vedolizumab was significantly lower than mean steady-state serum trough concentration of subcutaneous vedolizumab ($p = 0.002$) (Table 2). There was no significant difference between median C-reactive protein (CRP) and fecal calprotectin values or clinical scores (Harvey–Bradshaw index, HBI, or Partial Mayo score, PMS) prior to transition to subcutaneous vedolizumab and 6 months after the transition (Table 2). All patients were in clinical remission at the time of transition to subcutaneous vedolizumab, and 16 (66.7%) were in biochemical remission prior to transition. At follow-up, 87.5% (21/24) of patients were in clinical, and 54.2% (13/24) were in biochemical remission. In five patients who had fecal calprotectin >250 µg/g at follow-up, endoscopy was performed to confirm relapse. Endoscopic signs of disease flare were found in three patients (12.5%). There was no significant difference in the proportion of patients in clinical remission, biochemical remission or remission defined by fecal calprotectin <250 µg/g before and after the transition to subcutaneous vedolizumab ($p = 0.250$, $p = 0.453$, and $p = 1.000$, respectively; Figure 2). In four (16.7%) patients, two CD and two UC, therapy was changed during the follow-up period with a median of 5 months (minimum–maximum 4–6) from the transition to subcutaneous vedolizumab. In all patients, therapy was changed due to the loss of response. In two CD patients, vedolizumab dosing was optimized to every 4 weeks intravenously, and two UC patients started corticosteroids and were planned to switch to another biologic. No patient had surgery or was hospitalized due to IBD during the follow up period.

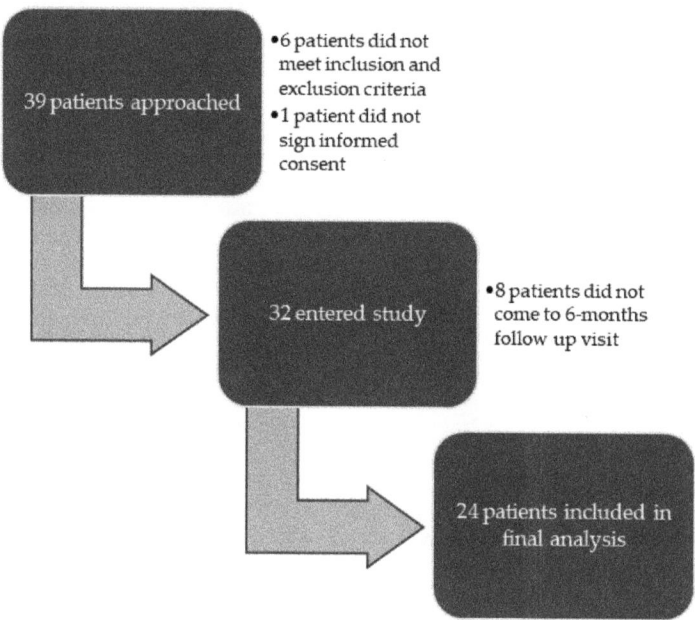

Figure 1. Algorithm of patients' enrolment in the study.

Table 1. Baseline patients' characteristics.

Patient Characteristics (N = 24)	
Female, n (%)	8 (33.3)
Age, years, median (minimum, maximum)	50 (25, 77)
Body mass, kilograms, median (minimum, maximum)	85 (55, 116)
Currently smoking, n (%)	2 (8.3)
Diagnosis, n (%)	
CD	11 (45.8)
UC	13 (54.2)
Duration of IV vedolizumab therapy, months, median (minimum, maximum)	11 (5–58)
Age at onset, CD, N = 11 (n, %)	
A1: <16 years	1 (9.1)
A2: 17–40 years	5 (45.45)
A3: >40 years	5 (45.45)
Disease location of CD, N = 11 (n, %)	
L1: Ileal	2 (18.2)
L2: Ileocolonic	7 (63.6)
L3: Colonic	2 (18.2)
L4: Upper gastrointestinal tract	1 (9.1)
CD behaviour, N = 11 (n, %)	
B1: Inflammatory	7 (63.6)
B2: Stricturing	3 (27.3)
B3: Fistulizing	1 (9.1)
P: Perianal disease	1 (9.1)

Table 1. *Cont.*

Patient Characteristics (N = 24)	
Age at onset, UC, N = 13 (n, %)	
A1: <16 years	0 (0)
A2: 17–40 years	6 (46.2)
A3: >40 years	7 (53.8)
Disease location of UC, N = 13 (n, %)	
E1: Proctitis	0 (0)
E2: Left-sided colitis	8 (61.5)
E3: Extensive colitis	5 (38.5)
Therapy prior to beginning of IV vedolizumab, n (%)	
Biologic-naïve	13 (54.2)
ASA, corticosteroids	8 (33.3)
AZA, MTX	5 (20.8)
Biologic-experienced	11 (45.8)
1	5 (20.8)
2 or more	6 (25.0)
Prior surgery due to IBD, (n, %)	
CD patients	
Bowel resection	5 (20.8)
Perianal disease	1 (4.2)
Liver transplantation due to PSC	1 (4.2)
UC patients	0 (0)
Concomitant therapy for IBD	
Corticosteroids, n (%)	1 (4.2)
AZA or MTX, n (%)	1 (4.2)
Disease activity	
HBI, n (median, minimum–maximum)	11 (0, 0–3)
PMS, n (median, minimum–maximum)	13 (0, 0–0)
Clinical remission, n (%)	24 (100)
CRP, mg/L, n (median, minimum–maximum)	23 (3.6, 0.4–23.1)
FC, µg/g, n (median, minimum–maximum)	16 (67, 16–772)
Biochemical remission, n (%)	16 (66.7)
Serum vedolizumab trough concentration during IV therapy (mg/L), mean (SD)	22.57 (15.42)

Abbreviations: IV—intravenous, CD—Crohn's disease, UC—ulcerative colitis, IBD—inflammatory bowel disease, ASA—aminosalycilates, AZA—azathioprine, MTX—methotrexate, PSC—primary sclerosing cholangitis, HBI—Harvey–Bradshaw index, PMS—Partial Mayo score, CRP—C-reactive protein, FC—fecal calprotectin, SD—standard deviation.

Table 2. Change in vedolizumab trough concentration, fecal calprotectin level, C-reactive protein level, Harvey–Bradshaw index, and Partial Mayo score before and after transition from intravenous vedolizumab to subcutaneous vedolizumab.

Outcome	Baseline	After 6 Months	p Value
Vedolizumab serum trough concentration (mg/L), n = 22, mean (SD)	22.86 (15.66)	35.62 (15.46)	0.002 *
Fecal calprotectin (µg/g), n = 15, median (minimum–maximum)	67 (16–772)	58.5 (16–1230)	0.570 **
C-reactive protein (mg/L), n = 19, median (minimum–maximum)	3.6 (0.4–23.1)	6.8 (0.6–34.5)	0.126 **
Harley-Bradshaw index, n = 11, median (minimum–maximum)	0 (0–3)	0 (0–3)	0.317 **
Partial Mayo score, n = 13, median (minimum–maximum)	0 (0)	0 (0–4)	0.102 **

Abbreviations: SD—standard deviation. * Student's t-test. ** Wilcoxon signed ranks test.

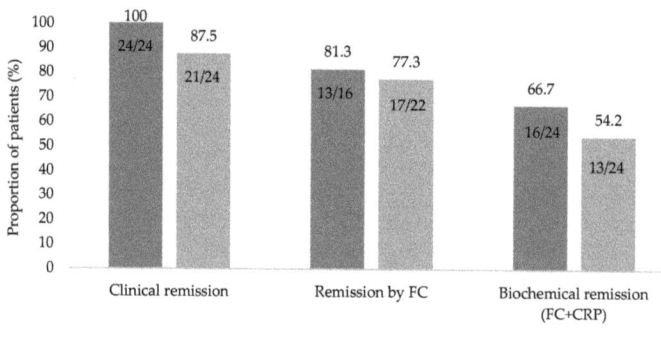

Figure 2. Proportion of patients in clinical remission, remission defined by fecal calprotectin (FC) < 250 µg/g, and biochemical remission, defined as C-reactive protein (CRP) ≤ 5 mg/L and/or FC < 250 µg/g, prior to transition to subcutaneous vedolizumab and after the transition.

In total, 13 (54.2%) treatment-emergent adverse events (TEAE) were reported by 11 patients, and the most common TEAE was COVID-19 (Table 3). One patient reported injection site reaction (erythema around the injection site), and no serious adverse events were reported.

Table 3. Incidence of treatment-emergent adverse events by system organ class and preferred term.

Treatment-Emergent Adverse Events (n, %)	All Patients (N = 24)
Infections and infestations	5 (20.8)
COVID-19	4 (16.6)
Fungal foot infection	1 (4.2)
Neoplasms benign, malignant and unspecified (incl cysts and polyps)	2 (8.4)
Anogenital warts	1 (4.2)
Bowen's disease	1 (4.2)
General disorders and administration site conditions	2 (8.4)
Pyrexia	1 (4.2)
Injection site erythema	1 (4.2)
Skin and subcutaneous tissue disorders	2 (8.4)
Urticaria	1 (4.2)
Pruritus	1 (4.2)
Blood and lymphatic system disorders	1 (4.2)
Iron deficiency anaemia	1 (4.2)
Musculoskeletal and connective tissue disorders	1 (4.2)
Arthritis	1 (4.2)

3. Discussion

Subcutaneous vedolizumab is a novel formulation of vedolizumab that can be used as a maintenance therapy in IBD patients as an alternative to the intravenous formulation. It is administered in a dosage of 108 mg every other week, compared to a dosing scheme of 300 mg every 8 weeks (or 4 weeks in optimized dosing) for intravenous formulation. Subcutaneous therapy has many advantages over intravenous administration of drugs. It requires less frequent visits to the hospital, and it is less time-consuming and therefore more convenient for patients. It also reduces the use of staff resources and the financial burden on a healthcare system. Subcutaneous therapy can also have some disadvantages, such as less control over patient's adherence to the therapy or potential local allergic reactions. As well, there is a possibility of an inappropriate storage of the drug at home, which can lead to lower effectiveness or adverse events. Some patients, moreover, dislike the idea of self-injecting or more frequent dosing of subcutaneous formulations [15]. In recent studies on patient acceptance of switching from intravenous infliximab or vedolizumab to subcutaneous formulations of the drug, the majority (58–78%) of the patients accepted the switch, and the main motivation was saving time [16,17].

Phase III trials, VISIBLE 1 and 2, presented data on the efficacy and safety of subcutaneous vedolizumab in patients with UC and CD in a controlled setting of a clinical trial. Our real-world study is assessing vedolizumab serum trough concentration, efficacy, and safety after the transition from intravenous to subcutaneous vedolizumab in patients that were on a prior stable maintenance therapy with intravenous vedolizumab. Median duration of prior intravenous vedolizumab therapy in our cohort is 11 months, with some patients receiving intravenous vedolizumab for almost 5 years (maximum of 58 months) prior to transition.

In our cohort, mean steady state serum vedolizumab trough concentration increased from 22.86 mg/L ($\pm$15.66 mg/L) for intravenous vedolizumab to 35.62 mg/L ($\pm$15.46 mg/L) for subcutaneous vedolizumab. Higher serum vedolizumab trough concentration after the transition to subcutaneous vedolizumab is comparable to data from the VISIBLE 1 and VISIBLE 2 studies. Initial pharmacokinetic modelling in the VISIBLE 1 trial estimated median serum trough concentration for subcutaneous vedolizumab at 34.6 mg/L (90% CI, 15.5–72.8 mg/L) [5]. In the VISIBLE 2 trial, median serum trough concentration at week 52 was 30.2 mg/L (0.78–70.1 mg/L) [6]. Our results are also in line with published real-world data. Volkers et al. [11] reported median serum vedolizumab trough concentration of 36 mg/L (IQR 29–39 mg/L) 24 weeks after transition from intravenous vedolizumab, although data on trough concentration were available from only eight patients. In the study by Wiken et al. [12], median vedolizumab plasma concentration was even higher, at 44 mg/L (IQR 28.9–64.7), but some patients were on a shorter dosing interval than the recommended 2-week dosing, and it is not evident whether the reported concentration is trough concentration. Two other studies [13,14] reported lower serum vedolizumab trough concentration in patients on subcutaneous vedolizumab (22.7 mg/L and 19 mg/L, respectively); in both, however, a comparable increase in serum vedolizumab trough concentration was seen after the switch from intravenous vedolizumab (Δ12.7 mg/L and Δ10.9 mg/L, compared to Δ12.8 mg/L in our study). As vedolizumab concentration in our and other real-life studies was measured using different ELISA-assays, differences in absolute values are probably due to low reproducibility and accuracy of the method. Although studies consistently show elevated trough levels of subcutaneous vedolizumab, the clinical significance of higher trough concentrations is not yet clear. Subcutaneous drugs have lower bioavailability, lower peak concentrations, and differences between peak and trough concentrations are smaller [18]. Therefore, two formulations cannot be directly compared. Total drug exposure for intravenous 8-week dosing and subcutaneous 2-week dosing of vedolizumab is shown to be similar [9], so increased trough levels for subcutaneous formulation are not expected to lead to better clinical outcomes. Further studies are needed to confirm or dismiss this statement. The exposure–response relationship was observed in studies for both formulations of vedolizumab [10,19,20]; however, exact cut-off values of vedolizumab trough levels for achieving positive clinical outcomes are still unknown [21].

A study by Ventress et al. [13] reported a significant, but not clinically important, rise in fecal calprotectin 12 weeks after the transition from intravenous vedolizumab. On the contrary, Bergqvist et al. [14] showed a decrease in median fecal calprotectin in all cohort subjects and in CD patients after the drug application type switch. In our patients, there was no significant difference between CRP, fecal calprotectin, or clinical scores prior to and after the transition to subcutaneous vedolizumab. Our results also showed that there was no significant difference in the proportion of patients in clinical and biochemical remission before and after the switch, implicating that patients on established vedolizumab therapy could be switched to subcutaneous vedolizumab without compromising the drug's efficacy.

Similar results were shown by two other real-life studies [11,12] further confirming the previous statement. During the 6 months follow-up, four patients (16.7%) discontinued subcutaneous vedolizumab because of loss of response, showing that drug persistence in our study is slightly lower than in patients on long-term maintenance therapy with intravenous vedolizumab [22,23]. In patients who switched to subcutaneous vedolizumab in other real-life studies, drug persistence was also slightly higher than in our cohort (88.1–95.5% at 6 months) [11,14].

No serious adverse events were reported during the follow-up, with COVID-19 being the most reported adverse event by patients. Injection site reactions are probably underreported due to predominantly mild reactions, as only one patient reported mild erythema around an injection site.

The main limitation of this study is the low number of patients included. However, as there are only a few real-world studies published so far, it will add valuable data to overall knowledge on efficacy and safety of subcutaneous vedolizumab as a maintenance therapy in a real-world setting, especially in patients that are already on established vedolizumab therapy. Due to the low number of patients included, we did not group our results according to diagnosis (CD and UC); instead, data are presented collectively. Moreover, there is no control group, as the study was designed to follow a cohort of patients prior to and after the switch to subcutaneous vedolizumab. Another potential limitation of this study is that we did not present data on vedolizumab immunogenicity, as there is no commercially available kit for detection of antidrug antibodies for vedolizumab. According to data from previous studies, immunogenicity of vedolizumab is low, so we do not expect that this data would be of clinical importance. Finally, endoscopy data prior to and after the switch were not presented, as only a few patients had data on endoscopy findings available.

4. Materials and Methods

4.1. Patients and Protocol Description

We approached CD and UC patients treated with vedolizumab at the Department of Gastroenterology and Hepatology in the University Hospital Centre Osijek. At our department, all patients that had a stable disease (based on clinical symptoms, fecal calprotectin, or endoscopy) and were not on corticosteroid therapy due to IBD or optimized vedolizumab dosing (every 4 weeks), were planned to transition to a subcutaneous form of vedolizumab after its approval in Croatia. Inclusion criteria for this study were: signed informed consent, diagnosis of IBD, age > 18 years, transition from intravenous to subcutaneous vedolizumab (prior or current), and at least four intravenous doses of vedolizumab received. Exclusion criteria were unwillingness to sign informed consent and continuation of intravenous vedolizumab. Data on age, gender, body mass, diagnosis, previous therapy for IBD, previous surgery due to IBD, comorbidities, concomitant therapy, CRP (at the time of the last intravenous dose of vedolizumab), HBI or PMS were gathered either from patients or from the electronic medical records. In patients that were still on intravenous vedolizumab, on the day of infusion, blood was taken for serum vedolizumab trough level. If patients were included in the study after they had already transitioned to subcutaneous vedolizumab, serum trough level of intravenous vedolizumab was taken from their medical records. The fecal calprotectin level was also collected from patients' medical records if it was recorded within six months prior to transition to subcutaneous vedolizumab, and only values from the Department of Laboratory Diagnostics of the University Hospital Centre Osijek were considered valid.

Patients were followed prospectively for 6 months from transition to subcutaneous vedolizumab or until a change in therapy. Data on a change in therapy (introduction of corticosteroids, vedolizumab optimization to every 4 weeks intravenously, or vedolizumab cessation), hospitalizations, surgery due to IBD, TEAE, CRP, and fecal calprotectin level, were taken at the 6-month visit. Data for HBI or PMS calculation were also taken. A four-week window was allowed around this timeline, as it was a real-world study. On the day of the dosing, blood was collected for subcutaneous vedolizumab serum trough level.

4.2. Outcomes

The primary outcome in this study was the change in serum vedolizumab trough level after the transition from intravenous to subcutaneous vedolizumab. The secondary outcomes were proportion of patients with change of therapy, change in CRP and fecal calprotectin level, change in clinical scores (HBI or PMS), remission rate, rate of hospitalizations or surgery due to IBD, and TEAE incidence after the transition to subcutaneous vedolizumab.

A change in therapy was defined as vedolizumab cessation, change to intravenous vedolizumab with a dosing schedule of every 4 weeks, or initiation of corticosteroids, due to loss of response or an adverse event. Clinical remission was defined as HBI < 5 and PMS < 2, and biochemical remission as CRP level $\leq$ 5 mg/L and/or fecal calprotectin < 250 µg/g [24,25]. TEAE were presented by system organ class and preferred term (Medical Dictionary for Regulatory Activities, MedDRA, version 25.1).

4.3. Vedolizumab Serum Trough Concentration

For vedolizumab serum concentration venous blood was sampled in a 4 mL tube without anticoagulant (BD Vacutainer, Becton, Dickinson, and Company, Franklin Lakes, NJ, USA). All blood samples for vedolizumab serum trough concentration were processed at the Department of Laboratory Diagnostics of University Hospital Centre Osijek. A blood sample from each patient was centrifuged for 10 min at $1370\times g$, and 2 mL of serum was separated and stored at -20 °C until analysis. In the serum sample, vedolizumab trough concentration was measured using a Promonitor VDZ sandwich enzyme-linked immunosorbent assay (ELISA) method (Progenika Biopharma S.A., Grifols, Barcelona, Spain) according to the manufacturer's protocol on an ELISA processor ETI-Max 3000 (DiaSorin S.p.A, Saluggia, Italy).

4.4. Statistics

Categorical variables are presented with absolute and relative frequencies. Numerical variables are presented as mean and standard deviation in case of normal distribution, or as a median and min-max range if data were not normally distributed. Differences between numerical variables of two dependent groups were calculated using paired Student's t-test or Wilcoxon test. Missing data are shown by presenting numbers of data points included in analysis in figures and tables. Differences between categorical variables were calculated using McNemar's test. All testing was two-tailed, and $p < 0.05$ was considered statistically significant. For statistical analysis, the MedCalc program was used (version 17.9.0, MedCalc Software, Osted, Belgium).

4.5. Ethical Considerations

The study was performed in accordance with the principles of the Declaration of Helsinki. The study was approved by the Ethics Committee of the Faculty of Medicine of the J. J. Strossmayer University of Osijek (602-04/22-08/02, 30 April 2022). Patients that agreed to participate in this study were included after they had signed the informed consent.

5. Conclusions

In conclusion, subcutaneous vedolizumab has been shown to be effective and safe in patients on previously established maintenance therapy with intravenous vedolizumab. Higher trough concentration of subcutaneous vedolizumab in our cohort did not lead to significant changes in clinical scores, CRP or fecal calprotectin level; however, further research is needed to establish whether it can lead to better clinical outcomes.

Author Contributions: Conceptualization, V.O.F., V.B., I.Š. and S.K.; methodology, V.O.F., V.B. and I.Š.; validation, V.O.F., V.B. and I.Š.; formal analysis, V.O.F.; investigation, V.O.F., V.B. and A.B.; resources, V.O.F. and V.B.; data curation, V.O.F. and A.B.; writing—original draft preparation, V.O.F. and A.B.; writing—review and editing, V.B., I.Š. and S.K.; visualization, V.O.F. and A.B.; supervision,

S.K.; project administration, S.K. All authors have read and agreed to the published version of the manuscript.

Funding: This research received no external funding.

Institutional Review Board Statement: The study was conducted in accordance with the Declaration of Helsinki and approved by the Ethics Committee of the Faculty of Medicine of the J. J. Strossmayer University of Osijek (Number of Approval 602-04/22-08/02).

Informed Consent Statement: Informed consent was obtained from all subjects involved in the study.

Data Availability Statement: Data is contained within the article.

Conflicts of Interest: V.O.F. has received speaker honoraria from Takeda, Janssen, Merck Sharp & Dohme, Sandoz, Ferring, Oktal Pharma, Abbvie, Viatris-Mylan and has been a member of advisory board for Janssen. V.B. has received speaker honoraria from Takeda, Janssen, Sandoz, Merck Sharp & Dohme, Abbvie, Oktal Pharma, Viatris-Mylan, Ferring and has been a member of advisory board for Takeda, Sandoz, Abbvie, Viatris-Mylan, Merck Sharp & Dohme. Other authors declare no conflict of interest.

References

1. Raine, T.; Bonovas, S.; Burisch, J.; Kucharzik, T.; Adamina, M.; Annese, V.; Bachmann, O.; Bettenworth, D.; Chaparro, M.; Czuber-Dochan, W.; et al. ECCO Guidelines on Therapeutics in Ulcerative Colitis: Medical Treatment. *J. Crohns Colitis* **2022**, *16*, 2–17. [CrossRef]
2. Torres, J.; Bonovas, S.; Doherty, G.; Kucharzik, T.; Gisbert, J.P.; Raine, T.; Adamina, M.; Armuzzi, A.; Bachmann, O.; Bager, P.; et al. ECCO Guidelines on Therapeutics in Crohn's Disease: Medical Treatment. *J. Crohns Colitis* **2020**, *14*, 4–22. [CrossRef]
3. Sandborn, W.J.; Feagan, B.G.; Rutgeerts, P.; Hanauer, S.; Colombel, J.-F.; Sands, B.E.; Lukas, M.; Fedorak, R.N.; Lee, S.; Bressler, B.; et al. Vedolizumab as Induction and Maintenance Therapy for Crohn's Disease. *N. Engl. J. Med.* **2013**, *369*, 711–721. [CrossRef] [PubMed]
4. Feagan, B.G.; Rutgeerts, P.; Sands, B.E.; Hanauer, S.; Colombel, J.-F.; Sandborn, W.J.; van Assche, G.; Axler, J.; Kim, H.-J.; Danese, S.; et al. Vedolizumab as Induction and Maintenance Therapy for Ulcerative Colitis. *N. Engl. J. Med.* **2013**, *369*, 699–710. [CrossRef] [PubMed]
5. Sandborn, W.J.; Baert, F.; Danese, S.; Krznarić, Ž.; Kobayashi, T.; Yao, X.; Chen, J.; Rosario, M.; Bhatia, S.; Kisfalvi, K.; et al. Efficacy and Safety of Vedolizumab Subcutaneous Formulation in a Randomized Trial of Patients With Ulcerative Colitis. *Gastroenterology* **2020**, *158*, 562–572. [CrossRef]
6. Vermeire, S.; D'Haens, G.; Baert, F.; Danese, S.; Kobayashi, T.; Loftus, E.V.; Bhatia, S.; Agboton, C.; Rosario, M.; Chen, C.; et al. Efficacy and Safety of Subcutaneous Vedolizumab in Patients With Moderately to Severely Active Crohn's Disease: Results From the VISIBLE 2 Randomised Trial. *J. Crohns Colitis* **2022**, *16*, 27–38. [CrossRef]
7. Restellini, S.; Afif, W. Update on TDM (Therapeutic Drug Monitoring) with Ustekinumab, Vedolizumab and Tofacitinib in Inflammatory Bowel Disease. *J. Clin. Med.* **2021**, *10*, 1242. [CrossRef]
8. Albader, F.; Golovics, P.A.; Gonczi, L.; Bessissow, T.; Afif, W.; Lakatos, P.L. Therapeutic Drug Monitoring in Inflammatory Bowel Disease: The Dawn of Reactive Monitoring. *World J. Gastroenterol.* **2021**, *27*, 6231–6247. [CrossRef]
9. Rosario, M.; Polhamus, D.G.; Chen, C.M.; Sun, W.; Dirks, N.L. P490 A Vedolizumab Population Pharmacokinetic Model Including Intravenous and Subcutaneous Formulations for Patients with Ulcerative Colitis. *J. Crohns Colitis* **2019**, *13*, S357. [CrossRef]
10. Rosario, M.; Polhamus, D.; Dirks, N.; Lock, R.; Yao, X.; Chen, J.; Chen, C.; Sun, W.; Feagan, B.; Sandborn, W.; et al. P529 Exposure–Response Relationship of Vedolizumab Subcutaneous Treatment in Patients with Ulcerative Colitis: VISIBLE 1. *J. Crohns Colitis* **2019**, *13*, S377–S378. [CrossRef]
11. Volkers, A.; Straatmijer, T.; Duijvestein, M.; Sales, A.; Levran, A.; van Schaik, F.; Maljaars, J.; Gecse, K.; Ponsioen, C.; Grootjans, J.; et al. Real-World Experience of Switching from Intravenous to Subcutaneous Vedolizumab Maintenance Treatment for Inflammatory Bowel Diseases. *Aliment Pharmacol. Ther.* **2022**, *56*, 1044–1054. [CrossRef] [PubMed]
12. Wiken, T.; Høivik, M.; Buer, L.; Bolstad, N.; Moum, B.; Medhus, A. P376 Switching from Intravenous to Subcutaneous Vedolizumab Maintenance Treatment; Feasibility, Safety and Clinical Outcome. *J. Crohns Colitis* **2022**, *16*, i378–i379. [CrossRef]
13. Ventress, E.; Young, D.; Rahmany, S.; Harris, C.; Bettey, M.; Smith, T.; Moyses, H.; Lech, M.; Gwiggner, M.; Felwick, R.; et al. Transitioning from Intravenous to Subcutaneous Vedolizumab in Patients with Inflammatory Bowel Disease [TRAVELESS]. *J. Crohns Colitis* **2022**, *16*, 911–921. [CrossRef]
14. Bergqvist, V.; Holmgren, J.; Klintman, D.; Marsal, J. Real-World Data on Switching from Intravenous to Subcutaneous Vedolizumab Treatment in Patients with Inflammatory Bowel Disease. *Aliment Pharmacol. Ther.* **2022**, *55*, 1389–1401. [CrossRef]
15. Jonaitis, L.; Marković, S.; Farkas, K.; Gheorghe, L.; Krznarić, Ž.; Salupere, R.; Mokricka, V.; Spassova, Z.; Gatev, D.; Grosu, I.; et al. Intravenous versus Subcutaneous Delivery of Biotherapeutics in IBD: An Expert's and Patient's Perspective. *BMC Proc.* **2021**, *15*, 25. [CrossRef] [PubMed]

16. Remy, C.; Caron, B.; Gouynou, C.; Haghnejad, V.; Jeanbert, E.; Netter, P.; Danese, S.; Peyrin-Biroulet, L. Inflammatory Bowel Disease Patients' Acceptance for Switching from Intravenous Infliximab or Vedolizumab to Subcutaneous Formulation: The Nancy Experience. *J. Clin. Med.* 2022, *11*, 7296. [CrossRef] [PubMed]
17. Burdge, G.; Hardman, A.; Carbery, I.; Broglio, G.; Greer, D.; Selinger, C.P. Uptake of a Switching Program for Patients Receiving Intravenous Infliximab and Vedolizumab to Subcutaneous Preparations. *J. Clin. Med.* 2022, *11*, 5669. [CrossRef]
18. Little, R.D.; Ward, M.G.; Wright, E.; Jois, A.J.; Boussioutas, A.; Hold, G.L.; Gibson, P.R.; Sparrow, M.P. Therapeutic Drug Monitoring of Subcutaneous Infliximab in Inflammatory Bowel Disease—Understanding Pharmacokinetics and Exposure Response Relationships in a New Era of Subcutaneous Biologics. *J. Clin. Med.* 2022, *11*, 6173. [CrossRef]
19. vande Casteele, N.; Sandborn, W.J.; Feagan, B.G.; Vermeire, S.; Dulai, P.S.; Yarur, A.; Roblin, X.; Ben-Horin, S.; Dotan, I.; Osterman, M.T.; et al. Real-world Multicentre Observational Study Including Population Pharmacokinetic Modelling to Evaluate the Exposure–Response Relationship of Vedolizumab in Inflammatory Bowel Disease: ERELATE Study. *Aliment Pharmacol. Ther.* 2022, *56*, 463–476. [CrossRef]
20. Löwenberg, M.; Vermeire, S.; Mostafavi, N.; Hoentjen, F.; Franchimont, D.; Bossuyt, P.; Hindryckx, P.; Rispens, T.; de Vries, A.; van der Woude, C.J.; et al. Vedolizumab Induces Endoscopic and Histologic Remission in Patients With Crohn's Disease. *Gastroenterology* 2019, *157*, 997–1006. [CrossRef]
21. Pouillon, L.; Vermeire, S.; Bossuyt, P. Vedolizumab Trough Level Monitoring in Inflammatory Bowel Disease: A State-of-the-Art Overview. *BMC Med.* 2019, *17*, 89. [CrossRef]
22. Danese, S.; Subramaniam, K.; van Zyl, J.; Adsul, S.; Lindner, D.; Roth, J.; Vermeire, S. Vedolizumab Treatment Persistence and Safety in a 2-Year Data Analysis of an Extended Access Programme. *Aliment Pharmacol. Ther.* 2021, *53*, 265–272. [CrossRef] [PubMed]
23. Amiot, A.; Serrero, M.; Peyrin-Biroulet, L.; Filippi, J.; Pariente, B.; Roblin, X.; Buisson, A.; Stefanescu, C.; Trang-Poisson, C.; Altwegg, R.; et al. Three-Year Effectiveness and Safety of Vedolizumab Therapy for Inflammatory Bowel Disease: A Prospective Multi-Centre Cohort Study. *Aliment Pharmacol. Ther.* 2019, *50*, 40–53. [CrossRef] [PubMed]
24. Harvey, R.F.; Bradshaw, J.M. A SIMPLE INDEX OF CROHN'S-DISEASE ACTIVITY. *Lancet* 1980, *315*, 514. [CrossRef]
25. Turner, D.; Ricciuto, A.; Lewis, A.; D'Amico, F.; Dhaliwal, J.; Griffiths, A.M.; Bettenworth, D.; Sandborn, W.J.; Sands, B.E.; Reinisch, W.; et al. STRIDE-II: An Update on the Selecting Therapeutic Targets in Inflammatory Bowel Disease (STRIDE) Initiative of the International Organization for the Study of IBD (IOIBD): Determining Therapeutic Goals for Treat-to-Target Strategies in IBD. *Gastroenterology* 2021, *160*, 1570–1583. [CrossRef] [PubMed]

Disclaimer/Publisher's Note: The statements, opinions and data contained in all publications are solely those of the individual author(s) and contributor(s) and not of MDPI and/or the editor(s). MDPI and/or the editor(s) disclaim responsibility for any injury to people or property resulting from any ideas, methods, instructions or products referred to in the content.

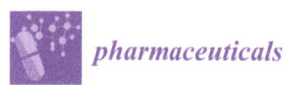

Article

MK2 Inhibitors as a Potential Crohn's Disease Treatment Approach for Regulating MMP Expression, Cleavage of Checkpoint Molecules and T Cell Activity

Eric J. Lebish, Natalie J. Morgan, John F. Valentine and Ellen J. Beswick *

Division of Gastroenterology, Hepatology and Nutrition, Department of Internal Medicine, University of Utah, Salt Lake City, UT 84112, USA
* Correspondence: ellen.beswick@hsc.utah.edu

Abstract: Crohn's Disease (CD) and Ulcerative Colitis (UC) are the two major forms of inflammatory bowel disease (IBD), which are incurable chronic immune-mediated diseases of the gastrointestinal tract. Both diseases present with chronic inflammation that leads to epithelial barrier dysfunction accompanied by loss of immune tolerance and inflammatory damage to the mucosa of the GI tract. Despite extensive research in the field, some of the mechanisms associated with the pathology in IBD remain elusive. Here, we identified a mechanism by which the MAPK-activated protein kinase 2 (MK2) pathway contributes to disease pathology in CD by regulating the expression of matrix metalloproteinases (MMPs), which cleave checkpoint molecules on immune cells and enhance T cell activity. By utilizing pharmaceuticals targeting MMPs and MK2, we show that the cleavage of checkpoint molecules and enhanced T cell responses may be reduced. The data presented here suggest the potential for MK2 inhibitors as a therapeutic approach for the treatment of CD.

Keywords: inflammatory bowel disease; Crohn's Disease; MK2; MAPKAPK2; checkpoint molecules; Lag3; PD-L1; matrix metalloproteinases (MMPs)

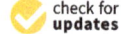

Citation: Lebish, E.J.; Morgan, N.J.; Valentine, J.F.; Beswick, E.J. MK2 Inhibitors as a Potential Crohn's Disease Treatment Approach for Regulating MMP Expression, Cleavage of Checkpoint Molecules and T Cell Activity. *Pharmaceuticals* 2022, 15, 1508. https://doi.org/10.3390/ph15121508

Academic Editors: Anderson Luiz-Ferreira and Carmine Stolfi

Received: 1 November 2022
Accepted: 1 December 2022
Published: 3 December 2022

Publisher's Note: MDPI stays neutral with regard to jurisdictional claims in published maps and institutional affiliations.

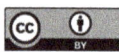

Copyright: © 2022 by the authors. Licensee MDPI, Basel, Switzerland. This article is an open access article distributed under the terms and conditions of the Creative Commons Attribution (CC BY) license (https://creativecommons.org/licenses/by/4.0/).

1. Introduction

The two major types of inflammatory bowel disease (IBD), Crohn's Disease (CD) and Ulcerative Colitis (UC), are incurable chronic immune-mediated diseases, but understanding the mechanisms of pathologic immune responses remains elusive. CD may affect the GI tract anywhere from the mouth to the anus, while UC is limited to the colon. These are life-long diseases that afflict over 1.6 million people in the US and have been increasing over the past decade worldwide [1]. Thus, in order to move forward in developing new effective treatment approaches, a better understanding of the mechanisms of inflammation are needed, with a focus on how CD and UC may differ in inflammatory mechanisms leading to pathogenesis of the GI tract.

One of the immune cell types that are known to be pathogenic, but are thought to differ between CD and UC, are CD4$^+$ T cell responses [2]. Specifically, CD is known to have increased Th1 and Th17 responses, which may not be as prominent in UC [3]. Checkpoint molecules are key regulators of the immune response and are critical for maintaining tolerance to keep the immune system in check. In IBD, there is a loss of tolerance and overactive immune responses to normal flora and other factors in the GI tract. In a hyperactive immune state, inhibitory checkpoint molecules may be dysregulated, leading to various pathologies. While the most well-studied inhibitory checkpoint molecule on T cells is the programmed cell death protein 1 (PD-1), there are other less well studied negative regulators of T cell responses. In particular, lymphocyte-activation gene 3 (Lag3) is expressed on activated T cells and binds to Class II MHC on antigen-presenting cells [4]. Lag3 plays a known role in negatively regulating T cell activation and has also been reported to promote the inhibitory activity of regulatory T cells (Tregs) [5]. During colitis, Lag3 is thought to be expressed by regulatory T cells and can restrain gut resident macrophages and innate lymphoid cells [6]. Thus, its regulation could be an important factor in IBD, and dysregulation of this molecule could lead to increased inflammatory damage. Another inhibitory checkpoint molecule expressed on T cells is B and T lymphocyte attenuator (BTLA), which is in the B7 family of checkpoint molecules. Upon BTLA binding to its receptor, herpes virus entry mediator (HVEM), which is expressed on a variety of cell types, this interaction plays an important role in regulating T cell proliferation and cytokine production [7]. In the intestine, BTLA has been suggested to play a critical role in preventing intestinal inflammation [8].

Other inhibitory checkpoint molecules may be expressed on antigen-presenting cells, fibroblasts, and epithelial cells of the GI tract. The programmed death-ligand-1 (PD-L1) has been a major focus for various diseases for maintaining tolerance in the intestine, inhibiting T cell responses, and promoting Tregs [9]. We previously found a difference in regulation of this molecule by fibroblasts in CD vs. UC, which directly affected T cell responses. In CD, PD-L1 was downregulated in association with increased Th1- and Th17-promoting cytokines [10], which may be partially responsible for the pathogenic $CD4^+$ T cell responses seen in CD.

Matrix metalloproteinases (MMPs) are enzymes that are critical in degrading proteins in the extra cellular matrix and play a major role in tissue remodeling and repair [11,12]. In IBD, MMPs 1, 2, 3, 7, 8, 9, 10, 12, and 13 have been documented to be produced and sustained during the disease course at multiple timepoints [13,14]. In CD in particular, MMPs are known to be increased in expression and play a role in fibrosis [15,16]. However, their overall effects and potential mechanisms associated with disease are not fully understood. We previously showed that several MMPs are produced by CD-derived fibroblasts and led to decreased PD-L1 expression in fibroblast cultures [10]. In particular, MMP7, MMP9, and MMP10 were found to be produced by CD-derived fibroblasts and have effects on PD-L1 expression, leading to increased Th1 and Th17 activity. Expression of MMPs are generally thought to be regulated by tissue inhibitors of metalloproteinases (TIMPs); however, here we found a novel regulator of MMP expression by the MK2 pathway. The MK2 pathway is known for the regulation of cytokine production and plays a critical role in inflammation and cancers [17,18]. Here, we found a novel function of this pathway in regulating MMP expression in CD tissues.

For this study, we sought to uncover the underlying mechanisms of MMP production and regulation of checkpoint molecules in IBD tissues. Their overall expression in IBD tissues was examined, resulting in observed differences between CD and UC, with multiple MMPs produced at significantly higher levels in CD than in UC tissues. MMP expression was further associated with the cleavage of several critical checkpoint molecules, including Lag3, BTLA, and PD-L1, which was specific to CD. We found these processes to rely on MMP1, MMP2, and MMP12. Furthermore, we found the MK2 pathway, an important pathway in cytokine regulation and colitis [19,20], to be highly expressed and activated in CD tissues, and found that MK2 inhibitors decreased MMP expression and checkpoint molecule cleavage. Finally, we identified that MMP1, MMP2, and MMP12 can cleave Lag3 and BTLA from T cells and PD-L1 from monocytes, suggesting that MK2 is a novel regulator of MMP expression and is a potential therapeutic target for CD.

2. Results

2.1. MK2 Expression and Activity Are Increased in CD

Because we have found the MK2 pathway to regulate inflammation, we examined its expression in CD tissues compared to normal tissues. Biopsies from patients with no known GI disease and from patients with active CD (visibly inflamed tissues) were stained for p-MK2 from multiple areas of the colon. Staining of p-MK2 was found to be very low in normal patient ascending colon (AC), descending colon (DC), and ileum, but drastically higher in active CD biopsies (Figure 1A). MK2 gene expression was also examined in panels of 12 samples where non-active CD showed a 1.78-fold increase compared to the mean of the panel of normal tissues, and active CD was found to have a mean of 7.52-fold increase (Figure 1B). UC tissues were found to have the same level of MK2 as normal tissues, suggesting that the MK2 pathway of inflammation may be specific to CD in IBD.

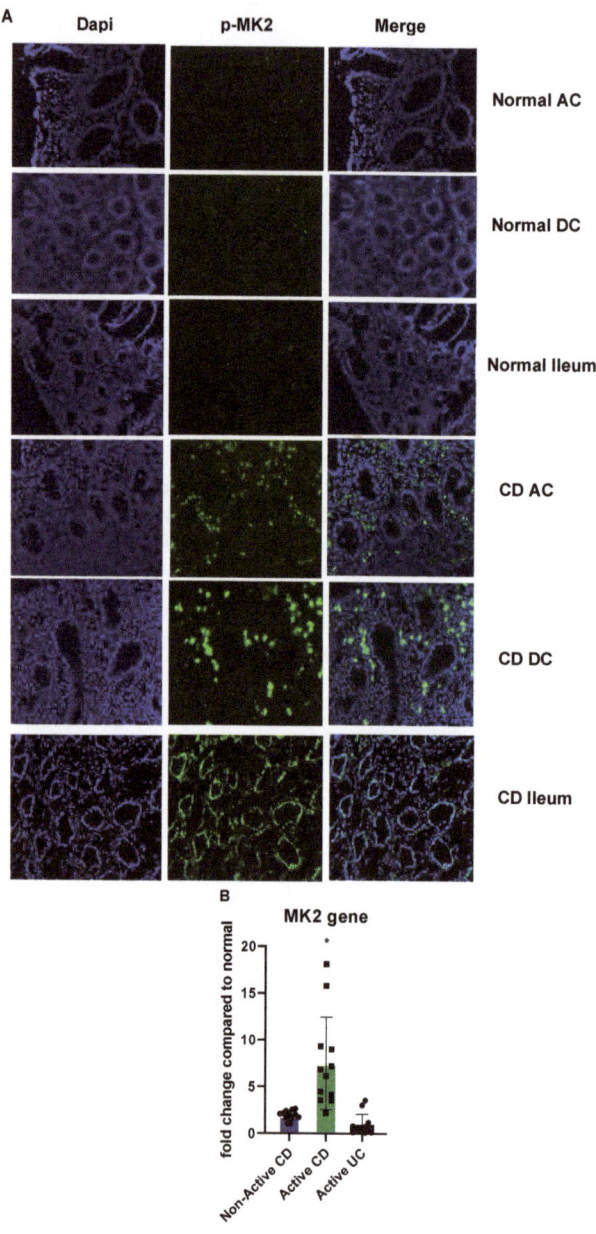

Figure 1. MK2 expression and activity are increased in CD tissues where (**A**) biopsies stained for p-MK2 show drastically increased staining in CD tissues compared to normal tissues and (**B**) MK2 gene expression is increased slightly in non-active CD tissues and much higher in active CD tissues, but not increased in active UC tissues. N = 12 for gene expression, * $p < 0.05$.

2.2. Checkpoint Molecules Are Cleaved from CD Tissues in an MK2-Dependent Manner

In IBD, there is evidence of soluble PD-L1 due to cleavage from fibroblasts [10], which led us to further examine this phenomenon. Tissues from CD and UC patients along with normal controls were divided into 4 mg sections and incubated with MK2i or vehicle control for 18 h. Supernatants were collected for analysis of checkpoint molecules by multiplex bead array. As shown in Figure 2A–D, BTLA, Lag3, PD-L1, and PD-L2 were found in supernatants in a soluble form from CD samples, but they were not significantly changed in supernatants from active UC tissues. To note, PD-1 was also examined, but not detected at significant levels in supernatants. These molecules were significantly decreased in supernatant from tissues incubated with MK2i in CD for BTLA, Lag3, and PD-L1, but not PD-L2, suggesting that MK2 may play a role in the regulation of checkpoint molecules in CD.

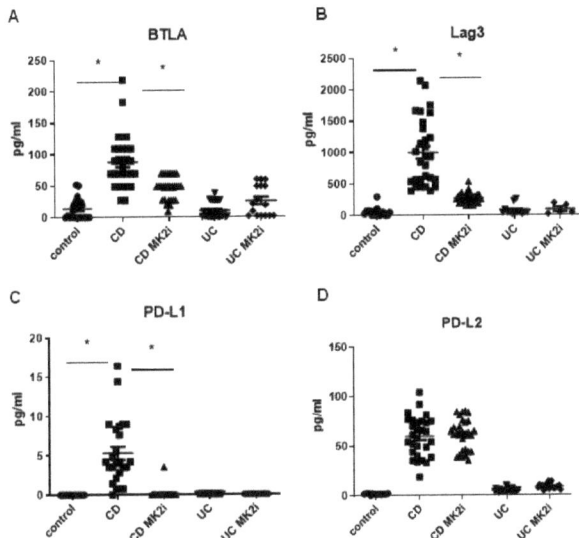

Figure 2. Checkpoint molecules are cleaved from CD tissues in an MK2-dependent manner where supernatants from 4 mg tissues pieces were incubated with MK2i or vehicle control and supernatants run on checkpoint multiplex array indicating that (**A**) BTLA, (**B**) Lag3, (**C**) PD-L1, and (**D**) PD-L2 were measured and shown to be cleaved into supernatants, which was reversed by MK2i treatment, but not with UC tissues. N = 23 for control, 29 for CD, and 27 for UC, * $p < 0.05$.

2.3. MMP Production Is Increased by CD Tissues in an MK2-Dependent Manner

Previous work has suggested that MMPs are able to cleave checkpoint molecules [10,21], so we sought to investigate a potential link between MMPs and MK2. Supernatants from normal, CD, and UC tissues mentioned above were also examined for MMP production by multiplex bead array. MMPs were found to be produced by both CD and UC tissues at higher levels than normal tissues (Figure 3A), with MMP1, MMP2, MMP10, and MMP12 produced at significantly higher levels in CD tissues than in UC tissues. These MMPs were decreased in the supernatants of samples that had been incubated with MK2 inhibitors compared to control. At the gene level, CD samples incubated with MK2i also showed decreased gene expression of these MMPs compared to control: MMP1 at 23-fold, MMP2 at 8-fold, MMP10 at 16-fold, and MMP12 at 28-fold (Figure 3B). Thus, taken together, we have demonstrated there is an MMP expression difference between CD and UC tissues, which may be directly regulated by MK2 activity.

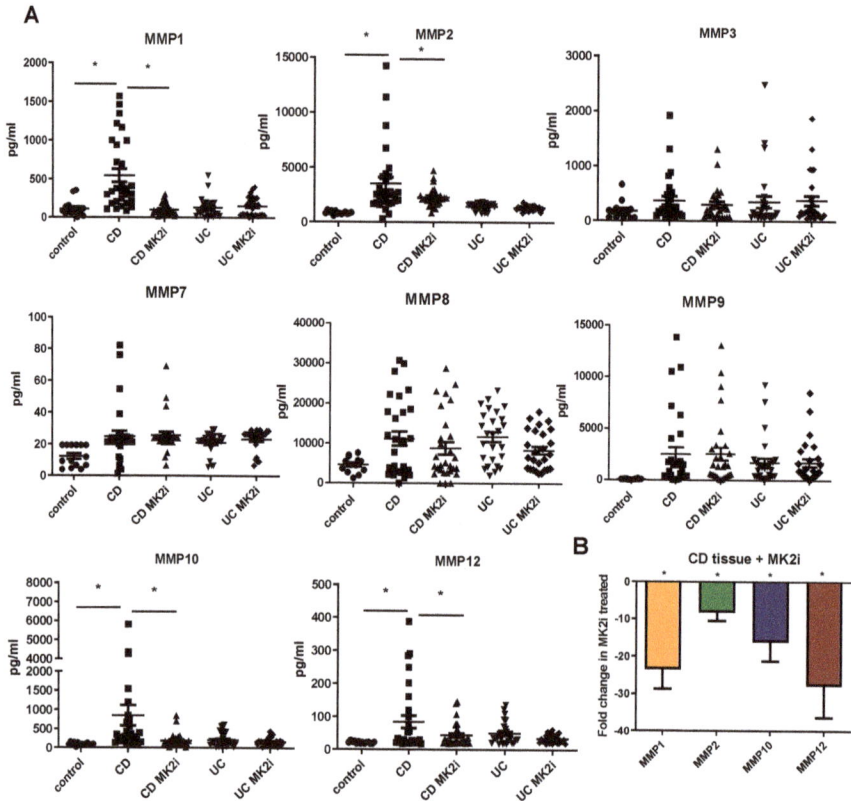

Figure 3. MMP production is increased in IBD tissues, but some are decreased by MK2 inhibition where (**A**) multiplex arrays of tissue supernatants indicate the MMP1, MMP2, MMP10, and MMP12 are produced by CD tissues and significantly decreased when tissues are treated with MK2 inhibitors and (**B**) gene expression of these MMP2 is also decreased by tissues incubated with MK2 inhibitors. N = 23 for control, 29 for CD, and 27 for UC, and 8 for gene expression * $p < 0.05$.

2.4. Checkpoint Molecules Are Cleaved from CD Tissues in an MMP-Dependent Manner

To investigate the direct role of MMPs in cleaving checkpoint molecules, a panel of CD tissues were incubated with the MMP inhibitor drug GM6001, in a similar approach as MK2 inhibitor described above and compared to the control. Supernatants were collected for analysis of checkpoint molecules. BTLA, Lag3, and PD-L1 were all found to be drastically decreased in the supernatants of tissues treated with GM6001 (Figure 4A–C), indicating that these molecules are cleaved in an MMP-dependent manner from CD tissues.

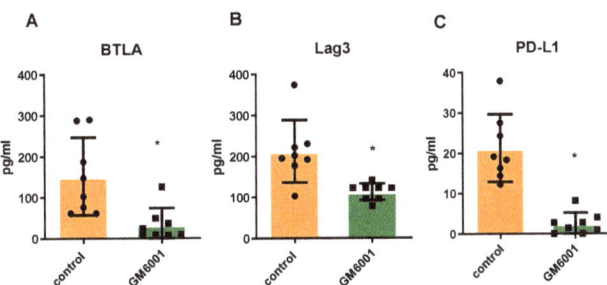

Figure 4. Checkpoint molecule cleavage from CD tissues is inhibited by GM6001 MMP inhibitor where the multiplex array of tissue supernatants indicates that (**A**) BTLA, (**B**) Lag2, and (**C**) PD-L1 are decreased when tissues are treated with GM6001. N = 8, * $p < 0.05$.

2.5. Recombinant MMPs Cleave Checkpoint Molecules from T Cells and Monocytes

In order to model the cell types involved in the pathogenesis of CD, Jurkat and THP-1 cells were utilized to examine the specific effect of the MMPs found in CD tissues, as shown in Figure 3A. Recombinant MMPs were incubated in an APMA-containing buffer for activation as previously described [21] and added to Jurkat cells treated with a cell stimulation cocktail for 24 h or THP-1 activated with LPS for 24 h to maximize checkpoint molecule surface expression. MMPs were added to cultures for 3 h for MMP1, MMP2, and MMP10 and 24 h for MMP12. Supernatants were analyzed for BTLA and Lag3 for Jurkat cells where MMP1, MMP2, and MMP12 were found to cleave these molecules (Figure 5A,B), but not MMP10. For THP-1 cells, PD-L1 was significantly increased in the supernatants by all four MMPs tested, which are specific to CD in our studies (Figure 5C). Taken together, these data show that MMPs have checkpoint cleavage capabilities on various immune cell types.

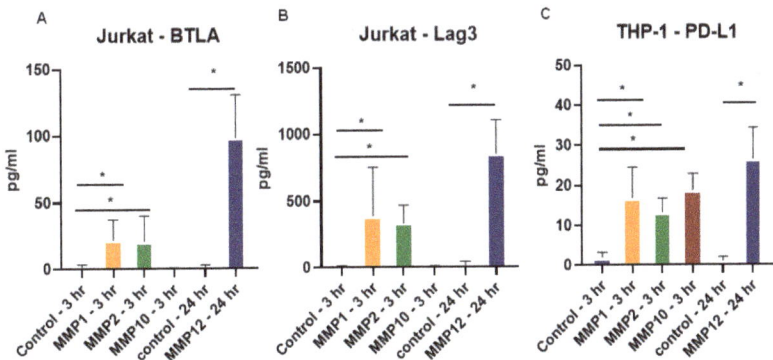

Figure 5. MMPs cleave checkpoint molecules from T cells and monocytes where cells are treated with recombinant MMPs activated in AMPA buffer and (**A**) BTLA and (**B**) Lag3 are cleaved from Jurkat T cell line, and (**C**) PD-L1 is cleaved from THP-1 cells in supernatants. N = 6, * $p < 0.05$.

2.6. T Cell Activation and Cytokine Production Are Dependent on MMPs

As checkpoint molecules are critical in T cell activation, proliferation, and cytokine production, the impact of MMPs on Jurkat cell activity was investigated. Jurkat cells were activated with a cell stimulation cocktail, and THP-1 cells were activated with LPS for 24 h. Supernatants from each cell type and co-cultures were examined for MMPs by multiplex array. MMP1, MMP2, and MMP10 (but not MMP12) were produced in cultures, with Jurkat cells treated with cell stimulation cocktail produced MMP2 and MMP10, but MMP1 required co-culture with THP-1 cells (Figure 6A). Furthermore, these cells were stained for CD69 as a marker of activation and found to express CD69 alone and in co-culture with THP-1 cells, which was decreased when exposed to the MMP inhibitor (Figure 6B). The supernatants from these cultures also showed increased IL-2 and IFNγ, which were significantly decreased in cultures with MMP inhibitors (Figure 6C,D). These data suggest an important role for MMPs in the regulation of T cell responses that are important in CD.

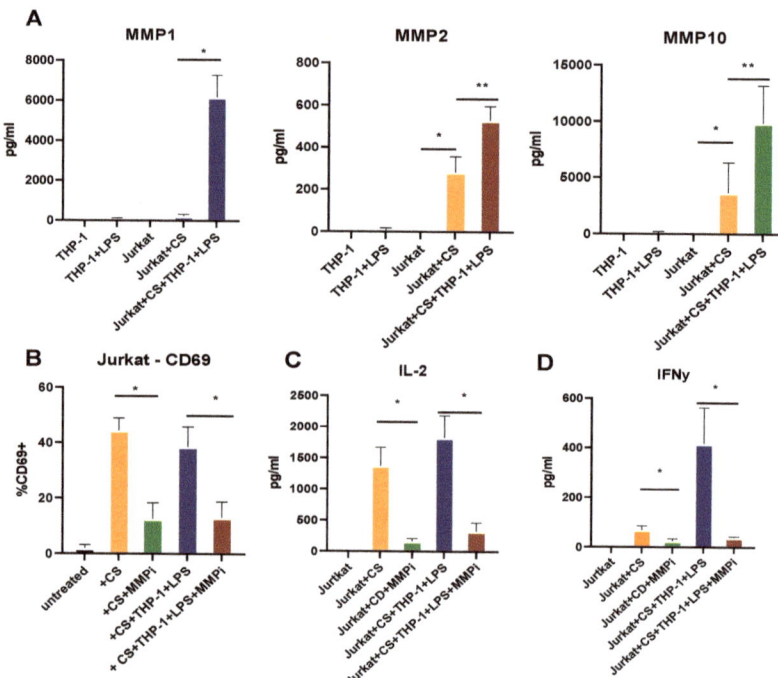

Figure 6. Activated T cells and T cells in co-culture with monocytes produce MMPs and are activated, which are decreased by GM6001 MMP inhibitor where (**A**) MMPs are produced and activated by Jurkat cells activated with a cell stimulation cocktail (CS) or activated in co-culture with THP-1 cells activated with LPS and (**B**) express CD69 as an activation marker that is decreased by cells treated with MMPi, as are (**C**) IL-2 and (**D**) IFNγ production. N = 6, * and ** $p < 0.05$.

2.7. CD Tissues Treated with MK2i or MMPi Have Decreased T Cell Activation Markers

In order to confirm the findings with Jurkat cells, indicating that MMPs cleave checkpoint molecules and increase activation and cytokine production, human 4 mg CD tissues were incubated with vehicle control, MK2i, or MMPi for 18 h. Tissues were examined for CD69 gene expression and MK2i was found to decrease expression by 3.64-fold, and MMPi similarly decreased expression by 4.03-fold, suggesting that the inhibitors may have an impact on T cell activation in tissue (Figure 7A). Furthermore, when supernatants were examined for cytokine production, IL-2 was significantly decreased as a marker of T cell activity (Figure 7B), and IL-17A and IFNγ were also decreased as markers of pathologic T cells in CD (Figure 7C,D). The known MK2 downstream cytokines IL-1β, IL-6, and TNFα, which also may be pathogenic in CD, were also significantly decreased with MK2i, but only IL-6 was decreased with MMPi (Figure 7E–G). Thus, confirming in vitro studies, T cell activity and inflammatory cytokine production were decreased ex vivo in CD tissues with inhibitors, suggesting that MK2i has therapeutic potential for CD.

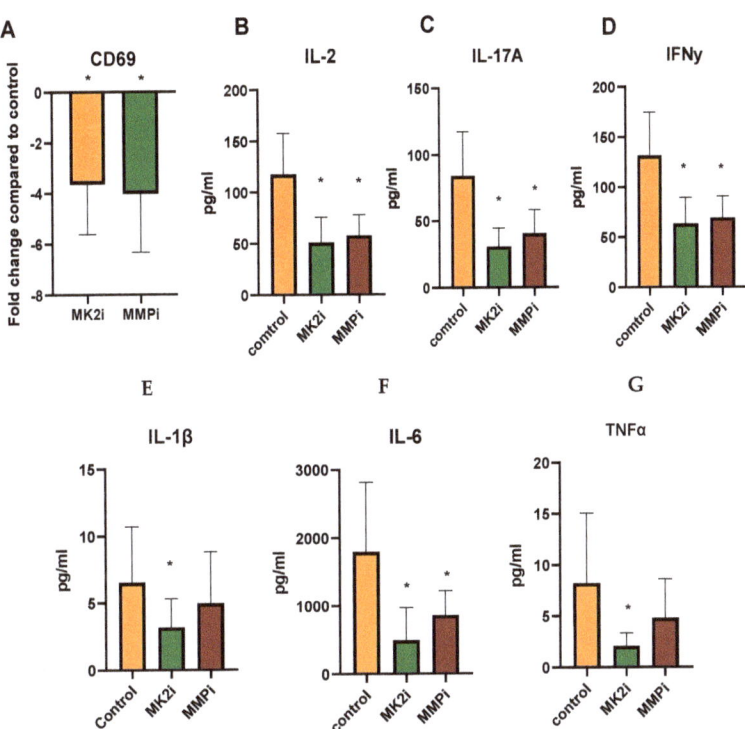

Figure 7. T cell activation markers are increased in active CD tissues but decreased when incubated with MK2i and MMPi where (**A**) CD69 gene expression is decreased in samples incubated with MK2i and MMPi compared to vehicle control and (**B**) IL-2, (**C**) IL-17A, (**D**) IFNγ, (**E**) IL-1β, (**F**) IL-6, and (**G**) TNFα are decreased in tissue supernatants incubated with inhibitors. N = 8, * $p < 0.05$.

3. Discussion

Although CD and UC are both diseases of chronic inflammation, there continue to be questions about differences in these two diseases that are puzzling. One difference in the immune response between the two diseases may be in the T cell responses, with CD having a stronger Th1 signature with IFNγ, but Th17 are also thought to play a role [22]. T cell responses in general are regulated by checkpoint molecules. Checkpoint molecules are in place to maintain tolerance, which is particularly important in the GI tract because of the vast microbial community. However, in CD, there is a loss of tolerance and an overactive T cell response, which leads to pathologies. Thus, dysregulation of checkpoint molecules is one area that needs further examination in order to understand IBD inflammatory pathologies.

The most well-studied checkpoint molecule expressed on antigen presenting cells and other cell types, such as fibroblasts, is PD-L1 [23]. Studies have shown that dysregulation of expression of PD-L1 promotes hyperactive T cell responses in IBD [9,24,25]. In previous work, we showed that PD-L1 expression by fibroblasts in CD could be cleaved by MMPs [10]. Here, we confirmed that this may also occur on monocytes/macrophages by examining the THP-1 cell line. Our work is in agreement with a study by Dezutter-Dambuyant et al. that showed MMP cleavage of PD-L1 by mesenchymal stromal cells. However, this study also indicated that PD-L2 was regulated by MMP9 and MMP13. We found soluble PD-L2 in CD tissue supernatants but did not examine this further because PD-L2 appeared to be regulated differently than PD-L1 in our system, in a non-MK2-dependent manner.

Checkpoint molecules expressed by T cells are also critical in regulating T cell activation, proliferation, and function. Lag3 is known to bind to class II MHC and suppress T cell function [4]. Early studies of Lag3 suggested that Lag3 inhibited T cell activation and that blocking Lag3 with antibodies led to increased CD69 expression and the production of Th1-associated cytokines [26]. Our study is in agreement with this study where we showed that, after incubation with MMPs, Lag3 was cleaved into supernatants and expression of CD69 and production of IL-2 and IFNγ were increased by Jurkat cells. Soluble Lag3 has also been shown in cancer studies to activate antigen-presenting cells [27]. Thus, there is potential that soluble Lag3 released from CD tissues could go on to exacerbate inflammation by activating macrophages and other APCs and thus promote further inflammation in IBD. Lag3 has also been suggested to be expressed by regulatory T cells and able to suppress gut macrophages and mucosal T cells in colitis [6], further suggesting that the cleavage of Lag3 in IBD is detrimental. BTLA is the other checkpoint molecule expressed by T cells that we investigated here. Less is known about the impact of the cleavage of this molecule from CD tissues; however, it has been suggested that is a critical molecule in protecting against mucosal damage in IBD [8]. In sepsis, soluble BTLA has been associated with disease severity [28], thus, more studies are needed to understand the impact of this molecule in IBD.

We have been examining the MK2 pathway for its role in inflammation and colitis-associated cancer [18]. Previous work by us and others has shown that MK2 regulated cytokine production implicated in CD inflammation, such as IL-1β, IL-6, and TNFα [17–19]. Here, we also show in ex vivo studies that treatment of tissue with MK2i leads to decreased IL-1β, IL-6, and TNFα, which is in line with our previous work as they are known to be involved in chronic inflammation in IBD. However, we also found a previously unrecognized role for MK2 in regulating MMP expression. We found that incubating CD tissues with MK2 inhibitors led to decreased MMP1, MMP2, MMP10, and MMP12, but other MMPs were not significantly changed. We also found this regulation to be at the gene level where tissues incubated with MK2 inhibitors had decreased MMP gene expression. Although this is the first study to suggest that MK2 may directly regulate expression of some MMPs, one group demonstrated that MK2 inhibition attenuated MMP2-dependent cancer cell migration [29]. Another group further confirmed the association of MK2 with MMP2 by transfecting cancer cells with constitutively active MK2, demonstrating that this was associated with high MMP2 activity [30], and one more study also suggested that MK2 is associated with MMP2 and MMP9 activity in bladder cancer [31]. However, to our knowledge this is the first study to suggest that MK2 is associated with MMP activity in CD.

The consequences of checkpoint cleavage were investigated by examining macrophage and T cell responses by cytokine production and the activation marker CD69. In culture with MMP inhibitors, THP-1 cells showed decreased PD-L1 cleavage, and Jurkat cells showed decreased BTLA and Lag3 cleavage. Furthermore, Jurkat cells also showed decreased CD69 expression and decreased production of IL-2 as T cell activation markers, and IFNγ indicative of a Th1 response. These responses are an important part of the pathogenesis seen in CD by contributing to the elevated levels of inflammatory cytokine production in active disease that disrupt barrier function. A limitation of the study is that cell lines had to be used as a tool to model T cell responses in CD. However, in our previous work, CD4$^+$ T cells from patient donors were examined, suggesting that the cell line model follows that Th1 and Th17 responses from the previous study [10]. We also performed experiments in an ex vivo approach, which may have some limitations and tissue may change over time, but because we were able to see cytokine changes that mimicked cell culture changes, the two approaches complement one another.

Our previous work also showed that MMP inhibition led to decreased Th1 and Th17 development from naïve CD4 T cells in primary cultures with fibroblasts from CD patients [10]. Furthermore, in ex vivo experiments, we showed that incubation of CD tissues with MK2i or MMPi have decreased T cell activity through CD69 expression and cytokine production. Thus, taken together, MMP inhibition has the potential to limit inflammation in CD, and overall MMPs have clearly been shown to promote pathogenesis in IBD [32,33]. However, drugs targeting MMPs have not shown much progress in clinical trials [13,34]. Despite those findings, MK2 inhibition may be a mor effective treatment approach because MK2 regulates MMP production and cytokine production. Here, we present evidence that MK2 regulates specific MMPs in CD and show that the cleavage of checkpoint molecules by specific MMPs (1, 2, 10, and 12) increases T cell activation and Th1-associated cytokine production. Given our data and the published information on MK2 regulation of inflammatory cytokine production and MMP expression, and the safety information on MK2 inhibitors in human trials [35,36], these pharmaceuticals should be considered as a novel therapeutic approach for CD.

4. Materials and Methods

4.1. Tissue Collection and Processing

CD and UC tissues were collected under IRB-approved protocols at the University of New Mexico (10-513) for discarded surgical resections and 00127500 for the use of biopsy samples from the GI and IBD Tissue Bank at the University of Utah. Samples were collected from patients with no GI pathologies or CD with active disease or in remission. Sample data are provided in a de-identified manner in Table 1. Tissue samples were divided into 4 mg +/− 0.3 mg and incubated in RPMI complete media for 18 h. Some samples were incubated with MK2 inhibitor (PF-3644022, Sigma Aldrich) at 50 µM, the MMP inhibitor GM6001 at 200 µM, or vehicle (DMSO) control for 18 h, and supernatants were collected for multiplex analysis.

Table 1. Sample number per location.

	Normal	UC	CD
Ileum	6	0	10
AC/transverse	6	7	6
DC/sigmoid	6	6	3
Rectum	5	5	6
Mixed	0	9	5
Total	23	27	29

4.2. Cell Lines

Jurkat and THP-1 cells were obtained from ATCC and maintained in RPMI supplemented with 10% FBS, 1% L-glutamine, and 1% Penicillin/Streptomycin (RPMI 10% complete media).

4.3. Immunofluorescence

Biopsy samples were snap frozen in optimal cutting temperature compound (OCT) and sliced to a 10-micron thickness using a cryostat. Sections were fixed with 4% PFA for 15–20 min at room temperature (RT) and left to air dry. After drying, sections were blocked with 2% BSA for 1 h and stained with anti-human MK2 overnight at 4 °C, followed by AF488 for 1 h at RT. Mounting media with DAPI was added to the section, and slides were imaged using an EVOS Auto2 microscope (ThermoFisher Scientific).

4.4. Multiplex Arrays

Tissue and cell supernatants were run in Milliplex arrays for soluble immune checkpoint molecules (Human Immune Oncology Panel), cytokines (Human Cytokine Panel 1), and MMPs (Human MMP1 and MMP2 panels) from MilliporeSigma according to the manufacturer's instructions. Plates were analyzed on a Luminex MagPix instrument.

4.5. Quantitative Real Time PCR

Tissue pieces were homogenized in TRIzol™ reagent (cat. 15596026, ThermoFisher Scientific, Waltham, MA, USA), and RNA extraction was performed according to the manufacturer's instructions. The quality and quantity of RNA were measured with a NanoDrop™ Lite Spectrophotometer (ThermoFisher Scientific, Waltham, MA, USA). Total RNA (100 ng/μL) was reverse transcribed using High-Capacity cDNA Reverse Transcription Kit (cat. 4368814, ThermoFisher Scientific, Waltham, MA, USA) with the following PCR settings: 25 °C for 10 min, 37 °C for 120 min, and 85°C for 5 min. Quantitation of mRNA was performed using real-time PCR with validated FAM dye-labeled TaqMan® probes (Applied Biosystems, Foster City, CA, USA) for *ACTB*, *MK2*, *MMP1*, *MMP2*, *MMP10*, *MMP12*, and *CD69*. The reaction mixture consisted of cDNA, TaqMan® Fast Advanced Master Mix (Applied Biosystems, Foster City, CA, USA), TaqMan® Assays, and RNase-free water in a total volume of 10 μL. Cycle parameters for TaqMan® assays were as follows: initial denaturation at 95 °C for 3 min, followed by 40 cycles of sequential incubations at 95 °C for 15 s and 60 °C for 1 min. Results were normalized to the expression of *Actb* gene, i.e., housekeeping gene. All experiments were performed as duplicates on QuantStudio™ 5 Real-Time PCR System (ThermoFisher Scientific, Waltham, MA, USA). The endpoint used in real-time PCR quantification, Ct parameter, was defined as the PCR cycle number that crossed the signal threshold. Quantification of gene expression was performed using the comparative CT method (Sequence Detector User Bulletin 2; Applied Biosystems) and reported as the fold change relative to the mRNA of the mouse housekeeping gene, *ACTB*.

4.6. MMP Cleavage Assays

Jurkat cells were stimulated with Cell Stimulation Cocktail (ThermoFisher Scientific) for 48 h in 10% RPMI complete media, while THP-1 cells were stimulated with 1 μg of LPS for 48 h. Cells were then fixed with 2% PFA for 15 min at RT then washed with 1X PBS. Human MMP1, 2, 10, and 12 were purchased from AnaSpec (Fremont, CA, USA) and resuspended in assay buffer containing 50 mM Tris, 10 mM CaCl2, 150 mM NaCL, and 0.05% w/v Brij-35 (TCNB) at pH 8.0 in a flat-bottom 96-well plate. MMPs were added to the cells to a final concentration of 200 ng/mL, along with 1 mM APMA, and MMPs 1, 2, and 10 were incubated for 3 h, while MMP12 was incubated for 24 h at 37 °C. Following the appropriate incubation period, the cells and TCNB media were centrifuged, and supernatants were collected and stored at -80 °C for further analysis.

4.7. Jurkat and THP-1 Co-Culture Assays

A total of 1×10^5 Jurkat and THP-1 cells were added at a 1:1 ratio in RPMI 10% complete media in flat-bottom 96-well plates. Jurkat cells were stained with Cell Trace Violet (CTV) (ThermoFisher Scientific) according to the manufacturer/s instructions. Some cells were added to media containing GM6001, a broad MMP inhibitor (MilliporeSigma), and incubated for 15 min at RT. Cell Stimulation Cocktail (ThermoFisher Scientific) and LPS (Enzo Life Sciences) were then added to cells, and media containing GM6001 and cells were incubated individually and in co-culture conditions at 37 °C for 24 h. Following 24 h incubation, media was collected for multiplex array analysis and cells were stained for CD69-APC clone FN50 (ThermoFisher Scientific) for flow cytometry. Flow cytometry analysis was performed using an Attune™ NxT Flow Cytometer and analyzed with Attune™ NxT Software (ThermoFisher Scientific, Waltham, MA, USA).

4.8. Statistical Analysis

Results were expressed as the mean ± SE of data obtained from at least three independent experiments, each performed in triplicate. Differences between means were evaluated by one-way ANOVA for multiple comparisons and Student's t-test for the analysis of the significance between two groups. Values of $p < 0.05$ were considered statistically significant. Association between MK2, MMPs, and cytokines were analyzed using Pearson correlation analysis.

5. Conclusions

The MK2 pathway was found to be increased at the gene and phosphorylation level in CD, but not in UC. MK2 was found to regulate MMP1, MMP2, MMP10, and MMP12 at the gene level and subsequently checkpoint molecule cleavage from tissues as indicated by incubating tissues with MK2 inhibitor drug. This cleavage was associated with increased T cell activation, and cytokine production was decreased by MMP inhibitor drug in culture and in tissues. Taken together, our data suggest that MK2 could be a novel therapeutic target for CD.

Author Contributions: E.J.L., N.J.M., J.F.V. and E.J.B. contributed to data collection, analysis, and review of the article and approved the submitted version. All authors have read and agreed to the published version of the manuscript.

Funding: This work was supported by the Department of Defense Peer Reviewed Medical Investigator Award W81XWH-22-1-0433.

Institutional Review Board Statement: This study was performed under the Institutional Review Board of Approval of the University of New Mexico, protocol number 10-513, and the University of Utah, protocol number 00127500.

Informed Consent Statement: Not applicable.

Data Availability Statement: All data is contained within the article.

Conflicts of Interest: The authors declare no conflict of interest.

References

1. Ng, S.C.; Shi, H.Y.; Hamidi, N.; Underwood, F.E.; Tang, W.; Benchimol, E.I.; Panaccione, R.; Ghosh, S.; Wu, J.C.Y.; Chan, F.K.L.; et al. Worldwide incidence and prevalence of inflammatory bowel disease in the 21st century: A systematic review of population-based studies. *Lancet* **2017**, *390*, 2769–2778. [CrossRef]
2. Imam, T.; Park, S.; Kaplan, M.H.; Olson, M.R. Effector T Helper Cell Subsets in Inflammatory Bowel Diseases. *Front. Immunol.* **2018**, *9*, 1212. [CrossRef]
3. Chen, M.L.; Sundrud, M.S. Cytokine Networks and T-Cell Subsets in Inflammatory Bowel Diseases. *Inflamm. Bowel Dis.* **2016**, *22*, 1157–1167. [CrossRef]
4. Maruhashi, T.; Sugiura, D.; Okazaki, I.-M.; Shimizu, K.; Maeda, T.K.; Ikubo, J.; Yoshikawa, H.; Maenaka, K.; Ishimaru, N.; Kosako, H.; et al. Binding of LAG-3 to stable peptide-MHC class II limits T cell function and suppresses autoimmunity and anti-cancer immunity. *Immunity* **2022**, *55*, 912–924.e8. [CrossRef] [PubMed]
5. Huang, C.-T.; Workman, C.J.; Flies, D.; Pan, X.; Marson, A.L.; Zhou, G.; Hipkiss, E.L.; Ravi, S.; Kowalski, J.; Levitsky, H.I.; et al. Role of LAG-3 in Regulatory T Cells. *Immunity* **2004**, *21*, 503–513. [CrossRef] [PubMed]
6. Bauché, D.; Joyce-Shaikh, B.; Jain, R.; Grein, J.; Ku, K.S.; Blumenschein, W.M.; Ganal-Vonarburg, S.C.; Wilson, D.C.; McClanahan, T.K.; Malefyt, R.D.W.; et al. LAG3+ Regulatory T Cells Restrain Interleukin-23-Producing CX3CR1+ Gut-Resident Macrophages during Group 3 Innate Lymphoid Cell-Driven Colitis. *Immunity* **2018**, *49*, 342–352.e5. [CrossRef] [PubMed]
7. Yu, X.; Zheng, Y.; Mao, R.; Su, Z.; Zhang, J. BTLA/HVEM Signaling: Milestones in Research and Role in Chronic Hepatitis B Virus Infection. *Front. Immunol.* **2019**, *10*, 617. [CrossRef]
8. Steinberg, M.W.; Turovskaya, O.; Shaikh, R.B.; Kim, G.; McCole, D.F.; Pfeffer, K.; Murphy, K.M.; Ware, C.F.; Kronenberg, M. A crucial role for HVEM and BTLA in preventing intestinal inflammation. *J. Exp. Med.* **2008**, *205*, 1463–1476. [CrossRef]
9. Chulkina, M.; Beswick, E.J.; Pinchuk, I.V. Role of PD-L1 in Gut Mucosa Tolerance and Chronic Inflammation. *Int. J. Mol. Sci.* **2020**, *21*, 9165. [CrossRef]
10. Aguirre, J.E.; Beswick, E.J.; Grim, C.; Uribe, G.; Tafoya, M.; Chacon Palma, G.; Samedi, V.; McKee, R.; Villeger, R.; Fofanov, Y.; et al. Matrix metalloproteinases cleave membrane-bound PD-L1 on CD90+ (myo-)fibroblasts in Crohn's disease and regulate Th1/Th17 cell responses. *Int. Immunol.* **2020**, *32*, 57–68. [CrossRef]
11. Rohani, M.G.; Parks, W.C. Matrix remodeling by MMPs during wound repair. *Matrix Biol.* **2015**, *44*, 113–121. [CrossRef] [PubMed]
12. Muller-Quernheim, J. MMPs are regulatory enzymes in pathways of inflammatory disorders, tissue injury, malignancies and remodelling of the lung. *Eur. Respir. J.* **2011**, *38*, 12–14. [CrossRef]
13. O'Sullivan, S.; Gilmer, J.F.; Medina, C. Matrix Metalloproteinases in Inflammatory Bowel Disease: An Update. *Mediat. Inflamm.* **2015**, *2015*, 1–19. [CrossRef] [PubMed]
14. Pedersen, G.; Saermark, T.; Kirkegaard, T.; Brynskov, J. Spontaneous and cytokine induced expression and activity of matrix metalloproteinases in human colonic epithelium. *Clin. Exp. Immunol.* **2008**, *155*, 257–265. [CrossRef] [PubMed]
15. Schuppan, D.; Freitag, T. Fistulising Crohn's disease: MMPs gone awry. *Gut* **2004**, *53*, 622–624. [CrossRef]
16. Rogler, G.; Hausmann, M. Factors Promoting Development of Fibrosis in Crohn's Disease. *Front. Med.* **2017**, *4*, 96. [CrossRef]

17. Liu, X.; Wu, T.; Chi, P. Inhibition of MK2 shows promise for preventing postoperative ileus in mice. *J. Surg. Res.* **2013**, *185*, 102–112. [CrossRef]
18. Ray, A.L.; Castillo, E.F.; Morris, K.T.; Nofchissey, R.A.; Weston, L.L.; Samedi, V.G.; Hanson, J.A.; Gaestel, M.; Pinchuk, I.V.; Beswick, E.J. Blockade of MK2 is protective in inflammation-associated colorectal cancer development. *Int. J. Cancer* **2015**, *138*, 770–775. [CrossRef]
19. Li, Y.Y.; Yuece, B.; MH, C.; Lv, S.; CJ, C.; Ochs, S.; Sibaev, A.; Deindl, E.; Schaefer, C.; Storr, M. Inhibition of p38/Mk2 signaling pathway improves the anti-inflammatory effect of WIN55 on mouse experimental colitis. *Lab. Investig.* **2013**, *93*, 322–333. [CrossRef]
20. Zhang, T.; Jiang, J.; Liu, J.; Xu, L.; Duan, S.; Sun, L.; Zhao, W.; Qian, F. MK2 Is Required for Neutrophil-Derived ROS Production and Inflammatory Bowel Disease. *Front. Med.* **2020**, *7*, 207. [CrossRef]
21. Dezutter-Dambuyant, C.; Durand, I.; Alberti, L.; Bendriss-Vermare, N.; Valladeau-Guilemond, J.; Duc, A.; Magron, A.; Morel, A.-P.; Sisirak, V.; Rodriguez, C.; et al. A novel regulation of PD-1 ligands on mesenchymal stromal cells through MMP-mediated proteolytic cleavage. *OncoImmunology* **2015**, *5*, e1091146. [CrossRef] [PubMed]
22. Tindemans, I.; Joosse, M.E.; Samsom, J.N. Dissecting the Heterogeneity in T-Cell Mediated Inflammation in IBD. *Cells* **2020**, *9*, 110. [CrossRef] [PubMed]
23. Pinchuk, I.V.; Saada, J.I.; Beswick, E.J.; Boya, G.; Qiu, S.M.; Mifflin, R.C.; Raju, G.S.; Reyes, V.E.; Powell, D.W. PD-1 ligand expression by human colonic myofibroblasts/fibroblasts regulates CD4+ T-cell activity. *Gastroenterology* **2008**, *135*, 1228–1237. [CrossRef] [PubMed]
24. Faleiro, R.; Liu, J.; Karunarathne, D.; Edmundson, A.; Winterford, C.; Nguyen, T.H.; Simms, L.A.; Radford-Smith, G.; Wykes, M. Crohn's disease is facilitated by a disturbance of programmed death-1 ligand 2 on blood dendritic cells. *Clin. Transl. Immunol.* **2019**, *8*, e01071. [CrossRef]
25. Nakazawa, A.; Dotan, I.; Brimnes, J.; Allez, M.; Shao, L.; Tsushima, F.; Azuma, M.; Mayer, L. The expression and function of costimulatory molecules B7H and B7-H1 on colonic epithelial cells. *Gastroenterology* **2004**, *126*, 1347–1357. [CrossRef] [PubMed]
26. Macon-Lemaitre, L.; Triebel, F. The negative regulatory function of the lymphocyte-activation gene-3 co-receptor (CD223) on human T cells. *Immunology* **2005**, *115*, 170–178. [CrossRef]
27. Wang, M.; Du, Q.; Jin, J.; Wei, Y.; Lu, Y.; Li, Q. LAG3 and its emerging role in cancer immunotherapy. *Clin. Transl. Med.* **2021**, *11*, e365. [CrossRef]
28. Lange, A.; Sundén-Cullberg, J.; Magnuson, A.; Hultgren, O. Soluble B and T Lymphocyte Attenuator Correlates to Disease Severity in Sepsis and High Levels Are Associated with an Increased Risk of Mortality. *PLoS ONE* **2017**, *12*, e0169176. [CrossRef]
29. Das, K.; Prasad, R.; Ansari, S.A.; Roy, A.; Mukherjee, A.; Sen, P. Matrix metalloproteinase-2: A key regulator in coagulation proteases mediated human breast cancer progression through autocrine signaling. *Biomed. Pharmacother.* **2018**, *105*, 395–406. [CrossRef]
30. Xu, L.; Bergan, R.C. Genistein inhibits matrix metalloproteinase type 2 activation and prostate cancer cell invasion by blocking the transforming growth factor beta-mediated activation of mitogen-activated protein kinase-activated protein kinase 2-27-kDa heat shock protein pathway. *Mol. Pharmacol.* **2006**, *70*, 869–877.
31. Kumar, B.; Koul, S.; Petersen, J.; Khandrika, L.; Hwa, J.S.; Meacham, R.B.; Wilson, S.; Koul, H.K. p38 Mitogen-Activated Protein Kinase–Driven MAPKAPK2 Regulates Invasion of Bladder Cancer by Modulation of MMP-2 and MMP-9 Activity. *Cancer Res.* **2010**, *70*, 832–841. [CrossRef] [PubMed]
32. Derkacz, A.; Olczyk, P.; Olczyk, K.; Komosinska-Vassev, K. The Role of Extracellular Matrix Components in Inflammatory Bowel Diseases. *J. Clin. Med.* **2021**, *10*, 1122. [CrossRef] [PubMed]
33. Marônek, M.; Marafini, I.; Gardlík, /.R.; Link, R.; Troncone, E.; Monteleone, G. Metalloproteinases in Inflammatory Bowel Diseases. *J. Inflamm. Res.* **2021**, *14*, 1029–1041. [CrossRef]
34. Schreiber, S.; Siegel, C.A.; Friedenberg, K.A.; Younes, Z.H.; Seidler, U.; Bhandari, B.R.; Wang, K.; Wendt, E.; McKevitt, M.; Zhao, S.; et al. A Phase 2, Randomized, Placebo-Controlled Study Evaluating Matrix Metalloproteinase-9 Inhibitor, Andecaliximab, in Patients With Moderately to Severely Active Crohn's Disease. *J. Crohn's Colitis* **2018**, *12*, 1014–1020. [CrossRef] [PubMed]
35. Gordon, D.; Hellriegel, E.T.; Hope, H.R.; Burt, D.; Monahan, J.B. Safety, Tolerability, Pharmacokinetics, and Pharmacodynamics of the MK2 Inhibitor ATI-450 in Healthy Subjects: A Placebo-Controlled Randomized Phase 1 Study. *Clin. Pharmacol. Adv. Appl.* **2021**, *13*, 123–134. [CrossRef]
36. Brown, D.I.; Cooley, B.C.; Quintana, M.T.; Lander, C.; Willis, M.S. Nebulized Delivery of the MAPKAP Kinase 2 Peptide Inhibitor MMI-0100 Protects Against Ischemia-Induced Systolic Dysfunction. *Int. J. Pept. Res. Ther.* **2016**, *22*, 317–324. [CrossRef] [PubMed]

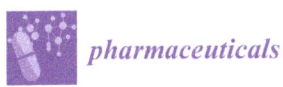

Article

(R,R)-BD-AcAc2 Mitigates Chronic Colitis in Rats: A Promising Multi-Pronged Approach Modulating Inflammasome Activity, Autophagy, and Pyroptosis

Sameh Saber [1], Mohannad Mohammad S. Alamri [2], Jaber Alfaifi [3], Lobna A. Saleh [4], Sameh Abdel-Ghany [5], Adel Mohamed Aboregela [6,7], Alshaimaa A. Farrag [8,9], Abdulrahman H. Almaeen [10], Masoud I. E. Adam [11], AbdulElah Al Jarallah AlQahtani [12], Ali M. S. Eleragi [13], Mustafa Ahmed Abdel-Reheim [14,15,*], Heba A. Ramadan [16] and Osama A. Mohammed [4,17,*]

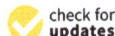

Citation: Saber, S.; Alamri, M.M.S.; Alfaifi, J.; Saleh, L.A.; Abdel-Ghany, S.; Aboregela, A.M.; Farrag, A.A.; Almaeen, A.H.; Adam, M.I.E.; AlQahtani, A.A.J.; et al. (R,R)-BD-AcAc2 Mitigates Chronic Colitis in Rats: A Promising Multi-Pronged Approach Modulating Inflammasome Activity, Autophagy, and Pyroptosis. *Pharmaceuticals* 2023, *16*, 953. https://doi.org/10.3390/ph16070953

Academic Editor: Réjean Couture

Received: 27 May 2023
Revised: 19 June 2023
Accepted: 29 June 2023
Published: 3 July 2023

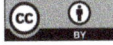

Copyright: © 2023 by the authors. Licensee MDPI, Basel, Switzerland. This article is an open access article distributed under the terms and conditions of the Creative Commons Attribution (CC BY) license (https://creativecommons.org/licenses/by/4.0/).

1. Department of Pharmacology, Faculty of Pharmacy, Delta University for Science and Technology, Gamasa 11152, Egypt; sampharm81@gmail.com
2. Department of Family Medicine, College of Medicine, University of Bisha, Bisha 61922, Saudi Arabia; malamri@ub.edu.sa
3. Department of Child Health, College of Medicine, University of Bisha, Bisha 61922, Saudi Arabia; jalfaifi@ub.edu.sa
4. Department of Clinical Pharmacology, Faculty of Medicine, Ain Shams University, Cairo 11566, Egypt; lobnasaleh_80@yahoo.ca
5. Department of Clinical Pharmacology, Faculty of Medicine, Mansoura University, Mansoura 35516, Egypt; samghany@mans.edu.eg
6. Human Anatomy and Embryology Department, Faculty of Medicine, Zagazig University, Zagazig 44519, Egypt; amaboregela@zu.edu.eg or aaboregela@ub.edu.sa
7. Basic Medical Sciences Department, College of Medicine, University of Bisha, Bisha 61922, Saudi Arabia
8. Department of Histology and Cell Biology, Faculty of Medicine, Assiut University, Assiut 71515, Egypt; alshaima@aun.edu.eg or afarraj@ub.edu.sa
9. Department of Anatomy, College of Medicine, University of Bisha, Bisha 61922, Saudi Arabia
10. Department of Pathology, College of Medicine, Jouf University, Sakaka 72388, Saudi Arabia; ahalmaeen@ju.edu.sa
11. Department of Medical Education and Internal Medicine, College of Medicine, University of Bisha, Bisha 61922, Saudi Arabia; mieadam@ub.edu.sa
12. Department of Internal Medicine, Division of Dermatology, College of Medicine, University of Bisha, Bisha 61922, Saudi Arabia; aaljarallah@ub.edu.sa
13. Department of Microbiology, College of Medicine, University of Bisha, Bisha 61922, Saudi Arabia; ameleragi@ub.edu.sa
14. Department of Pharmaceutical Sciences, College of Pharmacy, Shaqra University, Shaqra 11961, Saudi Arabia
15. Department of Pharmacology and Toxicology, Faculty of Pharmacy, Beni-Suef University, Beni Suef 62521, Egypt
16. Department of Microbiology and Immunology, Faculty of Pharmacy, Delta University for Science and Technology, Gamasa 11152, Egypt; hebaaa.aadel@gmail.com
17. Department of Clinical Pharmacology, College of Medicine, University of Bisha, Bisha 61922, Saudi Arabia
* Correspondence: m.ahmed@su.edu.sa or darshpharmacy@yahoo.com (M.A.A.-R.); oamohamed@ub.edu.sa or osamaabbass@med.asu.edu.eg (O.A.M.)

Abstract: Ulcerative colitis is a chronic and incurable form of inflammatory bowel disease that can increase the risk of colitis-associated cancer and mortality. Limited treatment options are available for this condition, and the existing ones often come with non-tolerable adverse effects. This study is the first to examine the potential benefits of consuming (R,R)-BD-AcAc2, a type of ketone ester (KE), and intermittent fasting in treating chronic colitis induced by dextran sodium sulfate (DSS) in rats. We selected both protocols to enhance the levels of β-hydroxybutyrate, mimicking a state of nutritional ketosis and early ketosis, respectively. Our findings revealed that only the former protocol, consuming the KE, improved disease activity and the macroscopic and microscopic features of the colon while reducing inflammation scores. Additionally, the KE counteracted the DSS-induced decrease in percentage of weight change, reduced the colonic weight-to-length ratio, and increased the survival rate of DSS-insulted rats. KE also showed potential antioxidant activities and improved the gut microbiome composition. Moreover, consuming KE increased the levels of tight junction proteins that protect against leaky gut and exhibited anti-inflammatory properties by reducing proinflammatory cytokine production. These effects were attributed to inhibiting NFκB and NLRP3 inflammasome activation and restraining pyroptosis and apoptosis while enhancing autophagy as revealed by reduced p62 and increased BECN1. Furthermore, the KE may have a positive impact on maintaining a healthy microbiome. To conclude, the potential clinical implications of our findings are promising, as (R,R)-BD-AcAc2 has a greater safety profile and can be easily translated to human subjects.

Keywords: ulcerative colitis; ketone esters; (R,R)-BD-AcAc2; NLRP3 inflammasome; pyroptosis; autophagy; gut dysbiosis

1. Introduction

Ulcerative colitis is a chronic inflammatory bowel disease (IBD) that affects a large number of people; unfortunately, it is not curable at present. According to an investigation into the worldwide impact of IBDs, there was a significant 47.45% increase in the estimated number of cases between 1990 and 2019 [1]. The total number of individuals living with IBDs globally is estimated to exceed 6.8 million [2]. The reported estimates indicate that the risk of colorectal cancer (CRC) in patients with ulcerative colitis (UC) is approximately 2% after 10 years, 8% after 20 years, and 18% after 30 years of having the disease [3]. According to a comprehensive cohort study conducted in Denmark, individuals with severe microscopic colitis were found to have a higher risk of mortality and colorectal cancer [4].

In addition to reducing the quality of life, patients with this condition are at a higher risk of colon cancer. While there are treatments available for this debilitating disease, they only provide temporary relief and patients are likely to experience relapses over time. Moreover, these treatments can have adverse effects and are often insufficient in achieving long-term remission without maintenance therapy. For many patients, surgery is also a reality, underscoring the urgent need for more effective treatments [5]. Risk factors for ulcerative colitis include genetic susceptibility and factors that influence the gut microbiota, such as antibiotic use and dietary changes, for example, extensive consumption of processed foods [6].

The abnormal activation of the nucleotide-binding oligomerization domain-like receptor protein 3 (NLRP3) inflammasome is a major contributor to the development of chronic colitis, and therapeutic interventions targeting NLRP3 have demonstrated significant efficacy in delaying or preventing disease onset [7]. Inflammasomes are a class of cytosolic protein complexes that can detect a variety of stressors, exogenous pathogens, and endogenous danger signals, triggering activation of caspase-1, and subsequent production of IL-1β and IL-18, thereby initiating the inflammatory process. The priming signal required for inflammasome activation converges on the activation of nuclear transcription factor kappa B (NFκB) and the transcriptional induction of NLRP3 and pro-IL-1β. The activating signal, which may be a danger signal, can directly activate inflammasome assembly [8]. Several mechanisms have been proposed to explain the activation of the NLRP3 inflammasome, including the generation of reactive oxygen species (ROS) [9]. Moreover, downstream of the NLRP3 inflammasome activation, gasdermin D (GSDMD) cleavage and membrane pore-formation has also been observed [10]. The process of pyroptosis, a highly inflammatory type of programmed cell death, is largely dependent on the cleavage of GSDMD, as this cleavage releases the gasdermin D N-terminal fragment (NGSDMD) which carries inherent pyroptosis-inducing capabilities [11]. In addition, The NLRP3 inflammasome has been identified as playing a significant role in coordinating host physiology and immunity, and researchers are actively studying its interactions with the gut microbiota [12]. Recent studies have suggested that dysregulation of the NLRP3 inflammasome in response to changes in the gut microbiota could contribute to the development of chronic colitis [13].

Autophagy is a vital cellular process that removes unnecessary or dysfunctional components through a regulated lysosome-dependent mechanism [14]. It is involved in several pathological processes and plays a significant role in various diseases [15]. Recent research indicates that autophagy dysregulation in intestinal epithelial cells (IECs) contributes to the development and progression of IBDs [16]. Additionally, autophagy has emerged as a potential drug target for managing colitis [17,18] and colitis-associated cancer [19,20]. In particular, targeting autophagy ablation in IECs increases epithelial apoptosis and aggravates inflammatory pathology [21]. These findings imply that manipulating autophagy may be a viable therapeutic approach for the management of chronic colitis.

β-hydroxybutyrate is a ketone body metabolite primarily produced by the brain, liver, heart, and skeletal muscles during caloric restriction, fasting, or a low-carbohydrate ketogenic diet (KD) [22]. Additionally, β-hydroxybutyrate and its producing stimuli, such as fasting and KD, have been shown to possess the ability to improve pro-inflammatory responses. Studies have demonstrated that β-hydroxybutyrate can alleviate pro-inflammatory responses in Parkinson's disease both in vitro and in vivo [23]. Several studies have shown the beneficial effects of intermittent fasting and calorie restriction on mitigating neuroinflammation and sickness behavior induced by lipopolysaccharide [24,25]. Moreover, a low-carbohydrate KD has been found to reduce tissue inflammatory responses in both juvenile and adult rats [26]. These effects are attributed to the ability of β-hydroxybutyrate to inhibit the NLRP3 inflammasome, which reduces the production of pro-inflammatory cytokines [22].

The brief half-life of β-hydroxybutyrate brings up concerns about its practicality as a potential treatment for humans. Moreover, the therapeutic use of this approach in a clinical environment may not be financially feasible. There have been cases where β-hydroxybutyrate was administered orally to two infants aged six months with persistent hyperinsulinemic hypoglycemia for 5 and 7 months. Despite receiving high doses of up to 32 g/day, these patients reportedly tolerated the treatment well without experiencing any adverse effects [27].

However, ketone esters (KEs), such as (R,R)-BD-AcAc2, offer an alternative source of ketones to boost blood β-hydroxybutyrate levels. Once ingested, KEs are broken down and metabolized, releasing ketone bodies into the bloodstream. This mimics the effects of fasting or adhering to a KD by increasing plasma β-hydroxybutyrate levels. Notably, KE supplementation can significantly enhance plasma β-hydroxybutyrate levels, even when consuming a regular diet. The effects of KEs appear to depend on the dosage and can endure for several hours after ingestion. Researchers are exploring the potential therapeutic benefits of KEs in conditions like epilepsy [28] and Alzheimer's disease [29], where increasing ketone levels could be advantageous. Some individuals also use KEs to achieve nutritional ketosis without following a strict ketogenic diet. Thus, consuming KEs can be an effective pharmacological approach to raising plasma β-hydroxybutyrate levels.

In addition, It has been suggested that β-hydroxybutyrate may regulate the gut microflora through indirect mechanisms that have yet to be fully understood [30]. While it is widely believed that β-hydroxybutyrate plays a crucial role in the gut microbiome, research directly studying its effects on the gut microflora is still very limited and its mechanism is not well characterized. However, studies have shown that KD can impact gut microbiota composition [31]. Therefore, it is possible that both intermittent fasting and KE consumption, as methods to boost β-hydroxybutyrate production, may lead to β-hydroxybutyrate-induced changes in the microbiome composition. Interestingly, the present study may help to shed light on the potential implications of these changes.

To avoid the need for dietary changes, supplements like KEs have been developed to mimic the effects of ketosis, as an alternative to KD. However, the use of exogenous ketone supplements for treating ulcerative colitis in humans and animals has not been thoroughly and directly evaluated in trials. Although the current evidence indicates that KDs can be a feasible approach, further research is urgently needed to determine the optimal methods, understand the underlying mechanisms, establish dosage and safety guidelines, and promote the widespread adoption of this strategy for treating colitis.

In this study, we have introduced a novel approach and potential treatment option that could improve the chances of long-lasting success against a prevalent type of IBD. Our research has presented preclinical data and explained the molecular mechanism behind utilizing the KE known as (R,R)-BD-AcAc2, for the development of a new IBD therapy. This treatment approach involves targeting the NLRP3 inflammasome and its downstream signaling molecules, inhibiting pyroptosis and inducing autophagy. We conducted preliminary trials to determine doses of (R,R)-BD-AcAc2 that successfully elevate blood levels of β-hydroxybutyrate to mimic a state of nutritional ketosis. Furthermore, 16 h of intermittent fasting in rats succeeded in boosting blood levels of β-hydroxybutyrate, mimicking a state of early ketosis.

This study is the first to examine the potential advantages of consuming (R,R)-BD-AcAc2, a type of KE, in comparison to intermittent fasting for treating chronic colitis induced by dextran sodium sulfate (DSS) in rats. Both protocols were selected to enhance the levels of β-hydroxybutyrate. Our findings provide important insights into a promising multi-pronged approach for achieving long-lasting remission in chronic colitis. The potential clinical implications of our findings are bolstered by the greater safety profile of KEs, which enhances their translatability to human subjects.

2. Results

2.1. The Impact of KE Ingestion and Intermittent Fasting on the Microscopic Characteristics of Chronic Colitis Induced by DSS

As depicted in Figure 1, the histopathological assessment of the N, N/F, and N/KE groups (A, B, and C) revealed regular rounded mucus-secreting colonic glands with goblet cells, indicating normal mucosal architecture with normal crypt bases and arrangement. In contrast, sections from the CC and CC/F groups (D and E) displayed submucosal edema, inflamed mucosa, distortion of architecture, complete destruction of colonic glands, and loss of goblet cells. Submucosal congestion and fibrotic tissue deposition were also observed, along with mucosal and submucosal focal and diffuse inflammatory infiltrates of lymphocytes, macrophages, eosinophils, and plasma cells. The ulcerated area from the CC/KE group (F) showed improvement in the structure of the mucosa, with the appearance of glands and crypts, a lower level of focal inflammatory cell infiltrate, and a clear submucosa of very low degree of inflammatory cell infiltration, while edema still existed. Less congestion and collagen deposition in the submucosa were also observed in this group. These findings were also confirmed upon the assessment of the inflammation score (G).

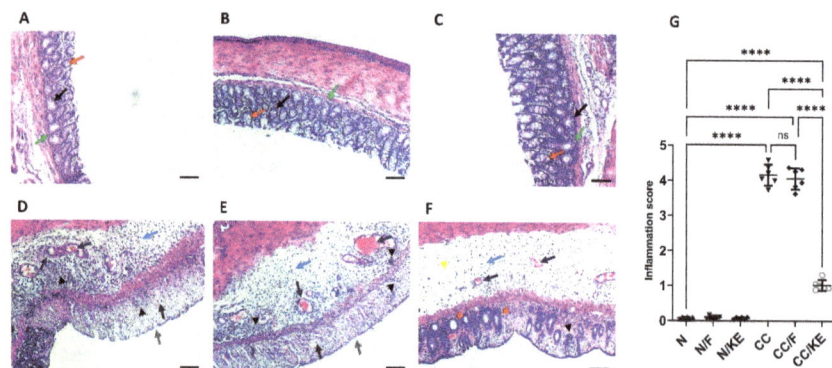

Figure 1. The impact of KE ingestion and intermittent fasting on the microscopic characteristics of chronic colitis induced by DSS. A histopathological evaluation was conducted on the N, N/F, and N/KE

groups (**A–C**, respectively), which demonstrate normal colonic gland structure characterized by rounded mucus-secreting glands (black arrows), with goblet cells present (red arrows). Additionally, normal mucosal architecture is observed with normal crypt bases and arrangement (green arrows). However, CC (**D**) and CC/F (**E**) groups exhibit submucosal edema (blue arrow), inflamed mucosa (light gray arrow), distorted architecture, great destruction of colonic glands, and loss of goblet cells (dark gray arrow). Submucosal congestion and deposition of fibrotic tissue are evident (dark blue arrows). Furthermore, there are focal and diffuse inflammatory infiltrates of lymphocytes, macrophages, eosinophils, and plasma cells in the mucosal and submucosal layers (black arrowheads). Panel (**F**) indicates an improvement in the structure of the mucosa in the ulcerated area of the CC/KE group. The appearance of glands and crypts (red arrowheads) indicates improved mucosal structure, with a lower level of focal inflammatory cell infiltration (black arrowhead) and clear submucosa with a very low degree of inflammatory cell infiltration (yellow arrowhead), although edema persisted (blue arrow). Additionally, there are less congestion and collagen deposition in the submucosa (black arrows). The scale bar is 100 μm. The inflammation score is shown in panel (**G**), with significance levels indicated by pairwise comparisons. ****, $p < 0.0001$; ns, non-significant.

2.2. The Impact of KE Ingestion and Intermittent Fasting on the Mean Percentage Body Weight Change and Colon Weight/Length Ratio

The percentage change in body weight in animal models can be a useful measure for determining the severity of colitis. This is due to the fact that colitis can promote weight loss through a number of processes, including decreased food intake, malabsorption, and increased energy expenditure as a result of inflammation. We can quantify the activity and severity of a disease objectively by tracking changes in body weight over time. Figure 2A illustrates the progressive body weight changes among different groups during the experimental period, while Figure 2B shows that both fasting and KE ingestion resulted in a significant decrease in body weight compared with normal rats. The study found that fasting resulted in a significant decrease in the percentage of body weight change in rats with chronic colitis when compared with the CC group. Similarly, the ingestion of KE, and not intermittent fasting, led to a significant reduction in the percentage of body weight change in rats with chronic colitis when compared with the CC group. These results suggest that KE ingestion may be effective in preventing body weight loss induced by chronic DSS administration. Additionally, the weight-to-length ratio of the colon is commonly used as an indicator of colitis severity in animal models, particularly in pre-clinical trials of new drugs for ulcerative colitis. Lower final ratios are associated with greater effectiveness in reducing severity. The results of the study demonstrated that KE consumption significantly decreased the final colon weight-to-length ratio in contrast to the CC group of rats, demonstrating KE's efficacy in lowering the severity of colitis (as shown in Figure 2C).

2.3. The Impact of KE Ingestion and Intermittent Fasting on the Disease Activity Index and Macroscopic Damage Index

The DAI provides a composite score of colitis severity based on the selected parameters of weight loss, stool consistency, and rectal bleeding. The DAI supplements other metrics like colon weight-to-length ratio and provides an aggregate quantitative measure of colitis severity from different perspectives to complement other evaluations. Based on our findings as shown in Figure 3A, we observed that the DAI significantly increased in the CC group of rats compared with the normal values. However, the rats from the CC/KE group displayed a significant reduction in the score compared with the CC group. On the other hand, the CC/F group did not show a significant change in the DAI compared with that of the CC group. These results indicate that the KE-induced increases in the β-hydroxybutyrate are significantly linked to a reduction in the colitis severity. This suggests that boosting ketone production helps reduce colitis severity as measured by the DAI.

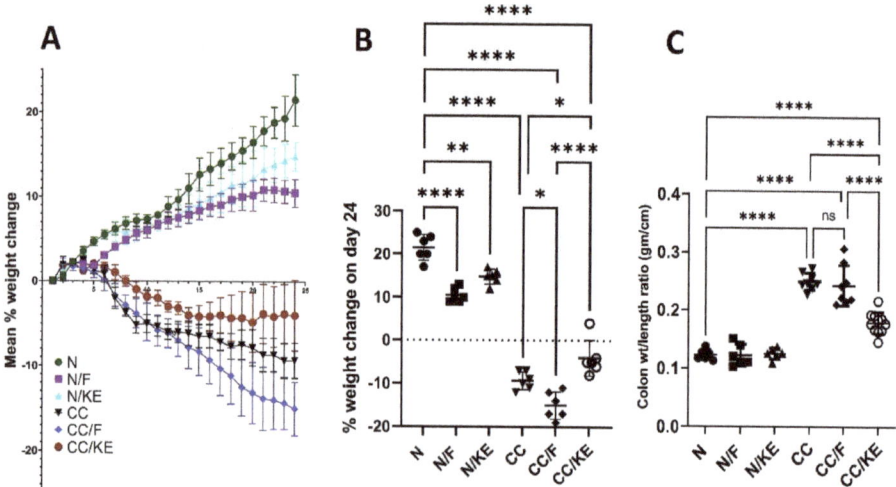

Figure 2. The impact of KE ingestion and intermittent fasting on three parameters: (**A**) the mean percentage body weight change, (**B**) the mean percentage body weight change on day 24, and (**C**) the colon weight/length ratio in rats with chronic colitis induced by DSS. Pairwise comparisons indicate significance levels between groups. *, $p < 0.05$; **, $p < 0.01$; ****, $p < 0.0001$; ns, non-significant.

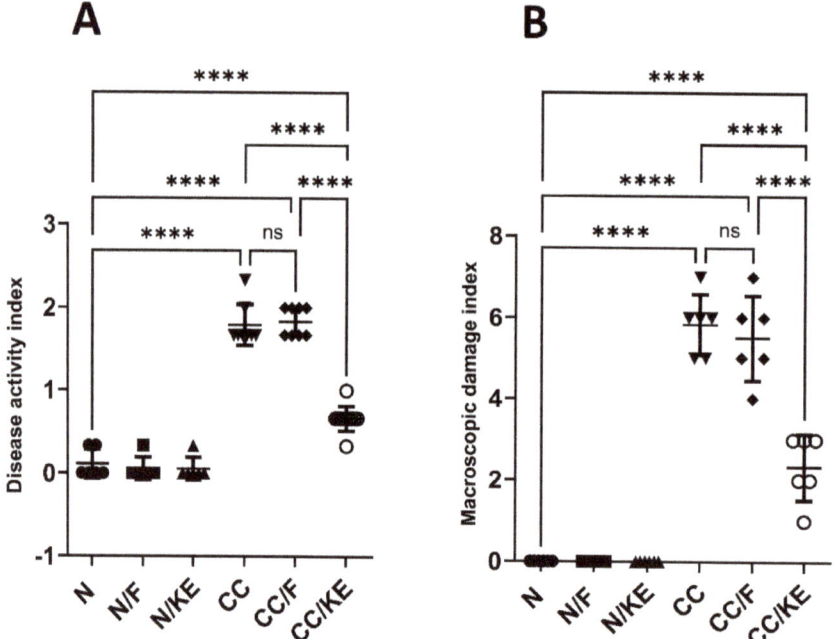

Figure 3. The impact of KE ingestion and intermittent fasting on the disease activity index (**A**) and macroscopic damage index (**B**) in rats with chronic colitis induced by DSS. Pairwise comparisons show the significance levels between the groups. ****, $p < 0.0001$; ns, non-significant.

In addition, the macroscopic damage index provides an additional objective measure of colonic damage that supplements other metrics. It evaluates colitis severity from the perspective of macroscopic colon abnormalities. Our findings (Figure 3B) showed that the MDI in the CC group of rats significantly increased compared with the normal values. When compared with the CC group, however, the rats from the CC/KE group showed a significant decline in scores. The MDI did not significantly vary between the CC group and the CC/F group, on the other hand. These findings suggest that a decrease in the severity of colitis is highly correlated with KE-induced elevations in the β-hydroxybutyrate.

2.4. The Impact of KE Ingestion and Intermittent Fasting on the Survival Property

Survival analysis is a significant statistical method for assessing the effectiveness of treatments for colitis. This approach analyzes the time it takes for an event to occur, and a longer time for the event with the experimental treatment indicates a higher level of effectiveness. Additionally, hazard ratios derived from survival analysis measure the risk of experiencing an adverse event, such as death, in one treatment group compared with another. The log-rank (Mantel–Cox) test was used to compare individual survival analyses between the DSS-exposed rats (CC group) and the CC/F or CC/KE groups of rats. The outcomes showed no statistically significant difference in the likelihood of survival between the CC group and the CC/F group (Figure 4A). Contrarily, our research showed that the DSS-exposed rats' survival rate considerably increased after receiving KE (Figure 4B; $p = 0.045$). Additionally, the CC and CC/KE groups' hazard ratio (log-rank) was 2.92 (95 percent CI of ratio 1.096 to 7.785). The increased survivability in colitic rats of KE-induced β-hydroxybutyrate plasma levels suggests that increasing ketone availability may be a viable treatment for colitis. The findings suggest that ketones may have anti-inflammatory, bioenergetic, and maybe protective cellular effects that could delay disease progression, lessen the severity, and prolong remission.

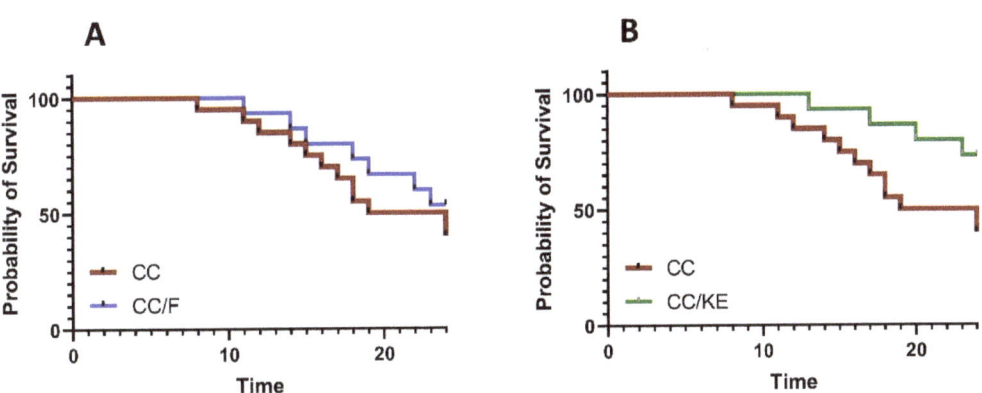

Figure 4. Survival analysis comparisons between the CC group and the CC/F group (**A**) and the CC group and CC/KE group (**B**), show the impact of KE ingestion and intermittent fasting on the survival property in rats with chronic colitis induced by DSS. The log-rank (Mantel–Cox) test was used to determine individual survival analyses. Pairwise comparisons indicate significance levels between groups.

2.5. The Impact of KE Ingestion and Intermittent Fasting on Oxidative Stress Parameters

Oxidative stress indicators can offer important insights into the severity and development of colitis. Lipids, proteins, DNA, and other molecules become oxidatively damaged when oxidants and antioxidants are out of equilibrium. Colitis severity is correlated with the degree of oxidative stress. Additionally, in colitis, the levels of lipid peroxidation products such as MDA are elevated. This increase in MDA is indicative of greater oxidative damage to the membranes, which suggests a more severe inflammatory response and compromise to the gastrointestinal barrier. Our results revealed a significant increase in the levels of ROS (Figure 5A) and MDA (Figure 5B) in response to DSS exposure compared with those of the normal rats. In contrast, KE ingestion significantly suppressed the DSS-induced increase in these levels. Enzymatic antioxidants, such as superoxide dismutase (SOD) play a critical role in regulating oxidant levels. Reduced activity of these enzymes impairs their ability to control reactive oxygen/nitrogen species levels, thereby worsening the severity of colitis. Also, during colitis, there is a depletion of the essential antioxidant glutathione (GSH). This results in increased susceptibility of cells to oxidative damage. We revealed a significant reduction in the levels of SOD (Figure 5C) and GSH (Figure 5D) in response to DSS exposure compared with those of the normal rats. In contrast, KE ingestion significantly suppressed the DSS-induced decrease in these levels.

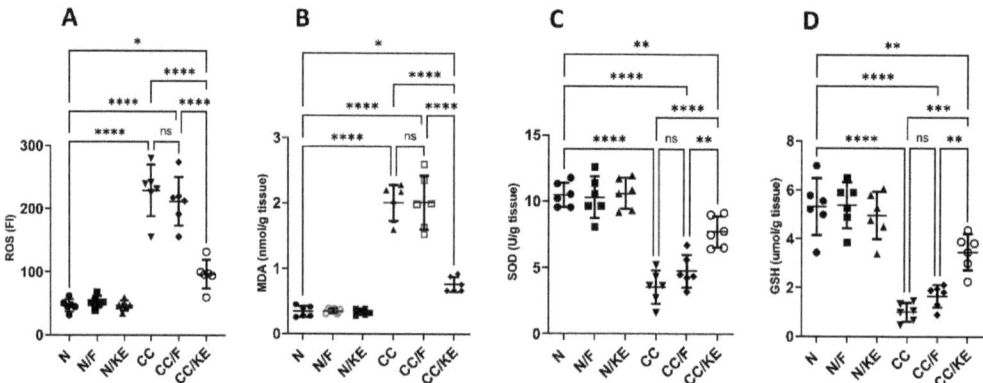

Figure 5. Impact of KE ingestion and intermittent fasting on oxidative stress markers: reactive oxygen species (ROS) (**A**), malondialdehyde (MDA) (**B**), superoxide dismutase (SOD) (**C**), and reduced glutathione (GSH) (**D**) in rats with chronic colitis induced by DSS. Pairwise comparisons indicate significance levels between groups. *, $p < 0.05$; **, $p < 0.01$; ***, $p < 0.001$; ****, $p < 0.0001$; ns, non-significant.

2.6. The Impact of KE Ingestion and Intermittent Fasting on the Plasma Levels of β-Hydroxybutyrate

At the end of the fasting period, the selected intermittent fasting protocol resulted in a significant increase in the β-hydroxybutyrate levels compared with normal non-fasting rats (adjusted p value = 0.043, 95% CI of difference −0.9895 to −0.01063), indicating a state resembling early ketosis. Conversely, ingestion of KE resulted in a significant increase in the β-hydroxybutyrate levels compared with normal non-fasting rats (adjusted p value < 0.0001, 95% CI of difference −3.525 to −2.546) indicating a state resembling nutritional ketosis. In contrast, chronic administration of DSS in the CC rat group did not significantly alter β-hydroxybutyrate levels compared with normal rats. Additionally, intermittent fasting in the CC/F rat group resulted in a significant increase in the levels of β-hydroxybutyrate compared with those of CC rats (adjusted p value = 0.02). Similarly, KE ingestion in CC/KE rat group resulted in a significant increase in the levels of β-hydroxybutyrate when compared with those of CC rats (adjusted p value < 0.0001). Overall, these findings (illustrated in Figure 6) suggest that both intermittent fasting for 16 h per day and KE ingestion elevated β-hydroxybutyrate levels beyond normal levels, inducing a state resembling early and nutritional ketosis, respectively.

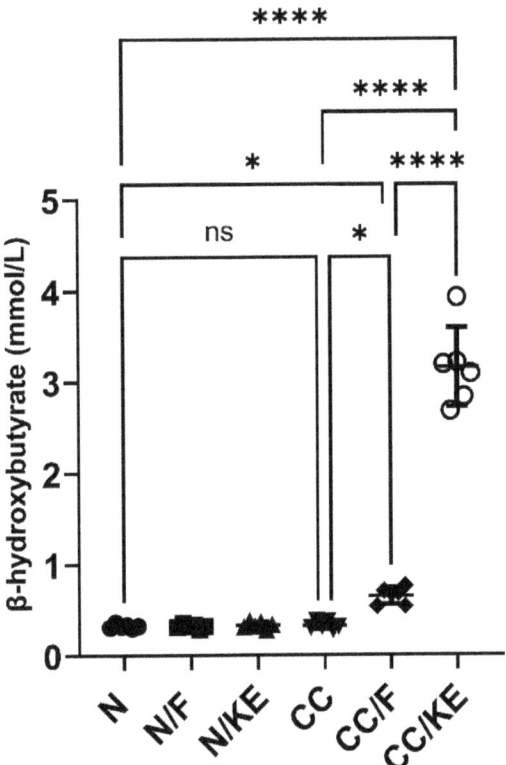

Figure 6. The impact of KE ingestion and intermittent fasting on plasma levels of β-hydroxybutyrate in rats with chronic colitis induced by DSS. Significance levels are indicated by pairwise comparisons. *, $p < 0.05$; ****, $p < 0.0001$; ns, non-significant.

2.7. The Impact of KE Ingestion and Intermittent Fasting on Different Cytokines as Inflammation Markers

In the CC group, chronic administration of DSS resulted in a significant increase in the levels of pro-inflammatory cytokines TNF-α (Figure 7A), IL-6 (Figure 7B), IL-1β (Figure 7C), and IL-18 (Figure 7D), and a significant increase in the levels of anti-inflammatory cytokines IL-10 (Figure 7E) and IL-4 (Figure 7F), compared with those in normal rats. However, the ingestion of KE had a significant impact on the reversal of DSS-induced changes in cytokine levels in the CC/KE groups, compared with the CC groups. Specifically, TNF-α, IL-6, IL-1β, IL-18, and IL-4 levels were significantly reduced, while IL-10 levels remained unchanged. Chronic colitis is known to be associated with an increase in pro-inflammatory cytokines, which contribute to persistent inflammation and colon tissue damage. The elevation of IL-1β and IL-18 levels suggests inflammasome activation, which is believed to be involved in chronic colitis. The higher levels of IL-10 and IL-4 in CC groups indicated a shift towards a Th2-mediated immune response. These cytokines are produced by various immune cells, including Th2 cells, Tregs, and macrophages, which are activated in chronic colitis. It is worth noting that cytokine levels were not significantly altered in rats that underwent intermittent fasting and were treated with DSS, compared with non-fasting rats that received DSS treatment.

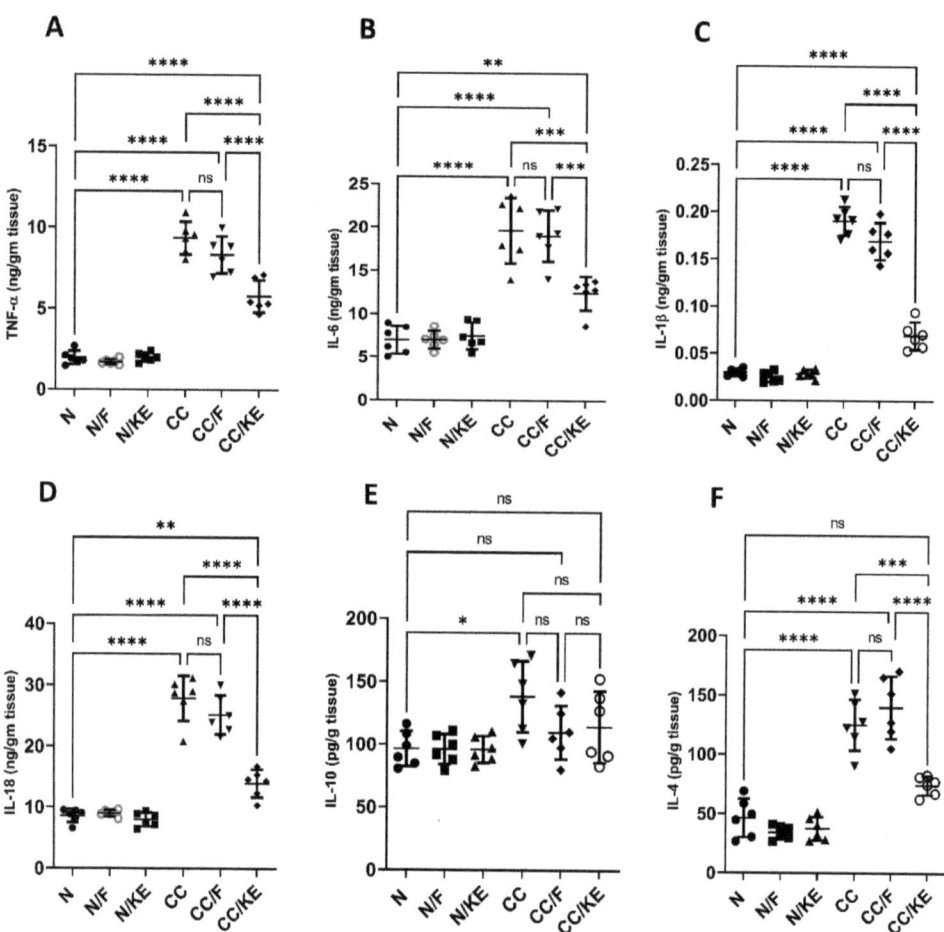

Figure 7. The impact of KE ingestion and intermittent fasting on tumor necrosis factor-alpha (TNF-α) (**A**), IL-6 (**B**), IL-1β (**C**), IL-18 (**D**), IL-10 (**E**), and IL-4 (**F**) levels in rats with chronic colitis induced by DSS. Significance levels are indicated by pairwise comparisons. *, $p < 0.05$; **, $p < 0.01$; ***, $p < 0.001$; ****, $p < 0.0001$; ns, non-significant.

2.8. The Impact of KE Ingestion and Intermittent Fasting on the Activities of Each Mpo, Nfκb Dna Binding, Caspase-1, and the Levels of Active Caspase-3

In chronic colitis, sustained activation of neutrophils leads to the release of MPO, which contributes to tissue damage by generating ROS and other reactive intermediates. The increased levels of NFκB in chronic colitis promote the sustained production of pro-inflammatory cytokines, thereby perpetuating the inflammatory response. NFκB activates the expression of genes involved in cytokine production, such as TNF-α, IL-6, and IL-1β, which recruit immune cells and further damage the tissue. In chronic colitis, increased activity of caspase-1 leads to the production of pro-inflammatory cytokines and the perpetuation of the inflammatory response. Caspase-1 processes the bioactivation of IL-1β and IL-18, which stimulate immune cells and promote tissue damage. Similarly, increased activity of caspase-3 in chronic colitis contributes to tissue damage and disease progression by inducing apoptosis and subsequent loss of epithelial cells. Apoptosis of intestinal epithelial cells leads to disruption of the intestinal barrier and increased permeability, allowing luminal antigens and bacteria to enter the mucosa and trigger further inflammation. Additionally, caspase-3-mediated apoptosis of immune cells can contribute to the dysregulation of the immune response and perpetuation of inflammation. Our results revealed that the activities of MPO (Figure 8A), NFκB DNA binding (Figure 8B), and caspase-1 (Figure 8C), and the levels of active caspase-3 (Figure 8D) were significantly increased in the chronic colitis rat group compared with normal rats. However, ingestion of KE significantly reversed the DSS-induced alterations in their levels, while intermittent fasting did not significantly alter their levels in the CC/F group compared with the CC group.

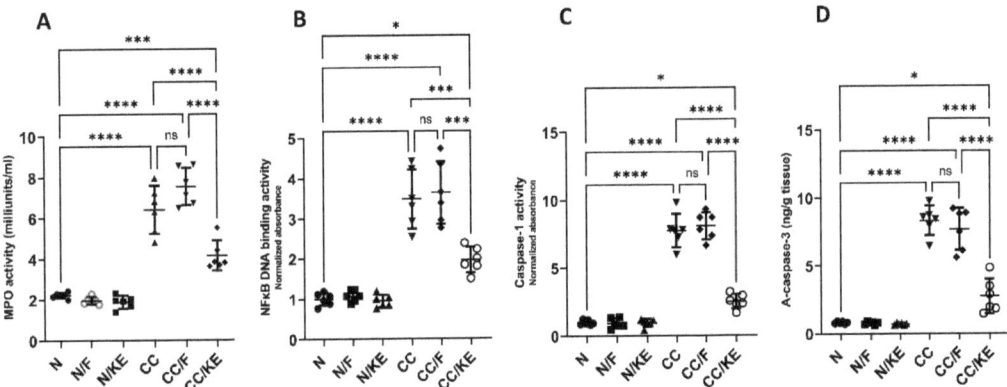

Figure 8. The impact of KE ingestion and intermittent fasting on the activities of each myeloperoxidase (MPO) (**A**), nuclear transcription factor kappa B (NFκB) DNA binding (**B**), caspase-1 (**C**), and the levels of active caspase-3 (**D**) in rats with chronic colitis induced by DSS. Significance levels are indicated by pairwise comparisons. *, $p < 0.05$; ***, $p < 0.001$; ****, $p < 0.0001$; ns, non-significant.

2.9. The Impact of KE Ingestion and Intermittent Fasting on the mRNA Expression of ASC and NLRP3

ASC acts as a linker protein, aiding in the assembly and activation of the inflammasome complex. The protein's N-terminus contains a caspase recruitment domain (CARD), which recruits and binds caspase-1 to the inflammasome complex, facilitating its activation. This process leads to the cleavage of pro-IL-1β and pro-IL-18 into their active forms. Additionally, ASC comprises a pyrin domain, which interacts with the NLRP3 sensor protein. The activation of the NLRP3 inflammasome occurs in two steps. First, the inflammasome undergoes priming through the activation of NFκB, which results in the upregulation of inflammasome components such as NLRP3. The second step involves the activation of NLRP3 by specific danger signals. This process leads to the assembly of the inflammasome complex and subsequent activation of caspase-1. Chronic colitis can be triggered by various factors that activate the NLRP3 inflammasome. These factors include the release of damage-associated molecular patterns (DAMPs) by damaged epithelial cells and the dysbiosis of the gut microbiome. The activation of the NLRP3 inflammasome results in an increased secretion of IL-1β and IL-18, promoting inflammation, epithelial damage, and the infiltration of immune cells into the colonic mucosa. This exacerbates the inflammation in chronic colitis. Our study found that in rats with chronic colitis, the mRNA expression of ASC (Figure 9A) and NLRP3 (Figure 9B) was significantly higher than in normal rats. However, ingestion of KE significantly reduced the mRNA expression of NLRP3, while ASC mRNA expression remained unchanged in the CC/KE group compared with the CC group. Additionally, there was no significant change in the mRNA expression of ASC and NLRP3 in the CC/F rat group compared with normal rats. These findings suggest that KE may have a therapeutic effect on chronic colitis by modulating the expression of NLRP3, a crucial component of the inflammasome complex.

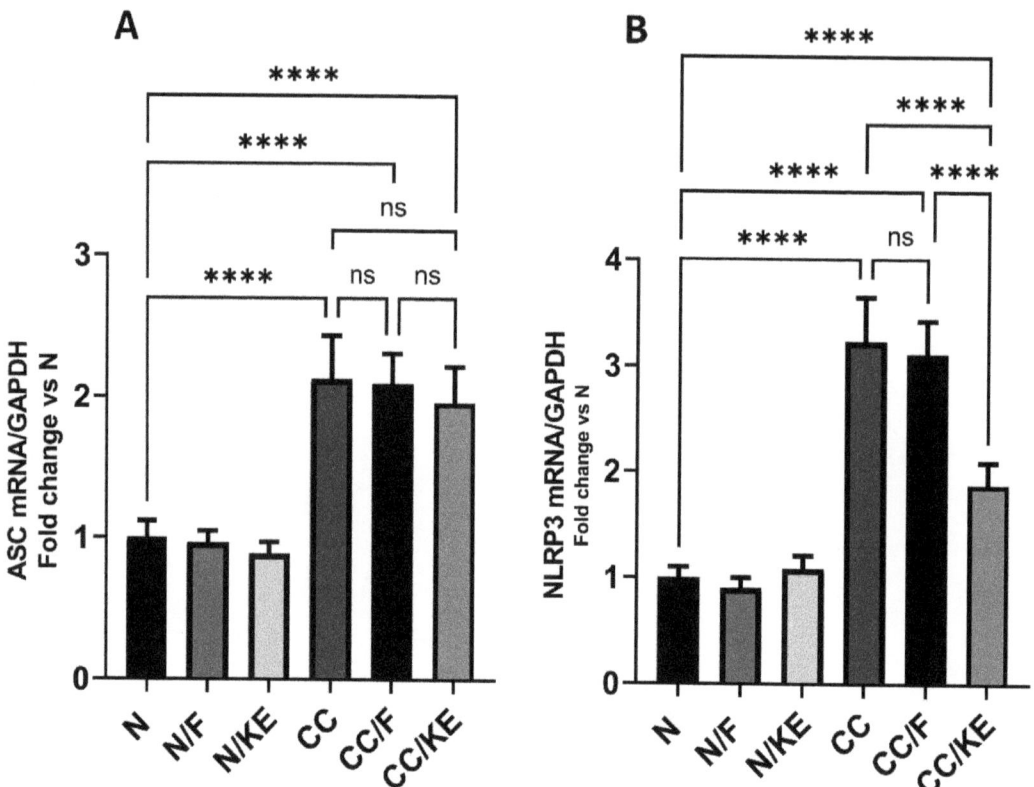

Figure 9. The impact of KE ingestion and intermittent fasting on the levels of the mRNA expression of apoptosis-associated speck-like protein containing a CARD (ASC) (**A**) and nucleotide-binding oligomerization domain-like receptor protein 3 (NLRP3) (**B**) in rats with chronic colitis induced by DSS. Significance levels are indicated by pairwise comparisons. ****, $p < 0.0001$; ns, non-significant.

2.10. The Impact of KE Ingestion and Intermittent Fasting on the Levels of NLRP3 and NGSDMD

The NLRP3 inflammasome is involved in activating caspase-1, which in turn cleaves GSDMD to generate its active N-terminal fragment known as NGSDMD. This fragment then oligomerizes to form membrane pores leading to cell swelling, membrane rupture, and pyroptotic cell death that allow the release of inflammatory cytokines. Excessive GSDMD cleavage has been linked to heightened pyroptosis, a form of programmed cell death, and inflammation in the colonic mucosa. Our study revealed a significant increase in both NLRP3 (Figure 10A) and NGSDMD (Figure 10B) levels in the CC group compared with the N group. However, the CC/KE group exhibited a significant reduction in these levels due to the consumption of KE compared with the CC group. Notably, intermittent fasting had no significant effect on these levels.

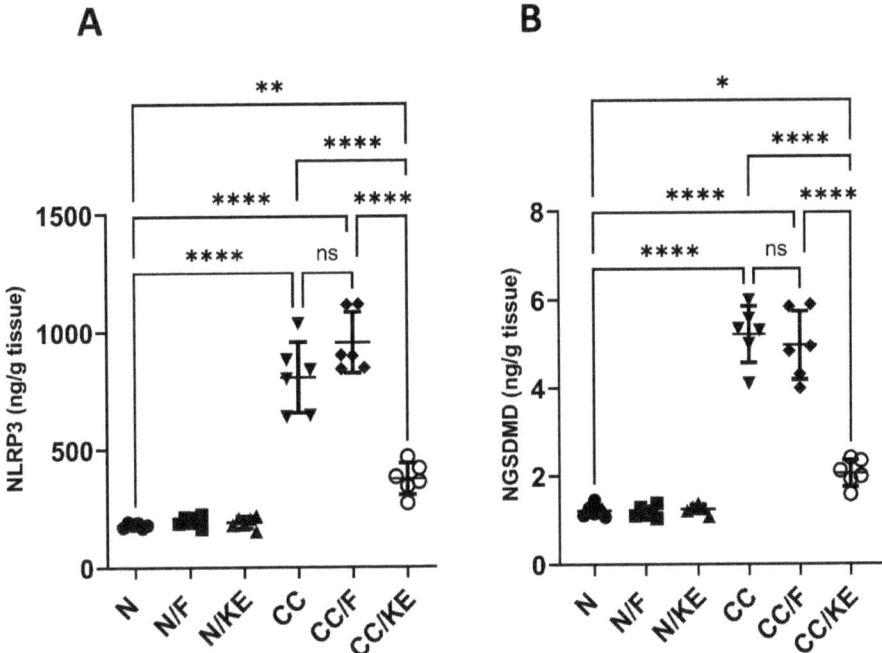

Figure 10. The impact of KE ingestion and intermittent fasting on the levels of nucleotide-binding oligomerization domain-like receptor protein 3 (NLRP3) (**A**) and gasdermin D N-terminal fragment (NGSDMD) (**B**) in rats with chronic colitis induced by DSS. Significance levels are indicated by pairwise comparisons. *, $p < 0.05$; **, $p < 0.01$; ****, $p < 0.0001$; ns, non-significant.

2.11. The Impact of KE Ingestion and Intermittent Fasting on the Macroautophagy Markers

The activation of macroautophagy in colitis is thought to be an adaptive response to help limit inflammation and tissue injury, indicating it plays a protective role. stimulating macroautophagy may have the potential as a treatment strategy. BECN1 is an important protein involved in the activation of macroautophagy. It forms a protein complex that is required for the initiation of macroautophagy by recruiting other proteins to form the isolation membrane that engulfs cellular components for degradation. BECN1 levels correlate with the activation of macroautophagy. Higher levels of BECN1 generally indicate more induction of the macroautophagy process. On the other hand, P62 is a protein that undergoes selective degradation through macroautophagy. Thus, its levels show an inverse correlation with macroautophagy activation. P62 binds to proteins and organelles that macroautophagy targets for degradation. It interacts with proteins on the autophagosome membrane to facilitate degradation. Once engulfed by the autophagosome, lysosomal enzymes break down p62 and the molecules it binds. Inducing macroautophagy leads to the degradation of more p62 and its targets, resulting in lower p62 levels in the cell. Conversely, impaired macroautophagy cannot effectively degrade p62, leading to its accumulation in the cell. In our study, we detected impaired macroautophagy in the CC rat group compared with normal rats. However, we observed macroautophagy activation in the CC/F group compared with the CC group (BECN1, $p < 0.02$; p62, $p < 0.0001$), as well as in the CC/KE group compared with the CC group (BECN1, $p < 0.0001$; p62, $p < 0.0001$). These findings (as shown in Figure 11A for BECN1 and Figure 11B for p62) suggest that both intermittent fasting and KE consumption induced macroautophagy activation, with KE consumption demonstrating a particularly strong effect.

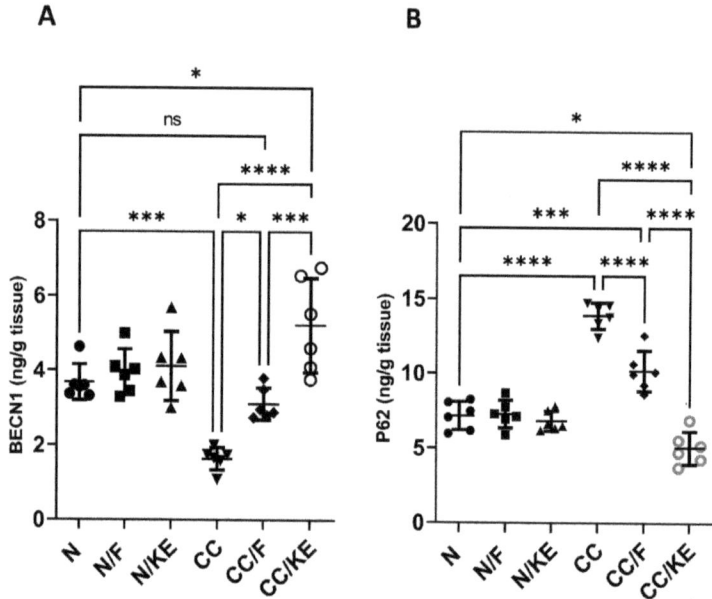

Figure 11. The impact of KE ingestion and intermittent fasting on Beclin-1 (BECN1) (**A**) and sequestosome-1 (p62) (**B**) in rats with chronic colitis induced by DSS. Significance levels are indicated by pairwise comparisons. *, $p < 0.05$; ***, $p < 0.001$; ****, $p < 0.0001$; ns, non-significant.

2.12. The Impact of KE Ingestion and Intermittent Fasting on Tight Junction Proteins

Maintaining the integrity and barrier function of the intestinal epithelium is a critical function of tight junction proteins. However, chronic colitis can disrupt these proteins, leading to increased intestinal permeability, bacterial translocation, and the release of inflammatory cytokines. In our study, we administered DSS to rats in the CC group, which resulted in a significant decrease in the levels of tight junction proteins ZO-1 (Figure 12A), OCLN (Figure 12B), and CLDN5 (Figure 12C) compared with their baseline levels. Interestingly, KE consumption, rather than intermittent fasting, resulted in significant increases in the levels of these proteins compared with the DSS-treated CC rat group.

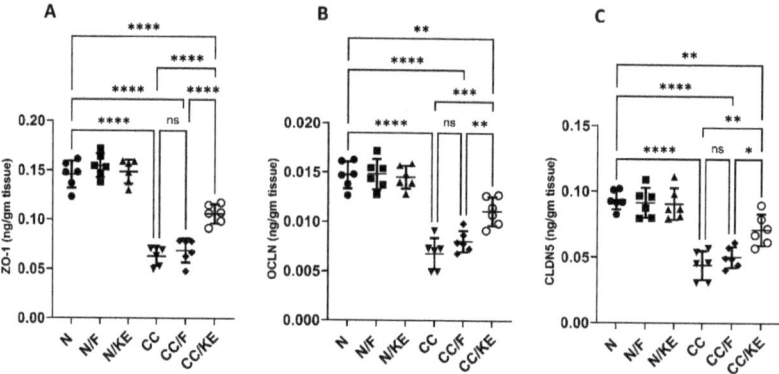

Figure 12. The impact of KE ingestion and intermittent fasting on tight junction proteins zonula occludens-1 (ZO-1) (**A**), occludin (OCLN) (**B**), and claudin-5 (CLDN5) (**C**) in rats with chronic colitis induced by DSS. Significance levels are indicated by pairwise comparisons. *, $p < 0.05$; **, $p < 0.01$; ***, $p < 0.001$; ****, $p < 0.0001$; ns, non-significant.

2.13. Correlation Analysis of the Measured Parameters

As shown in Figure 13, our research findings demonstrate a positive correlation between the levels of β-hydroxybutyrate in rats with chronic colitis and the tight junction proteins OCLN and CLDN5, with a strong tendency towards a positive correlation with ZO-1. This suggests that increasing the levels of β-hydroxybutyrate could be beneficial in reducing gut permeability. In addition, β-hydroxybutyrate may help manage colitis symptoms by stabilizing or upregulating these key barrier proteins. This potential mechanism may explain the beneficial effects of ketogenic diets or ketone supplementation in managing colitis and other forms of intestinal inflammation.

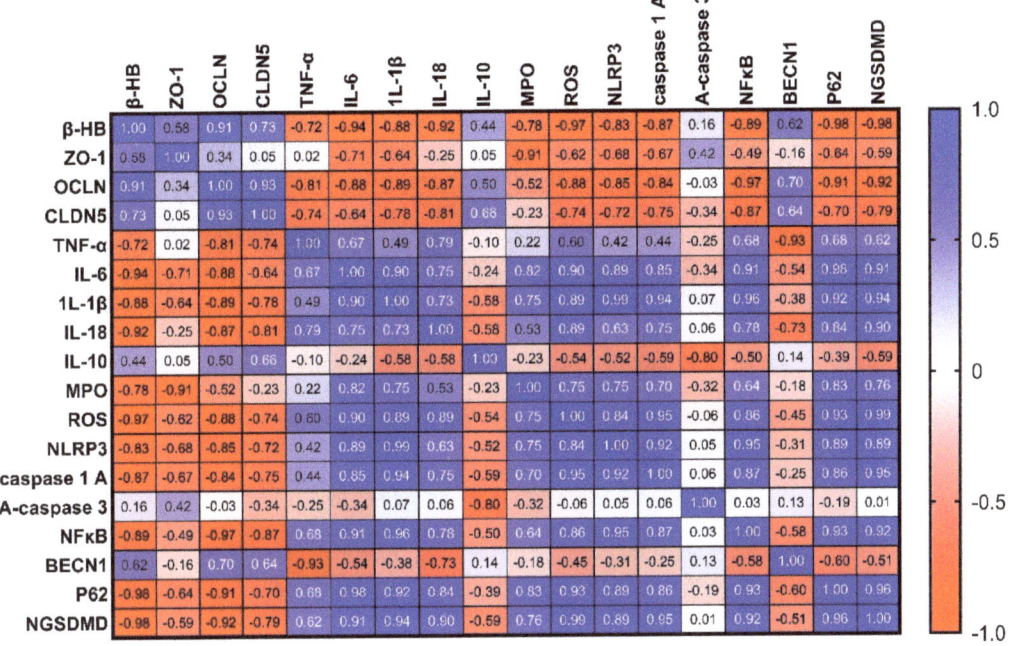

Figure 13. Correlation analysis of the measured parameters in rats with chronic colitis induced by DSS.

In addition, our study revealed a negative correlation between the levels of β-hydroxybutyrate in rats with chronic colitis and proinflammatory cytokines such as TNF-α, IL-6, IL-1β, and IL-18, with a strong tendency towards a positive correlation with IL-10 levels. This suggests that β-hydroxybutyrate may have anti-inflammatory effects in chronic colitis by reducing the production of proinflammatory cytokines and mitigating the inflammatory response. Additionally, β-hydroxybutyrate may increase the levels of the anti-inflammatory cytokine IL-10 to suppress inflammation and facilitate intestinal healing.

Furthermore, our investigation revealed a negative correlation between the levels of β-hydroxybutyrate in rats with chronic colitis and several inflammatory markers, including MPO activity, ROS production, NLRP3 levels, caspase-1 activity, NFκB DNA binding activity, and the NGSDMD. However, we did not find a significant correlation with active caspase-3 levels. These findings suggest that β-hydroxybutyrate may help mitigate gut inflammation in chronic colitis by inhibiting inflammasome activation and oxidative stress through various mechanisms. Specifically, MPO activity and ROS production were negatively correlated with β-hydroxybutyrate levels, implying that β-hydroxybutyrate may reduce oxidative stress, which is often increased in colitis and contributes to gut inflammation. Moreover, NLRP3 levels, caspase-1 activity, and NFκB DNA binding activity were all negatively correlated with β-hydroxybutyrate levels. These components play a role in the NLRP3 inflammasome activation, which drives intestinal inflammation in colitis by consequent production of IL-1β and IL-18. Thus, the negative correlations suggest that β-hydroxybutyrate may suppress NLRP3 inflammasome activation. In addition, NGSDMD levels were also negatively correlated with β-hydroxybutyrate. NGSDMD release is associated with pyroptosis, a proinflammatory form of programmed cell death. Therefore, lower levels of NGSDMD with higher β-hydroxybutyrate suggest that β-hydroxybutyrate may inhibit pyroptosis. However, our results did not show a significant correlation between caspase-3 activity and β-hydroxybutyrate levels. This indicates that β-hydroxybutyrate's effects may be specific to inflammasome-related pathways rather than overall apoptosis.

Finally, we revealed a negative correlation between levels of β-hydroxybutyrate and p62, while there is a positive correlation with BECN1. This suggests that β-hydroxybutyrate may have a modulating effect on autophagy in chronic colitis. The negative correlation between β-hydroxybutyrate and p62 indicates that higher levels of β-hydroxybutyrate are associated with lower levels of p62 protein, which is a marker of autophagic flux. Increased levels of p62 typically indicate impaired autophagy, so the lower p62 levels observed with higher β-hydroxybutyrate suggest that β-hydroxybutyrate may enhance autophagy. The positive correlation between β-hydroxybutyrate and BECN1 further supports this idea, as BECN1 is important for initiating autophagy and higher levels of BECN1 promote autophagy. Therefore, the positive correlation between β-hydroxybutyrate and BECN1 suggests that β-hydroxybutyrate may stimulate autophagy by upregulating BECN1. Autophagy helps remove damaged organelles and aggregates to maintain cellular homeostasis, and its impairment has been linked to chronic inflammation, including colitis. By potentially enhancing autophagy through reducing p62 and increasing BECN1, β-hydroxybutyrate may help resolve gut inflammation in colitis. Although the correlations provide insight into potential mechanisms, the observational nature of the correlation means that causation cannot be definitively established.

2.14. The Impact of KE Ingestion and Intermittent Fasting on Microbiome Composition

Chronic colitis is associated with elevated levels of *Fusobacterium* species, which may contribute to inflammation by invading intestinal cells, activating the NLRP3 inflammasome, and dysregulating the microbiome. Additionally, increased levels of *Bacteroides* have been implicated in some inflammatory bowel diseases such as chronic colitis. The overgrowth of certain *Clostridium* species may also trigger and sustain chronic inflammation in colitis by affecting the intestinal environment and immune system. On the other hand, *Bifidobacteria* are a beneficial bacteria genus that constitutes a significant proportion of the gut microbiota, particularly in the colon. Reduction in *Bifidobacteria* is linked to increased disease severity and poorer outcomes in colitis. Lactobacillus bacteria are generally considered probiotics that may have potential health benefits. However, patients with ulcerative colitis and Crohn's disease often exhibit lower levels of Lactobacillus than healthy individuals. This observation suggests that lower abundances of *Lactobacillus* may be associated with dysbiosis and chronic inflammation in the gut. In our study, we revealed a significant disruption in the gut composition of the abovementioned bacteria species in the CC rat group. While both intermittent fasting and KE ingestion caused a significant reversal in the relative abundance of these bacteria species compared with the CC group (except for KE in the case of *Bacteroides*), neither regimen could fully restore the normal relative abundance of these bacteria, except for *Lactobacillus*, as depicted in Figure 14A (*Fusobacterium*), B (*Bacteroides*), C (*Clostridium*), D (*Bifidobacteria*), and E (*Lactobacillus*).

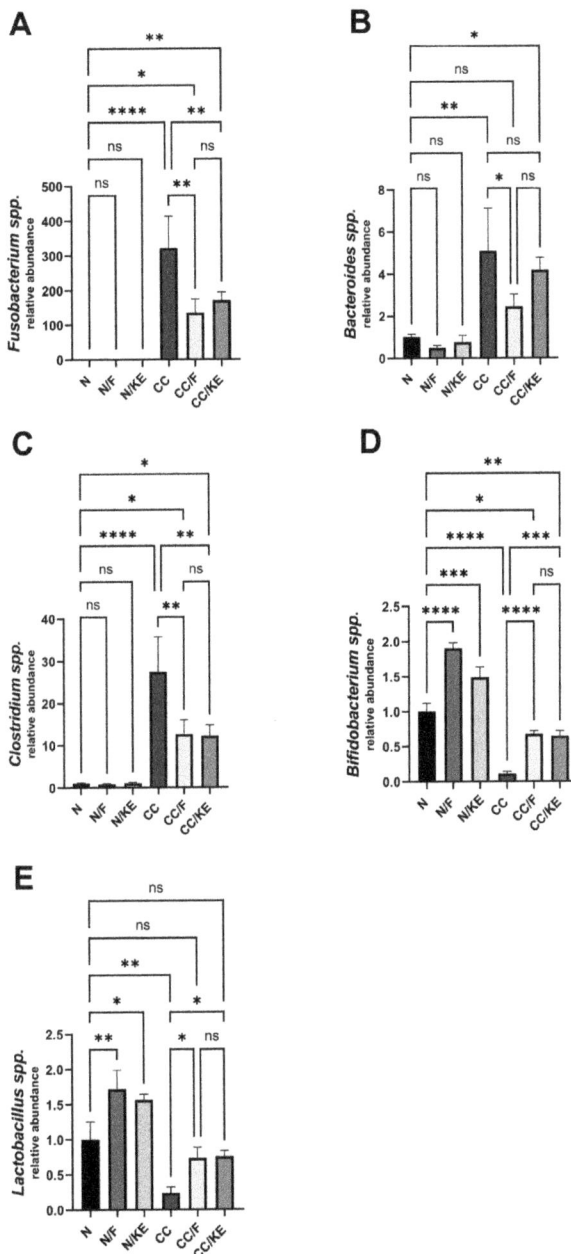

Figure 14. The impact of KE ingestion and intermittent fasting on microbiome composition in rats with chronic colitis induced by DSS: This figure depicts the changes in the microbiome composition of five bacterial species, *Fusobacterium* spp. (**A**), *Bacteroids* spp. (**B**), *Clostridium* spp. (**C**), *Bifidobacterium* spp. (**D**), and *Lactobacillus* spp. (**E**), in response to KE ingestion and intermittent fasting. The significance levels are indicated by pairwise comparisons, and the results suggest significant changes associated with β-hydroxybutyrate boosting on the microbiome composition of these bacterial species. *, $p < 0.05$; **, $p < 0.01$; ***, $p < 0.001$; ****, $p < 0.0001$; ns, non-significant.

3. Discussion

Ulcerative colitis is a chronic and incurable form of IBDs that can significantly impair quality of life and increase the risk of colitis-associated cancer and mortality. One major challenge associated with ulcerative colitis is the limited treatment options available, which often come with non-tolerable adverse effects.

In this study, we aimed to shed light on the potential therapeutic value of ketosis/ketone production in managing IBD. Specifically, we investigated the benefits of ketone-based medications or supplements that can increase ketone levels without requiring a restrictive diet. This approach has the potential to improve compliance and safety in the treatment of chronic colitis. To examine this novel treatment method, we investigated the effects of two regimens that increase β-hydroxybutyrate levels: intermittent fasting and the consumption of a specific type of KE called (R,R)-BD-AcAc2. We evaluated their effectiveness in managing chronic colitis induced by DSS in rats.

In accordance with our protocol, rats were administered the KE, resulting in elevated levels of β-hydroxybutyrate, indicating a state resembling nutritional ketosis. Additionally, 16 h of intermittent fasting led to increased levels of β-hydroxybutyrate, suggesting the onset of early ketosis. Interestingly, despite exhibiting modulation of autophagy and correction of dysbiosis, rats subjected to 24 days of intermittent fasting did not show significant coloprotective effects against chronic DSS administration. In contrast, the consumption of KE demonstrated a notable coloprotective property, primarily by modulating the NLRP3 inflammasome and its downstream inflammatory pyroptotic cell death. These results indicate that achieving a state of nutritional ketosis, as opposed to early ketosis, is necessary to confer a coloprotective effect.

It is noteworthy that both protocols demonstrated almost the same impact on the relative abundance of the tested bacteria. This suggests that the correction of dysbiosis is not the primary mechanism through which β-hydroxybutyrate alleviates colitis. Although the intermittent fasting protocol induced only a small increase in autophagy, it seems that this minor change has a negligible effect on colon inflammation. On the other hand, KE consumption was more effective than the intermittent fasting protocol as it exhibited stronger autophagy-inducing capabilities in addition to demonstrating the inactivation of the NLRP3 inflammasome.

In addition to improving disease activity, the consumption of KE resulted in the improvement of colonic macroscopic and microscopic features, as well as a decrease in inflammation scores. Furthermore, KE counteracted the DSS-induced decrease in the percentage of weight change upon experiment completion, reduced the colonic weight-to-length ratio, and increased the survival rate of DSS-insulted rats. Although oxidative stress parameters were not normalized, KE ingestion showed potential antioxidant activities. Along with improving gut microbiome composition, KE consumption improved the levels of tight junction proteins, which protect against leaky gut. Moreover, KE consumption exhibited anti-inflammatory properties by reducing proinflammatory cytokine production.

It is worth noting that our results revealed an increase in the levels of IL-10 and IL-4 in non-treated chronic colitis rats. This result suggests that the body mounts an immunoregulatory response involving IL-10 and IL-4 against chronic colitis, but this response is inadequate to resolve the inflammation. Additionally, this result indicated a shift towards a Th2-mediated immune response, confirming the chronic nature of our model.

The transcriptional regulation of IL-1β and IL-18 is mediated by NFκB, which acts as the priming signal for the activation of the NLRP3 inflammasome. The assembly of the inflammasome complex and subsequent activation of caspase-1 leads to the bioactivation of IL-1β and IL-18, making them key players in the pyroptosis process. The coloprotective effect of KE can be attributed to its ability to inhibit both the priming and activation signals of the NLRP3 inflammasome, thus preventing highly inflammatory pyroptotic cell death. Importantly, KE consumption was found to decrease NFκB DNA binding and downregulate NLRP3, which is also transcriptionally regulated by NFκB. This results in a reduction in caspase-1 activity, ultimately leading to the inhibition of IL-1β and IL-18 bioactivation. This was further confirmed by a reduction in the gasdermin D N-terminal fragment, which is indicative of curbed pyroptosis. During pyroptosis, inflammatory cytokines such as IL-1β and IL-18 are released from the dying cell, which can stimulate the production of ROS and recruit immune cells such as neutrophils that release MPO during inflammation. The decrease in MPO activity observed after KE consumption can, therefore, be explained by the inhibited release of IL-1β and IL-18, which in turn reduces the production of ROS and the recruitment of immune cells.

Furthermore, the administration of KE has been shown to significantly repress active caspase-3, confirming its antiapoptotic effects. Specifically, oxidative stress resulting from excessive ROS production in the damaged colon can overwhelm the cell's antioxidant defenses, leading to DNA damage and mitochondrial dysfunction that trigger apoptosis. The release of cytochrome c from the mitochondria activates caspases and triggers the apoptotic pathway. Therefore, KE's anti-apoptotic function may be attributed, at least in part, to its ability to improve the antioxidant defense machinery in the cell.

Our study shows that increased levels of β-hydroxybutyrate in rats with chronic colitis are positively correlated with tight junction proteins OCLN and CLDN5, with a strong tendency towards a positive correlation with ZO-1, indicating that increasing β-hydroxybutyrate levels could be beneficial in reducing gut permeability. Therefore, β-hydroxybutyrate may help manage colitis symptoms by stabilizing or upregulating these key barrier proteins, which may explain the beneficial effects of ketogenic diets or ketone supplementation in managing colitis and other forms of intestinal inflammation. Our analysis also revealed that β-hydroxybutyrate is negatively correlated with the measured proinflammatory cytokines in our study. Indicating that β-hydroxybutyrate may have anti-inflammatory effects in chronic colitis by reducing the production of proinflammatory cytokines and mitigating the inflammatory response. Furthermore, we found that β-hydroxybutyrate may help mitigate gut inflammation in chronic colitis by inhibiting NFκB and NLRP3 inflammasome activation and restraining oxidative stress as revealed also by correlation analysis. β-hydroxybutyrate may also enhance autophagy as revealed by reduced p62 and increased BECN1, which may help resolve gut inflammation in colitis. Finally, β-hydroxybutyrate may have a positive impact on maintaining a healthy microbiome.

In conclusion, this preclinical study indicates a potential therapeutic benefit of ketosis and ketone production in the management of various inflammatory diseases, particularly in the context of IBDs.

Our encouraging results provide a strong rationale for conducting further clinical research to explore the efficacy of β-hydroxybutyrate boosting compounds such as KEs in treating these conditions. If successful, these novel treatment approaches could significantly improve the lives of patients suffering from inflammatory diseases with the greatest safety. However, our study has limitations, including the use of an animal model that may not fully capture the intricate complexities of human pathophysiology, potentially limiting generalizability. The specific experimental conditions and the focus on short-term outcomes also restrict the applicability and understanding of the long-term effects of (R,R)-BD-AcAc2. Additionally, despite rigorous methodologies and blinded assessments, uncontrolled confounding variables should be considered. Therefore, more investment in clinical research is needed to fully realize the therapeutic potential of (R,R)-BD-AcAc2 and other KEs or ketone salts.

4. Materials and Methods

4.1. Drugs and Chemicals

(R)-3-Hydroxybutyl (R)-3-hydroxybutyrate ketone ester known as (R,R)-BD-AcAc2 with the formula $C_8H_{16}O_4$ was obtained from MCE (Monmouth Junction, NJ, USA). Dextran sodium sulfate was supplied by Sigma-Aldrich (St. Louis, MO, USA; Mw = ~40,000). Fine chemicals and reagents were supplied by Sigma-Aldrich unless indicated else.

4.2. Animals

We obtained male Sprague Dawley (SD) rats from TBRI, aged seven weeks and weighing 180–200 g. The rats were given a two-week period to acclimate to the laboratory before the commencement of the experiment. They were kept in controlled environmental conditions since birth, with a temperature of 22 ± 2 °C, a relative humidity of $50 \pm 10\%$, and a 12 h light/dark cycle (lights on from 09:00 a.m. to 09:00 p.m.). The rats were provided with ad libitum feeding and drinking. The protocol was approved by the IACUC at FPDU under FPDU24120,2. All animals were treated and sacrificed according to the corresponding guidelines.

4.3. Induction of Chronic Colitis in Rats

According to the procedure outlined by Hoffmann, et al. [32], chronic colitis was induced in the experimental animals by administering 2% DSS for seven days, followed by 1% DSS for ten days, and finally, another seven days of 2% DSS treatment. Throughout the experiment, the animals were monitored daily for changes in body weight, and the percentage of body weight loss was determined relative to their initial body weight on the first day of the study.

4.4. Experimental Design

Table 1 shows that the rats were randomly divided into six groups. The N group (n = 8) served as the control group. The N/F group (n = 8) consisted of rats that were subjected to 16 h of fasting including the dark cycle (from 05:00 p.m. to 09:00 a.m.) while being fed standard rodent food ad libitum at other times. The N/KE group (n = 8) consisted of rats that were given a mixture of KE and standard rodent food ad libitum. The CC group (n = 20) consisted of rats that received DSS. The CC/F group (n = 15) consisted of rats that received DSS and were subjected to the intermittent fasting protocol. The CC/KE group (n = 15) consisted of rats that received DSS and the KE/standard food mixture. On the start of day 25 at 09:00 a.m., all animals were sacrificed while under anesthesia (thiopental sodium 40 mg/kg).

Table 1. Experimental design.

Exp. Groups	Days 1–7	Days 8–17	Days 18–24	Day 25
N group (n = 8)	Non-fasting	Non-fasting	Non-fasting	
N/F (n = 8)	Fasting—16 h	Fasting—16 h	Fasting—16 h	
N/KE (n = 8)	Non-fasting KE	Non-fasting KE	Non-fasting KE	Sacrifice day
CC (n = 20)	Non-fasting 2% DSS	Non-fasting 1% DSS	Non-fasting 2% DSS	
CC/F (n = 15)	Fasting—16 h 2% DSS	Fasting—16 h 1% DSS	Fasting—16 h 2% DSS	
CC/KE (n = 15)	Non-fasting 2% DSS KE	Non-fasting 1% DSS KE	Non-fasting 2% DSS KE	

CC, chronic colitis; DSS, dextran sodium sulfate; F, fasting; KE, ketone ester.

In this experiment, blood samples were collected from all animal groups to determine β-hydroxybutyrate levels after 8 h of the fasting period, which begins at 5:00 p.m. on day 24. This occurred before the end of the day at 1:00 a.m. The animal groups were then allowed free access to food to prevent discrepancies in disease activity and body weight changes on the final day of the experiment. One hour after the end of the fasting period (at 10:00 a.m.), disease activity and body weight changes were assessed in all animal groups, followed by animal sacrifice and tissue sample collection. Throughout the experiment, body weight changes were monitored in all animal groups one hour after breakfast (at 10:00 a.m.) on previous days. It is worth noting that our preliminary trials revealed levels of β-hydroxybutyrate.

4.5. Rational of KE Dosing and Fasting Protocol

The normal control group of rats was given free access to standard rodent food (FPDU rodent food). In contrast, the groups receiving the KE were given (R,R)-BD-AcAc2 mixed with their standard rodent food ad libitum. Our pilot experiment showed that a 200 g SD rat in our lab typically consumes an amount of food equivalent to 7.5% of its body weight. Therefore, the rats in the KE group were given standard rodent food mixed with 4% (R,R)-BD-AcAc2 and 1% saccharin for palatability, as previously described [33], This mixture helped prevent food aversion in the rats. After conducting a preliminary trial, it was determined that the combination of KE and food resulted in increased plasma levels of β-hydroxybutyrate to >3 mmol/L after one week of continuous feeding. The amount of KE used in this experiment was then calculated accordingly. A plasma β-hydroxybutyrate level of >3 mmol/L indicates that the body is in a state of ketosis, this can occur in several situations, including during prolonged fasting and low-carbohydrate diets (such as the ketogenic diet). All animal groups received standard rodent food containing 1% saccharin. It is worth noting that our initial trials showed that the levels of β-hydroxybutyrate, measured at the end of the fasting period in both the fasting rat groups (N/F and CC/F), did not exceed 1 mmol/L. Moreover, there was no significant difference between these levels and those measured 8 h after the start of the fasting period. These findings indicate that a state of early ketosis was maintained until the end of the fasting period.

4.6. Assessment of the Weight/Length Colonic Ratio

To effectively evaluate the severity of colitis progression, one commonly used method is to calculate the weight/length colonic ratio. This approach involves measuring the entire colon that has been well-evacuated of feces and calculating the ratio of its weight to length. The resulting colon weight/length ratio is expressed in grams per centimeter of colonic tissue.

4.7. Assessment of the Disease Activity Score (DAI)

The Disease Activity Index (DAI) is an important tool used to evaluate the severity of colitis in preclinical studies. It provides a quantitative assessment of clinical signs associated with colitis, including alterations in body weight, consistency of stool, and blood in the stool. On the 25th day of the experiment, a blinded gastroenterologist determined the DAI. For each rat, the DAI was calculated as the average score for percentage body weight loss, diarrhea, and bloody stool. The evaluation criteria for body weight changes were: 0 for no weight loss, 1 for 1–5% loss, 2 for 6–10% loss, 3 for 11–15% loss, and 4 for 16–20% loss. For diarrhea, the evaluation criteria were: 0 for normal stool, 1 for soft stool, 2 for very soft stool, and 3 for watery diarrhea. The criteria for evaluating bloody stool were: 0 for negative hemoccult, 1 for positive hemoccult, 2 for traces of blood, and 3 for gross rectal bleeding.

4.8. Assessment of the Macroscopic Damage Index (MDI)

A blinded pathologist experienced in gastroenterology visualized the macroscopic features of colon tissue injury in the longitudinally opened colon segments. The MDI was determined for each rat using the following scoring criteria: a score of zero indicated no damage, a score of one indicated hyperemia without ulcers, a score of two indicated the presence of a linear ulcer without significant inflammation, a score of three indicated a linear ulcer with inflammation at one site, a score of four indicated the presence of two or more sites with inflammation or ulceration, a score of five indicated the presence of two or more major sites of inflammation or ulceration or one site with inflammation or ulceration extending $\geq$ 1 cm along the length of the colon, and a score of six-ten was assigned if the damage covered ≥ 2 cm along the length of the colon, with the score increasing by one for each additional centimeter of involvement.

4.9. Sample Collection and Preparation

After completing the experiment, the colons were weighed after being dissected and measured for length. Blood collected was used to isolate plasma for β-hydroxybutyrate analysis. The fresh colons were cleaned using ice-cold saline and dried using sterile towels. The colons were then partitioned into two parts. The first one, which included specimens from the distal colon, was kept in 4% neutral-buffered formalin to be histopathologically examined. The second part was instantly frozen in liquid nitrogen and stored at −80 °C for qRT-PCR, ELISA, and colorimetry. Additionally, 300 mg stool samples from the cecum were collected from each rat promptly after dissecting colons. DNA was extracted from the stool samples using the QIAamp DNA Stool Mini Kit (Qiagen Inc., Hilden, Germany) following the guidelines of the manufacturer. The extracted DNA was analyzed for concentration using a NanoDrop instrument (OPTIZEN NanoQ, Mecasys) via spectrophotometry.

4.10. Histological Examination

The colon tissues were washed with distilled water and then dehydrated using serial dilutions of alcohol. After that, the sections were washed in xylene and embedded in paraffin at 56 °C. Paraffin beeswax tissue blocks were then cut into 4–5-μm thicknesses using a microtome. The specimens were deparaffinized, rehydrated, and stained with hematoxylin and eosin stain. The standard histology procedures were performed blindly by a histologist, and the specimens were examined using a Leica DFC camera. The microscopic criteria of the histological scoring system of inflammation were applied as follows: 0 represented normal colonic tissue, 1 represented inflammation or focal ulceration limited to the mucosa, 2 represented focal or extensive ulceration and inflammation limited to the mucosa and submucosa, 3 represented focal or extensive ulceration and inflammation with involvement of the muscularis propria, 4 represented focal ulceration and transmural inflammation with involvement of the serosa, 5 represented extensive ulceration and transmural inflammation with involvement of the serosa, and 6 represented focal or extensive ulceration and transmural inflammation and perforation.

4.11. Determination of ROS, Malondialdehyde (MDA), Superoxide Dismutase (SOD), and Reduced Glutathione (GSH)

To investigate the presence of ROS in colon tissues, we followed a previously described methodology [13]. Initially, we homogenized 200 mg of fresh colon samples in ice-cold Tris-HCl buffer (40 mM, pH = 7.4) at a 1:10 w/v ratio. Afterward, we mixed 100 μL of homogenates with 1 mL of Tris-HCl buffer and added 10 μM of 2′,7′-dichlorofluorescin diacetate (Sigma). The reaction mixtures were incubated at 37 °C for 30 min, followed by measuring fluorescence intensity (FI) using a SpectraFluor Plus Microplate Reader (Tecan, Mainz, Germany) with excitation at 485 nm and emission at 525 nm.

To determine the concentration of MDA in colon tissue homogenate, a reaction was carried out with thiobarbituric acid (TBA) at 95 °C for 30 min under acidic conditions. This reaction produced a thiobarbituric acid reactive product, which was measured colorimetrically at 534 nm to determine the absorbance of the resulting pink product. For this procedure, a kit was utilized which was obtained from Bio-diagnostic (Giza, Egypt), and the analysis was conducted following the instructions provided by the manufacturer.

The SOD assay was performed by following the manufacturer's instructions (Bio-diagnostic). This assay involved inhibiting the reduction of nitroblue tetrazolium dye mediated by phenazine methosulphate through the enzyme's activity.

The method employed to determine GSH levels involved the reduction of 5,5′ dithiobis (2-nitrobenzoic acid) (DTNB) using GSH to yield a yellow-colored compound. The concentration of GSH was determined by measuring the absorbance of the reduced chromogen at

405 nm. The absorbance was directly proportional to the GSH concentration. All assays of oxidative stress markers were determined in duplicate.

4.12. Determination of Plasma β-Hydroxybutyrate

Plasma samples were centrifuged at $10,000 \times g$ for 10 min followed by centrifuging the supernatants at $10,000 \times g$ with a 50 KD ultrafiltration tube for 15 min. In this assay (Elabscience, Wuhan, China), β-hydroxybutyrate dehydrogenase catalyzes the oxidative dehydrogenation of β-hydroxybutyrate. Meanwhile, NAD^+ is reduced to NADH which under the action of the hydrogen transmitter, transfers electrons to WST-8 to produce a yellow product. The content of β-hydroxybutyrate can be calculated by measuring the change of absorbance value at 450 nm. The β-hydroxybutyrate assay was determined in duplicate.

4.13. Determination of Tumor Necrosis Factor-Alpha (TNF-α), IL-6, IL-1β, IL-18, IL-10, and IL-4 Levels in Colon Tissue

The TNF-α and IL-10 levels were determined using ELISA kits purchased from LifeSpanBioSciences, Inc. (Seattle, WA, USA), while the IL-6 and IL-4 levels were assessed by kits from R&D System (Minneapolis, MN, USA). The IL-1β levels were measured by an ELISA kit obtained from BioLegend (San Diego, CA, USA), while the measurement of IL-18 was conducted using a kit obtained from eBioscience (Vienna, Austria). All protocols used in the assays strictly adhered to the manufacturer's instructions. All cytokine assays were determined in duplicate.

4.14. Determination of Myeloperoxidase (MPO) Activity, NFκB DNA Binding Activity, Caspase-1 Activity, and Active Caspase-3

Myeloperoxidase is predominantly expressed in neutrophil granulocytes and is believed to mirror the level of neutrophil activation and infiltration into tissues. To determine the activity of MPO in the colonic tissue, we used an MPO assay obtained from Sigma-Aldrich. In this assay, hypochlorous acid produced by MPO reacts with taurine to form taurine chloramine, which subsequently reacts with TNB to produce DTNB. The activity of MPO was quantified as the amount of MPO enzyme required to hydrolyze the substrate and generate taurine chloramine that could consume 1.0 µmole of TNB per minute at 25 °C. We conducted the MPO assay in duplicate.

To evaluate the nuclear translocation of the p65 subunit, we utilized an assay kit obtained from Abcam that allowed for the analysis of nuclear extracts. The kit contained a specific double-stranded DNA sequence with the NFκB p65 consensus binding site (5′–GGGACTTTCC–3′) to selectively bind to active NFκB p65. We then used a primary antibody to detect an epitope of NFκB p65, which is only accessible when the protein is active and bound to its target DNA [34]. The NFκB p65 activity was determined in duplicate.

To assess the activity of caspase-1, we employed a caspase-1 colorimetric assay kit obtained from R&D Systems. This involved detecting the chromophore p-nitroanilide (p-NA) following its cleavage from the labeled substrate YVAD-p-NA, and quantifying the resulting p-NA light emission at 405 nm with a microtiter plate reader. Cytosolic extracts were obtained by preparing tissue lysates with chilled lysis buffer and then centrifuging them at $10,000 \times g$. The protein concentration of the cytosolic extracts was determined, and 100 mg of protein was diluted in 50 µL of lysis buffer. Then, 50 µL of 2× reaction buffer (containing 10 mM DTT) and 5 µL of YVAD-p-NA substrate were added to each sample, and they were incubated at 37 °C for 1–2 h. Finally, we performed duplicate assays of the samples and read them at 405 nm in a microtiter plate reader.

We measured the levels of active caspase-3 using a kit obtained from MyBioSource Inc. (San Diego, CA, USA). The kit utilized a polyclonal anti-active caspase-3 antibody and an active caspase-3-HRP conjugate, and the color intensity obtained was inversely proportional to the amount of active caspase-3 present in the samples. The competition between the active caspase-3 from the samples and the active caspase-3-HRP conjugate for binding sites on the anti-active caspase-3 antibody was restricted by the limited number of available binding sites. As a result, as more binding sites were occupied by active caspase-3 from the sample, fewer binding sites remained available for active caspase-3-HRP conjugate to bind [35]. The determination of active caspase-3 was conducted in duplicate.

4.15. qRT-PCR Analysis for the mRNA Expression of Apoptosis-Associated Speck-like Protein Containing a CARD (ASC) and NLRP3

The extraction of total RNA from colonic tissues was performed using a Qiagen kit (Venlo, The Netherlands), following the supplier's recommendations. RNA quality and purity were evaluated at 260 nm using a NanoDrop (Thermo Fisher Scientific, Waltham, MA, USA). To reverse transcribe RNA, the RevertAid First Strand cDNA synthesis kit was utilized. We conducted qRT-PCR using the StepOne™ Real-Time PCR System (Thermo Fisher Scientific). To determine relative expression, we calculated using the comparative cycle threshold (Ct) ($2^{-\Delta\Delta CT}$) method, normalized to the GAPDH gene. The PCR primer pairs used are described below: For ASC, F: 5′-CTCTGTATGGCAATGTGCTGAC-3′ and R: 5′-GAACAAGTTCTTGCAGGTCAG-3′. For NLRP3, F: 5′-GAGCTGGACCTCAGTGACAATGC-3′ and R: 5′-ACCAATGCGAGATCCTGACAACAC-3′. For GAPDH, F: 5′-TCAAGAAGGTGGTGAAGCAG-3′ R: 5′-AGGTGGAAGAATGGGAGTTG-3′.

4.16. Determination of NLRP3 and NGSDMD

Kits supplied by MyBioSource Inc. (San Diego, CA, USA) were used for the determination of NLRP3 and NGSDMD in colon tissue homogenates according to the manufacturer's instructions. The NGSDMD ELISA kit utilizes a competitive enzyme immunoassay technique. The assay involves incubating the assay sample and buffer with an NGSDMD-HRP conjugate and an anti-NGSDMD antibody in a pre-coated plate for one hour. Following incubation, the wells are decanted and washed five times before adding a substrate for the HRP enzyme. The enzyme-substrate reaction produces a blue-colored complex, which is stopped by the addition of a stop solution, resulting in a yellow solution. The intensity of the color is measured spectrophotometrically at 450 nm in a microplate reader. The intensity of the color is inversely proportional to the concentration of NGSDMD, as both the NGSDMD from the sample and NGSDMD-HRP conjugate compete for binding sites on the anti-NGSDMD antibody. Since the binding sites are limited, the more NGSDMD from the sample that binds to the antibody, the fewer sites are available for NGSDMD-HRP conjugate to bind. By plotting a standard curve relating the intensity of the color to the concentration of standards, the NGSDMD concentration in each sample can be interpolated.

4.17. Determination of Beclin-1 (BECN1) and Sequestosome-1 (p62)

BECN1 and p62 colon tissue levels were determined using ELISA kits supplied by CUSABIO (Wuhan, China) and MyBioSource, respectively. All protocols followed the manufacturer's instructions.

4.18. Determination of Zonula Occludens-1 (ZO-1), Occludin (OCLN), and Claudin-5 (CLDN5)

ZO-1, OCLN, and CLDN5 levels were determined following instructions given by CUSABIO.

4.19. Detection of Gut Microbiota Using Conventional PCR

To prepare the DNA samples for thermal cycling, we followed a protocol that involved creating reaction mixtures of 25 µL. The mixtures were prepared by combining 12.5 µL of my Taq red mix (Bioline Co., UK), 1 µL of each primer (10 µM each), 2.5 µL of DNA, and nuclease-free water. The PCR amplification protocol consisted of an initial denaturation step at 94 °C for 5 min, followed by 35 cycles at 94 °C for 30 s, annealing at a temperature that was calculated for each primer mix (as indicated in Table 2) for 30 s, extension at 72 °C for 45 s, and a final termination step at 72 °C for 3 min. To detect the expected PCR amplicons, we conducted electrophoretic separation on a 1.5% agarose gel and compared the results with a GeneRuler 100 bp plus DNA ladder (Thermo Scientific, USA). The gels were then stained with ethidium bromide and visualized using a UV transilluminator. For each type of bacteria, specific primer sequences are listed in Table 2.

Table 2. Primer sequences for the detection of different species of bacteria.

Primer Name		Primer Sequence	Ta (°C)	bp
(16S)	F	GAGTTTGATCCTGGCTCAG	51	312
	R	GCTGCCTCCCGTAGGAGT		
Fusobacterium	F	GGATTTATTGGGCGTAAAGC	51.5	162
	R	GGCATTCCTACAAATATCTACGAA		
Bacteroides spp.	F	AAGGGAGCGTAGATGGATGTTTA	55	193
	R	CGAGCCTCAATGTCAGTTGC		
Clostridium spp.	F	CGGTACCTGACTAAGAAGC	50	429
	R	AGTTTGATTCTTGCGAACG		
Bifidobacterium	F	CTCCTGGAAACGGGTGG	51	551
	R	GGTGTTCTTCCCGATATCTACA		
Lactobacillus spp.	F	AGCAGTAGGGAATCTTCCA	50	334
	R	CACCGCTACACATGGAG		

4.20. qRT-PCR for the Detection of the Relative Abundance of Fusobacteria, Bifidobacteria, Bacteroides, Clostridium, and Lactobacillus

In order to evaluate the quantity of specific bacteria in the gut, we employed primers for the 16S rDNA housekeeping gene. Fecal DNA (40–80 ng) was extracted and combined with 12.5 µL (2 × SYBR Green PCR master mix (Willowfort Co., Birmingham, UK), 1.5 µL of each forward and reverse primer (10 µmol), and 7.5 µL of nuclease-free water, resulting in a final volume of 25 µL. Real-time PCR was performed on a MyGo machine using the following cycling protocol: an initial 5 min denaturation step at 95 °C, followed by 45 cycles of 95 °C for 20 s, annealing for 20 s, and 72 °C for 40 s. The Ct values and melting curves were obtained using MyGo software. The relative abundance of each bacterial species was calculated as a relative unit normalized to the total bacteria in the corresponding sample, using the $2^{-\Delta\Delta Ct}$ method (where ΔCt represents the average Ct value of each target minus the average Ct value of total bacteria). The primer sequences for detecting the various bacterial strains are listed in Table 2.

4.21. Statistical Analysis

The statistical analysis was carried out using the GraphPad Prism software version 9 (GraphPad Software Inc., La Jolla, CA, USA). The results were expressed as mean ± standard deviation (SD). One-way analysis of variance (ANOVA) was performed followed by Tukey's post hoc test to determine the differences between groups. To investigate the correlation between multiple variables, Pearson correlation analysis was conducted. Survival probability was assessed by survival analysis comparisons, and survival curves were generated using the log-rank (Mantel–Cox) test. All statistical tests were performed at a significance level of less than 0.05.

Author Contributions: Data curation, S.S.; Formal analysis, S.S.; Funding acquisition, M.A.A.-R. and O.A.M.; Investigation, S.S.; Methodology, S.S., M.M.S.A., J.A., L.A.S., S.A.-G., A.M.A., A.A.F., A.H.A., M.I.E.A., A.A.J.A., A.M.S.E., M.A.A.-R., H.A.R. and O.A.M.; Project administration, S.S. and O.A.M.; Resources, O.A.M.; Software, S.S.; Supervision, S.S.; Validation, S.S.; Visualization, S.S.; Writing—original draft, S.S.; Writing—review and editing, S.S., M.M.S.A., J.A., L.A.S., S.A.-G., A.M.A., A.A.F., A.H.A., M.I.E.A., A.A.J.A., A.M.S.E., M.A.A.-R., H.A.R. and O.A.M. All authors have read and agreed to the published version of the manuscript.

Funding: This research received no external funding.

Institutional Review Board Statement: All the in vivo protocols were approved by the IACUC at the Faculty of Pharmacy, Delta University for Science and Technology, Egypt, (approval number, FPDU24120).

Informed Consent Statement: Not applicable.

Data Availability Statement: Data is contained within the article.

Acknowledgments: The authors would like to thank the Deanship of Scientific Research at Shaqra University for supporting this work. Osama Mohammed's contribution is greatly appreciated. We acknowledge his efforts in coordinating the project and ensuring its smooth progression.

Conflicts of Interest: The authors declare no conflict of interest.

Abbreviations

(R,R)-BD-AcAc2, (R)-3-Hydroxybutyl (R)-3-hydroxybutyrate ketone ester; ASC, apoptosis-associated speck-like protein containing a CARD; BECN1, Beclin-1; CLDN5, claudin-5; DAI, disease activity score; DSS, dextran sodium sulfate; GSDMD, gasdermin D; GSH, reduced glutathione; IBD, inflammatory bowel disease; KD, ketogenic diet; KE, ketone ester; MDA, malondialdehyde; MDI, macroscopic damage index; MPO, myeloperoxidase; NFκB, nuclear transcription factor kappa B; NGSDMD, gasdermin D N-terminal fragment; NLRP3, nucleotide-binding oligomerization domain-like receptor protein 3; OCLN, occludin; p62, sequestosome-1; ROS, reactive oxygen species; SOD, superoxide dismutase; TNF-α, tumor necrosis factor-alpha; ZO-1, zonula occludens-1.

References

1. Wang, R.; Li, Z.; Liu, S.; Zhang, D. Global, regional and national burden of inflammatory bowel disease in 204 countries and territories from 1990 to 2019: A systematic analysis based on the Global Burden of Disease Study 2019. *BMJ Open* **2023**, *13*, e065186. [CrossRef]
2. Jairath, V.; Feagan, B.G. Global burden of inflammatory bowel disease. *Lancet. Gastroenterol. Hepatol.* **2020**, *5*, 2–3. [CrossRef] [PubMed]
3. Eaden, J.A.; Abrams, K.R.; Mayberry, J.F. The risk of colorectal cancer in ulcerative colitis: A meta-analysis. *Gut* **2001**, *48*, 526. [CrossRef] [PubMed]
4. Weimers, P.; Vedel Ankersen, D.; Lophaven, S.; Bonderup, O.K.; Münch, A.; Løkkegaard, E.C.L.; Munkholm, P.; Burisch, J. Disease Activity Patterns, Mortality, and Colorectal Cancer Risk in Microscopic Colitis: A Danish Nationwide Cohort Study, 2001 to 2016. *J. Crohn's Colitis* **2020**, *15*, 594–602. [CrossRef] [PubMed]
5. Ramos, L.; Teo-Loy, J.; Barreiro-de Acosta, M. Disease clearance in ulcerative colitis: Setting the therapeutic goals for future in the treatment of ulcerative colitis. *Front. Med.* **2022**, *9*, 1102420. [CrossRef]
6. Cavalu, S.; Sharaf, H.; Saber, S.; Youssef, M.E.; Abdelhamid, A.M.; Mourad, A.A.E.; Ibrahim, S.; Allam, S.; Elgharabawy, R.M.; El-Ahwany, E.; et al. Ambroxol, a mucolytic agent, boosts HO-1, suppresses NF-κB, and decreases the susceptibility of the inflamed rat colon to apoptosis: A new treatment option for treating ulcerative colitis. *FASEB J.* **2022**, *36*, e22496. [CrossRef]
7. Liu, L.; Dong, Y.; Ye, M.; Jin, S.; Yang, J.; Joosse, M.E.; Sun, Y.; Zhang, J.; Lazarev, M.; Brant, S.R.; et al. The Pathogenic Role of NLRP3 Inflammasome Activation in Inflammatory Bowel Diseases of Both Mice and Humans. *J. Crohn's Colitis* **2017**, *11*, 737–750. [CrossRef]
8. Franchi, L.; Muñoz-Planillo, R.; Núñez, G. Sensing and reacting to microbes through the inflammasomes. *Nat. Immunol.* **2012**, *13*, 325–332. [CrossRef]
9. Zhou, R.; Tardivel, A.; Thorens, B.; Choi, I.; Tschopp, J. Thioredoxin-interacting protein links oxidative stress to inflammasome activation. *Nat. Immunol.* **2010**, *11*, 136–140. [CrossRef]
10. Kayagaki, N.; Stowe, I.B.; Lee, B.L.; O'Rourke, K.; Anderson, K.; Warming, S.; Cuellar, T.; Haley, B.; Roose-Girma, M.; Phung, Q.T.; et al. Caspase-11 cleaves gasdermin D for non-canonical inflammasome signalling. *Nature* **2015**, *526*, 666–671. [CrossRef]
11. Shi, J.; Zhao, Y.; Wang, K.; Shi, X.; Wang, Y.; Huang, H.; Zhuang, Y.; Cai, T.; Wang, F.; Shao, F. Cleavage of GSDMD by inflammatory caspases determines pyroptotic cell death. *Nature* **2015**, *526*, 660–665. [CrossRef] [PubMed]
12. Yang, D.; Wang, Z.; Chen, Y.; Guo, Q.; Dong, Y. Interactions between gut microbes and NLRP3 inflammasome in the gut-brain axis. *Comput. Struct. Biotechnol. J.* **2023**, *21*, 2215–2227. [CrossRef]

13. Saber, S.; Abd El-Fattah, E.E.; Yahya, G.; Gobba, N.A.; Maghmomeh, A.O.; Khodir, A.E.; Mourad, A.A.E.; Saad, A.S.; Mohammed, H.G.; Nouh, N.A.; et al. A Novel Combination Therapy Using Rosuvastatin and Lactobacillus Combats Dextran Sodium Sulfate-Induced Colitis in High-Fat Diet-Fed Rats by Targeting the TXNIP/NLRP3 Interaction and Influencing Gut Microbiome Composition. *Pharmaceuticals* **2021**, *14*, 341. [CrossRef]
14. Kobayashi, S. Choose Delicately and Reuse Adequately: The Newly Revealed Process of Autophagy. *Biol. Pharm. Bull.* **2015**, *38*, 1098–1103. [CrossRef] [PubMed]
15. Abd El-Fattah, E.E.; Saber, S.; Youssef, M.E.; Eissa, H.; El-Ahwany, E.; Amin, N.A.; Alqarni, M.; Batiha, G.E.-S.; Obaidullah, A.J.; Kaddah, M.M.Y.; et al. AKT-AMPKα-mTOR-dependent HIF-1α Activation is a New Therapeutic Target for Cancer Treatment: A Novel Approach to Repositioning the Antidiabetic Drug Sitagliptin for the Management of Hepatocellular Carcinoma. *Front. Pharmacol.* **2022**, *12*, 4018. [CrossRef] [PubMed]
16. Macias-Ceja, D.C.; Barrachina, M.D.; Ortiz-Masià, D. Autophagy in intestinal fibrosis: Relevance in inflammatory bowel disease. *Front. Pharmacol.* **2023**, *14*, 1170436. [CrossRef]
17. Youssef, M.E.; Abd El-Fattah, E.E.; Abdelhamid, A.M.; Eissa, H.; El-Ahwany, E.; Amin, N.A.; Hetta, H.F.; Mahmoud, M.H.; Batiha, G.E.-S.; Gobba, N.; et al. Interference With the AMPKα/mTOR/NLRP3 Signaling and the IL-23/IL-17 Axis Effectively Protects Against the Dextran Sulfate Sodium Intoxication in Rats: A New Paradigm in Empagliflozin and Metformin Reprofiling for the Management of Ulcerative Colitis. *Front. Pharmacol.* **2021**, *12*, 719984. [CrossRef]
18. Nasr, M.; Cavalu, S.; Saber, S.; Youssef, M.E.; Abdelhamid, A.M.; Elagamy, H.I.; Kamal, I.; Gaafar, A.G.A.; El-Ahwany, E.; Amin, N.A.; et al. Canagliflozin-loaded chitosan-hyaluronic acid microspheres modulate AMPK/NF-κB/NLRP3 axis: A new paradigm in the rectal therapy of ulcerative colitis. *Biomed. Pharmacother.* **2022**, *153*, 113409. [CrossRef]
19. Devenport, S.N.; Shah, Y.M. Functions and Implications of Autophagy in Colon Cancer. *Cells* **2019**, *8*, 1349. [CrossRef]
20. Sheng, Y.H.; Giri, R.; Davies, J.; Schreiber, V.; Alabbas, S.; Movva, R.; He, Y.; Wu, A.; Hooper, J.; McWhinney, B.; et al. A Nucleotide Analog Prevents Colitis-Associated Cancer via Beta-Catenin Independently of Inflammation and Autophagy. *Cell. Mol. Gastroenterol. Hepatol.* **2021**, *11*, 33–53. [CrossRef]
21. Pott, J.; Maloy, K.J. Epithelial autophagy controls chronic colitis by reducing TNF-induced apoptosis. *Autophagy* **2018**, *14*, 1460–1461. [CrossRef]
22. Youm, Y.-H.; Nguyen, K.Y.; Grant, R.W.; Goldberg, E.L.; Bodogai, M.; Kim, D.; D'Agostino, D.; Planavsky, N.; Lupfer, C.; Kanneganti, T.D.; et al. The ketone metabolite β-hydroxybutyrate blocks NLRP3 inflammasome–mediated inflammatory disease. *Nat. Med.* **2015**, *21*, 263–269. [CrossRef] [PubMed]
23. Fu, S.-P.; Wang, J.-F.; Xue, W.-J.; Liu, H.-M.; Liu, B.-r.; Zeng, Y.-L.; Li, S.-N.; Huang, B.-X.; Lv, Q.-K.; Wang, W.; et al. Anti-inflammatory effects of BHBA in both in vivo and in vitro Parkinson's disease models are mediated by GPR109A-dependent mechanisms. *J. Neuroinflamm.* **2015**, *12*, 9. [CrossRef] [PubMed]
24. Vasconcelos, A.R.; Yshii, L.M.; Viel, T.A.; Buck, H.S.; Mattson, M.P.; Scavone, C.; Kawamoto, E.M. Intermittent fasting attenuates lipopolysaccharide-induced neuroinflammation and memory impairment. *J. Neuroinflamm.* **2014**, *11*, 85. [CrossRef] [PubMed]
25. MacDonald, L.; Hazi, A.; Paolini, A.G.; Kent, S. Calorie restriction dose-dependently abates lipopolysaccharide-induced fever, sickness behavior, and circulating interleukin-6 while increasing corticosterone. *Brain Behav. Immun.* **2014**, *40*, 18–26. [CrossRef] [PubMed]
26. Ruskin, D.N.; Kawamura, M.; Masino, S.A. Reduced pain and inflammation in juvenile and adult rats fed a ketogenic diet. *PLoS ONE* **2009**, *4*, e8349. [CrossRef]
27. Plecko, B.; Stoeckler-Ipsiroglu, S.; Schober, E.; Harrer, G.; Mlynarik, V.; Gruber, S.; Moser, E.; Moeslinger, D.; Silgoner, H.; Ipsiroglu, O. Oral β-Hydroxybutyrate Supplementation in Two Patients with Hyperinsulinemic Hypoglycemia: Monitoring of β-Hydroxybutyrate Levels in Blood and Cerebrospinal Fluid, and in the Brain by In Vivo Magnetic Resonance Spectroscopy. *Pediatr. Res.* **2002**, *52*, 301–306. [CrossRef]
28. Poff, A.M.; Rho, J.M.; D'Agostino, D.P. Ketone Administration for Seizure Disorders: History and Rationale for Ketone Esters and Metabolic Alternatives. *Front. Neurosci.* **2019**, *13*, 1041. [CrossRef]
29. Pawlosky, R.J.; Kashiwaya, Y.; King, M.T.; Veech, R.L. A Dietary Ketone Ester Normalizes Abnormal Behavior in a Mouse Model of Alzheimer's Disease. *Int. J. Mol. Sci.* **2020**, *21*, 1044. [CrossRef]
30. Cabrera-Mulero, A.; Tinahones, A.; Bandera, B.; Moreno-Indias, I.; Macías-González, M.; Tinahones, F.J. Keto microbiota: A powerful contributor to host disease recovery. *Rev. Endocr. Metab. Disord.* **2019**, *20*, 415–425. [CrossRef]
31. Qi, J.; Gan, L.; Fang, J.; Zhang, J.; Yu, X.; Guo, H.; Cai, D.; Cui, H.; Gou, L.; Deng, J.; et al. Beta-Hydroxybutyrate: A Dual Function Molecular and Immunological Barrier Function Regulator. *Front. Immunol.* **2022**, *13*, 805881. [CrossRef]
32. Hoffmann, M.; Schwertassek, U.; Seydel, A.; Weber, K.; Falk, W.; Hauschildt, S.; Lehmann, J. A refined and translationally relevant model of chronic DSS colitis in BALB/c mice. *Lab. Anim.* **2017**, *52*, 240–252. [CrossRef]
33. Poff, A.M.; Ari, C.; Arnold, P.; Seyfried, T.N.; D'Agostino, D.P. Ketone supplementation decreases tumor cell viability and prolongs survival of mice with metastatic cancer. *Int. J. Cancer* **2014**, *135*, 1711–1720. [CrossRef]

34. Abdelhamid, A.M.; Youssef, M.E.; Abd El-Fattah, E.E.; Gobba, N.A.; Gaafar, A.G.A.; Girgis, S.; Shata, A.; Hafez, A.-M.; El-Ahwany, E.; Amin, N.A.; et al. Blunting p38 MAPKα and ERK1/2 activities by empagliflozin enhances the antifibrotic effect of metformin and augments its AMPK-induced NF-κB inactivation in mice intoxicated with carbon tetrachloride. *Life Sci.* **2021**, *286*, 120070. [CrossRef]
35. Saber, S.; Nasr, M.; Saad, A.S.; Mourad, A.A.E.; Gobba, N.A.; Shata, A.; Hafez, A.-M.; Elsergany, R.N.; Elagamy, H.I.; El-Ahwany, E.; et al. Albendazole-loaded cubosomes interrupt the ERK1/2-HIF-1α-p300/CREB axis in mice intoxicated with diethylnitrosamine: A new paradigm in drug repurposing for the inhibition of hepatocellular carcinoma progression. *Biomed. Pharmacother.* **2021**, *142*, 112029. [CrossRef]

Disclaimer/Publisher's Note: The statements, opinions and data contained in all publications are solely those of the individual author(s) and contributor(s) and not of MDPI and/or the editor(s). MDPI and/or the editor(s) disclaim responsibility for any injury to people or property resulting from any ideas, methods, instructions or products referred to in the content.

Super Carbonate Apatite-miR-497a-5p Complex Is a Promising Therapeutic Option against Inflammatory Bowel Disease

Naoto Tsujimura [1], Takayuki Ogino [1], Masayuki Hiraki [2], Taisei Kai [3], Hiroyuki Yamamoto [3], Haruka Hirose [4], Yuhki Yokoyama [3], Yuki Sekido [1], Tsuyoshi Hata [1], Norikatsu Miyoshi [1], Hidekazu Takahashi [1], Mamoru Uemura [1], Tsunekazu Mizushima [5], Yuichiro Doki [1], Hidetoshi Eguchi [1] and Hirofumi Yamamoto [1,3,*]

[1] Department of Gastroenterological Surgery, Graduate School of Medicine, Osaka University, Yamadaoka 2-2, Suita City 565-0871, Japan; togino04@gesurg.med.osaka-u.ac.jp (T.O.); ysekido@gesurg.med.osaka-u.ac.jp (Y.S.); tsuyoshihata@gesurg.med.osaka-u.ac.jp (T.H.); nmiyoshi@gesurg.med.osaka-u.ac.jp (N.M.); htakahashi@gesurg.med.osaka-u.ac.jp (H.T.); muemura@gesurg.med.osaka-u.ac.jp (M.U.); ydoki@gesurg.med.osaka-u.ac.jp (Y.D.); heguchi@gesurg.med.osaka-u.ac.jp (H.E.)
[2] Department of Gastroenterological Surgery, Kansai Rosai Hospital, 3-1-69 Inabaso, Amagasaki 660-8511, Japan
[3] Department of Molecular Pathology, Division of Health Sciences, Graduate School of Medicine, Osaka University, Yamadaoka 1-7, Suita City 565-0871, Japan; yyokoyama@sahs.med.osaka-u.ac.jp (Y.Y.)
[4] Division of Systems Biology, Nagoya University Graduate School of Medicine, Nagoya 466-8550, Japan
[5] Department of Gastroenterological Surgery, Osaka Police Hospital, Osaka 543-0035, Japan; tmizushima@oph.gr.jp
* Correspondence: hyamamoto@sahs.med.osaka-u.ac.jp; Tel.: +81-6-6879-2591; Fax: +81-6-6879-2591

Abstract: The incidence of inflammatory bowel disease (IBD) is increasing worldwide. It is reported that TGF-β/Smad signal pathway is inactivated in patients with Crohn's disease by overexpression of Smad 7. With expectation of multiple molecular targeting by microRNAs (miRNAs), we currently attempted to identify certain miRNAs that activate TGF-β/Smad signal pathway and aimed to prove in vivo therapeutic efficacy in mouse model. Through Smad binding element (SBE) reporter assays, we focused on miR-497a-5p. This miRNA is common between mouse and human species and enhanced the activity of TGF-β/Smad signal pathway, decreased Smad 7 and/or increased phosphorylated Smad 3 expression in non-tumor cell line HEK293, colorectal cancer cell line HCT116 and mouse macrophage J774a.1 cells. MiR-497a-5p also suppressed the production of inflammatory cytokines TNF-α, IL-12p40, a subunit of IL-23, and IL-6 when J774a.1 cells were stimulated by lipopolysaccharides (LPS). In a long-term therapeutic model for mouse dextran sodium sulfate (DSS)-induced colitis, systemic delivery of miR-497a-5p load on super carbonate apatite (sCA) nanoparticle as a vehicle restored epithelial structure of the colonic mucosa and suppressed bowel inflammation compared with negative control miRNA treatment. Our data suggest that sCA-miR-497a-5p may potentially have a therapeutic ability against IBD although further investigation is essential.

Keywords: inflammatory bowel disease; miR-497a-5p; TGF-β; macrophage

1. Introduction

Inflammatory bowel disease (IBD) such as ulcerative colitis (UC) and Crohn's disease (CD) is an intractable chronic inflammatory disease, and the number of patients is increasing in the world year by year [1–3]. Medical treatments such as 5-aminosalicylic acid (5-ASA), corticosteroids, and anti-tumor necrosis factor-α (TNF-α) antibody are first line-therapies against IBD, but remissions and relapses are often repeated [4,5]. In recent years, anti-interleukin 12/23 antibody, JAK inhibitors, and anti-α4β7 integrin antibody emerged as new molecular-targeted drugs [6–9], but they carry the risk of immunocompromise, allergy and other side effects and they still cannot cure IBD. Therefore, continuous effort to develop novel therapy is required against IBD.

Although the cause of IBD has not been fully clarified, involvement of genetic factors and environmental factors is suggested [10–12]. When the barrier mechanism of the intestinal mucosa is destroyed, food residues and intestinal bacteria are phagocytosed by antigen presenting dendritic cell which present antigen to Naïve T cells and induce differentiation into regulatory T lymphocytes (Treg) and inflammatory T lymphocytes (Th17) [13,14]. In IBD patients, Th17 becomes dominant and Treg declines, so that inflammatory cytokines, TNF-α, and interferon-γ (IFN-γ) increase, and an anti-inflammatory cytokine transforming growth factor-β (TGF-β) decreases [15]. It is reported that TGF-β/Smad signal pathway is suppressed in IBD patients [16–18]. Smads involved in this pathway are classified into three types: Inhibitory Smads (I-Smad: Smad 6/7) that inhibit the signal pathway, Common mediator Smad (Co-Smad: Smad 4) that forms a complex with Smad 2/3, and Receptor-regulated Smads (R-Smads: Smad 2/3 and others) that activate the signal pathway [19,20]. It is reported that Smad 7 was highly expressed in mononuclear cells at intestinal lamina propria in patients with IBD [17,18,21]. Intestinal macrophages also play an important role in IBD [22–24]. It is reported that intestinal-specific macrophages subset $CD14^+$ macrophages produce a large amount of inflammatory cytokines IL-23, TNF-α and IL-6, leading to chronic inflammation in Crohn's disease [25].

MicroRNA (miRNA) is a single-stranded non-cording RNA of 21 to 25 bases MiRNA that binds to the 3′ UTR of the target mRNA to suppress translation, or control gene expression by cleaving mRNA [26,27]. Although limited numbers of siRNA- and miRNA-based therapeutic options have advanced to clinical stages [28–35], venous infusion of nucleic acid medicine is expected as a powerful therapeutic option especially against severe IBD at acute exacerbation. Using IBD models considerable efforts have been made for systemic delivery of various miRNAs [36–43], but it still remains an unsolved clinical challenge mainly due to lack of suitable delivery system. Thus, miRNA and siRNA are rapidly degraded when administered to the blood stream, which made it difficult to supply sufficient amount of nucleic acid to target lesions.

sCA nanoparticle is a pH-sensitive in vivo delivery system for miRNA and siRNA with no significant immune activation based on modified calcium phosphate method [44]. We had previously reported that systemic administration of sCA incorporating siRNA and miRNA showed antitumor effects in various carcinomas and anti-inflammatory effects in IBD model [44–55].

A phase II clinical trial showed that oral Smad 7 antisense oligonucleotides improved clinical symptoms in patients with Crohn's disease [21], but the phase III clinical study was unfortunately discontinued [56]. Some reports suspect insufficient quality of nucleic acid prepared in the phase III study [56–59]. Unlike antisense oligonucleotides, miRNA can bind to and regulate multiple genes [26,27]. Instead of single molecule targeting, we currently attempted to identify certain miRNAs based on TGF-β/Smad signal activity, which should exert multiple function. Finally, we investigated therapeutic efficacy of miR-497a-5p in mouse dextran sodium sulfate (DSS)-induced colitis using super carbonate apatite as a systemic delivery vehicle.

2. Results and Discussion

2.1. Selection of microRNAs That Up-Regulate TGF-β/Smad Signal Pathway

Using a public database TargetScan [60] miRbase [61], 18 mmu miRNAs were selected as candidates which may potentially bind and inhibit expression of negative regulators in TGF-β/Smad signal pathway such as Smad 6, Smad 7, SMURF1, SMURF2, LTBP1, TGIF (Supplementary Figure S1, Point 1). Among 18 miRNAs we chose 13 miRNAs which conserve identical sequences also in human species (Supplementary Figure S1, Point 2). Potential binding combination between 3′ UTR mRNA of the negative regulators and mmu miRNAs are summarized in Table 1.

Table 1. Potential binding combination between inhibitors of TGF-β/SMAD signal pathway and mmu miRNAs.

Gene	mmu miRNA	Position in the UTR	Seed Match Count
SMURF1	125a-5p	2315–2322	8mer
	125b-5p	2315–2322	8mer
	15a-5p	2628–2634	7mer-m8
	15b-5p	2628–2634	7mer-m8
	16-5p	2628–2634	7mer-m8
	19a-3p	642–649	8mer
	19b-3p	642–649	8mer
SMURF2	497a-5p	205–211	7mer-1A
	322-5p	205–211	7mer-1A
	15a-5p	205–211	7mer-1A
	15b-5p	205–211	7mer-1A
	16-5p	205–211	7mer-1A
	195a-5p	205–211	7mer-1A
	19b-3p	2572–2578	7mer-m8
	19a-3p	2572–2578	7mer-m8
	148a-3p	2574–2580	7mer-m8
	152-3p	2574–2580	7mer-m8
	186-5p	2441–2447	7mer-m8
LTBP1	152-3p	37–43	7mer-m8
	148a-3p	37–43	7mer-m8
	148b-3p	37–43	7mer-m8
SMAD6	196b-5p	102–108	7mer-1A
	196a-5p	102–108	7mer-1A
	186-5p	248–254	7mer-m8
SMAD7	15a-5p	69–76	8mer
	497a-5p	69–76	8mer
	195a-5p	69–76	8mer
	15b-5p	69–76	8mer
	16-5p	69–76	8mer
	322-5p	69–76	8mer
TGIF	19a-3p	625–632	8mer
	19b-5p	543–549	7mer-1A
	6965-5p	192–198	7mer-m8
	7075-5p	195–202	8mer
	148b-3p	126–132	7mer-m8
	148a-3p	126–132	7mer-m8
	15a-5p	1709–1715	7mer-m8
	16-5p	1709–1715	7mer-m8
	152-3p	1678–1685	8mer
	195a-5p	1709–1715	7mer-m8
	322-5p	1709–1715	7mer-m8
	497a-5p	1709–1715	7mer-m8

All mmu miRNAs except for miR-15b-5p-, miR-125b-5p, miR-322-5p-, miR-6965-5p, miR-7075-5p are identical to human hsa miRNAs.

To find certain miRNAs that activate TGF-β/Smad signal pathway, SBE reporter assays were performed using the two different systems (Supplementary Figure S1, Point 3,4). Supplementary Figure S2 shows the principle of this reporter assay. Thus, once Smad 3/Smad 4 binds to SBE together with various transcriptional factors, luciferase signal comes out.

In the first screening, we examined the ability of 13 miRNAs in activation of TGF-β/Smad signal pathway using HEK293 cells where the SBE reporter plasmid was initially transduced. The experimental time schedule is shown in Figure 1A. Thus, cells were exposed with TGF-β at 0.5 ng/mL for 18 h in the assay medium (DMEM supplemented with 0.5% FBS, 1% non-essential amino acids, 1 mM Na pyruvate), and SBE reporter assay was performed. Treatment with TGF-β significantly enhanced SBE activity in parental cells and miR-NC-treated cells (* $p < 0.05$ for each, Figure 1B). We found that 7 of 13 miRNAs activated the TGF-β/Smad signal pathway by TGF-β treatment when compared with miR-NC (* $p < 0.05$, Figure 1B).

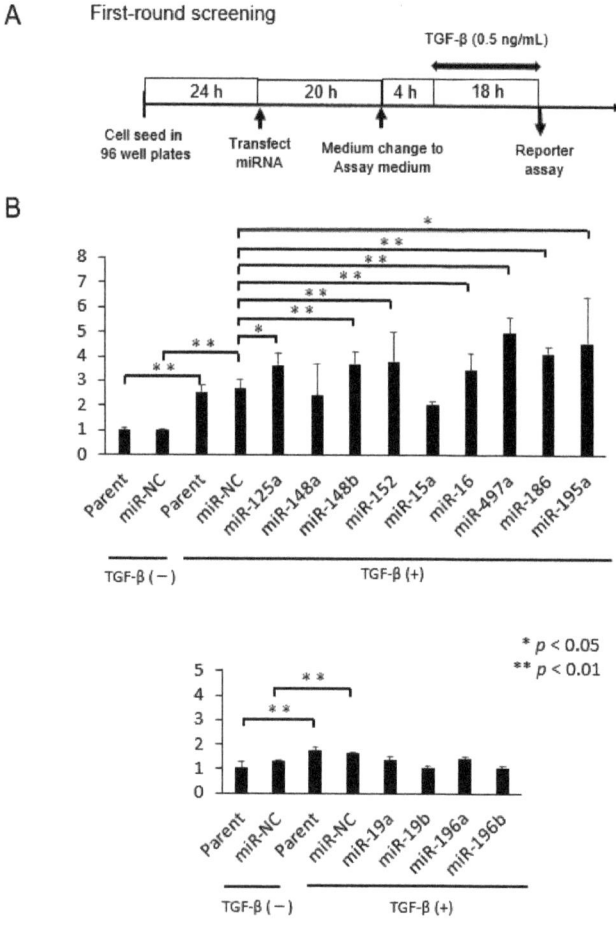

Figure 1. The first-round screening. (**A**) The experimental time schedule is shown here. (**B**) Of the 13 candidate miRNAs, 7 miRNAs significantly activated SBE reporter activity when compared to miR-NC (** $p < 0.01$,* $p < 0.05$, miR-NC vs. miR-125a-5p, $p = 0.043$; miR-NC vs. miR-148b-3p, $p = 0.005$; miR-NC vs. miR-152-3p, $p = 0.005$; miR-NC vs. miR-16-5p, $p = 0.005$; miR-NC vs. miR-497a-5p, $p = 0.003$; miR-NC vs. miR-186-5p, $p = 0.001$; miR-NC vs. miR-195a-5p, $p = 0.016$).

In the second screening, we employed a dual luciferase assay system in which SBE activity is normalized by expression of co-transfected Renilla luciferase vector, thus providing more accurate data. Seven miRNAs selected in the first-round screening were transfected 24 h prior to transfection of the plasmids. Then cells were exposed in the assay medium containing 0.5 ng/mL TGF-β for 24 h (Figure 2A). As results, we found that 3 miRNAs (miR-497a-5p, miR-186-5p, miR-195a-5p) again significantly activated the SBE activity when compared with miR-NC (* $p < 0.05$) (Figure 2B). Because miR-195a-5p had already been reported as a potential treatment option for IBD by promoting intestinal barrier integrity and restoration of the intestinal epithelium [62,63], we focused on miR-479a-5p and miR-186-5p in the subsequent experiments.

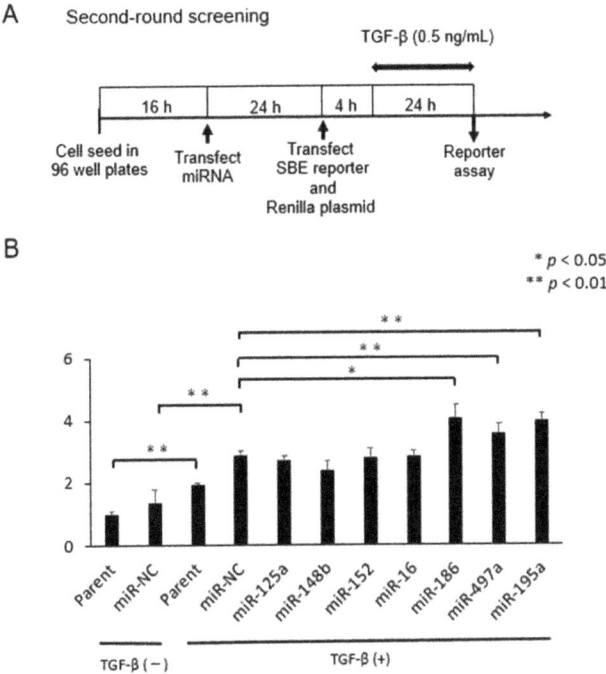

Figure 2. The second-round screening. (A) The experimental time schedule is shown here. (B) Of the 7 miRNAs, 3miRNAs (miR-497a-5p, miR-186-5p, miR-195a-5p) significantly activated SBE reporter activity when compared to miR-NC (** $p < 0.01$, * $p < 0.05$, miR-NC vs. miR-497a-5p, $p = 0.016$; miR-NC vs. miR-186-5p, $p = 0.001$; miR-NC vs. miR-195a-5p, $p = 0.001$).

2.2. Effect of miRNA Treatment on Smad Expression

The sequences of miR-186 and miR-497a-5p were conserved between mouse and human species [60]. HEK 293 cells were transfected with miR-NCs, miR-186, and miR-497a-5p, grown for 24 h or 48 h under treatment with TGF-β at 0.5ng/mL for 1 h, as previously reported [17,64–66] (Figure 3A). MiR-497a-5p treatment increased the expression of phosphorylated-Smad 2 (p-Smad 2) and decreased Smad 7 expression compared with parental HEK293 cells, miR-NC1, and miR-NC2-treated cells 48 h after transfection (Figure 3B). By contrast, treatment with miR-186 did not affect p-Smad 2 or Smad 7 expression. In colorectal cancer (CRC) cell line HCT116 under TGF-β treatment, miR-497a-5p up-regulated p-Smad 2 largely and p-Smad 3 to some extent, and decreased Smad 7 24 h after transfection (Figure 3C). In mouse macrophage J774a.1 cells, miR-497a-5p treatment decreased Smad 7 expression 48 h after transfection, although p-Smad 2 and p-Smad 3 levels were maintained as well (Figure 3D).

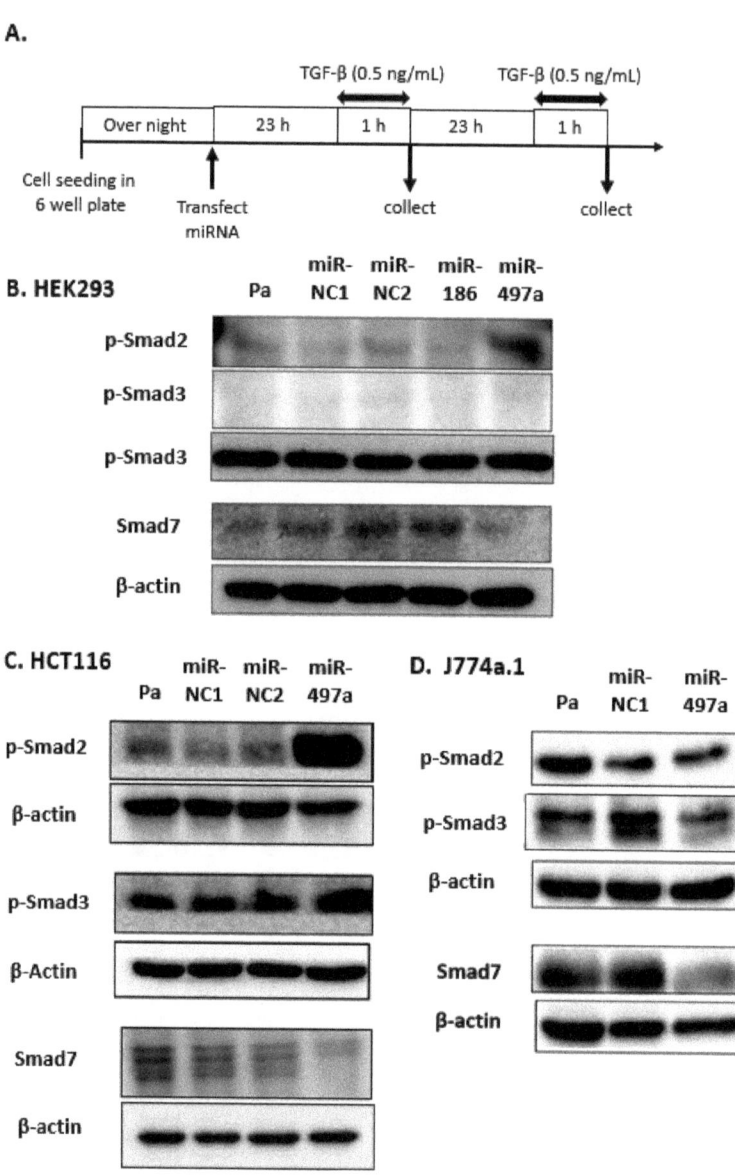

Figure 3. Western blot analyses for Smads in TGF-β/Smad signal pathway. (**A**) Experimental time schedule is shown here. (**B**) In HEK293cells, miR-497a-5p suppressed the expression of Smad 7 and increased the expression of p-Smad 2 48 h after transfection. The expression of p-Smad 3 was not detected. (**C**) In CRC line HCT116, miR-497a-5p suppressed the expression of Smad 7 and increased the expression of p-Smad 2 and p-Smad 3 24 h after transfection. (**D**) In mouse macrophage cell line J774a.1, miR-497a-5p suppressed the expression of Smad 7 miR-NC 48 h after transfection. The expressions of p-Smad 2 and p-Smad 3 were not affected much.

2.3. Smad 7 Is a Direct Target of miR-497a-5p

Based on the findings of western blots, we preferentially focused on miR-497a-5p. It is reported that miR-497-5p indirectly activated latent TGF-β via reversion-inducible cysteine-rich protein (Reck) in lung fibrosis model [67]. Here we show that miR-497a-5p directly inhibit Smad 7 expression. In silico survey showed that mouse Smad 7 mRNA has the binding site of miR-497a-5p in its 3′ UTR (Figure 4A). Seed sequence of human miR-497-5p and its binding site in 3′ UTR of human Smad 7 mRNA are both well conserved between mouse and human species (Supplementary Figure S3). We constructed a luciferase reporter plasmid containing the miR-497a-5p binding sites in the 3′ UTR of Smad 7 (Figure 4B). When luciferase assay was performed using HCT116 cells, it was revealed that miR-497a-5p significantly suppressed luciferase activity compared with miR-NC ($p < 0.05$), indicating the direct binding between miR-497a-5p and the 3′ UTR of Smad 7 (Figure 4C).

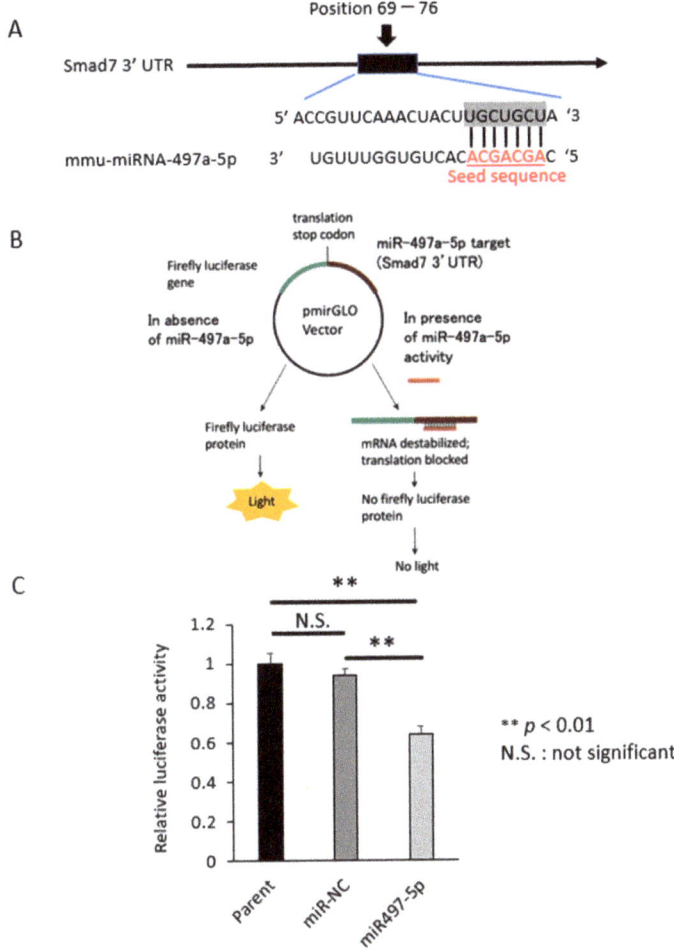

Figure 4. Binding assay of miR-497a-5p and 3′ UTR of Smad 7. (**A**) TargetScan was used to identify a binding site at position 69–76 of the Smad 7 mRNA 3′ UTR that was complementary to the seed sequence of miR-497a-5p. (**B**) Schematic illustration for binding assay. PmirGLO plasmid vector expresses luminescence according to luciferase activity. When miR-497a-5p binds to the cloning site of the 3′ UTR of Smad 7, luciferase luminescence reduces. At 24 h after transfection, firefly and Renilla luciferase activities were measured. (**C**) In CRC cell lines HCT116, miR-497a-5p significantly suppressed the luciferase activities as compared to miR-NC or parental cells (** $p < 0.01$, miR-NC vs. miR-497a-5p, $p = 0.0007$), indicating a direct binding of miR-497a-5p to the sequence of 3′ UTR of Smad 7.

2.4. MiR-497a-5p Suppressed Expression of Inflammatory Cytokines in Mouse Macrophage J774a.1

It is reported that Smad 7 was highly expressed in mononuclear cells in lamina propria of intestinal mucosa in patients with IBD [16–18,21]. A part of mononuclear cells turns into macrophages which produce a large number of inflammatory cytokines such as IL-23, TNF-α, and IL-6 by stimulation of intestinal bacteria, leading to chronic inflammation [23–25]. Co-culture of macrophages and intestinal epithelial cells is also used as a colitis model in vitro [68]. Therefore, we examined whether miR-497a-5p would suppress the production of inflammatory cytokines TNF-a, IL-6, and IL-12p40 (a subunit of IL-23), when lipopolysaccharides (LPS) at 100 ng/mL was added to mouse macrophage cell line J774a.1 according to the time schedule shown in Figure 5A. qRT-PCR assays showed that miR-497a-5p suppressed the production of TNF-α, IL-6, and IL-12p40 compared with miR-NC at the indicated time points with asterisks (* $p < 0.05$, Figure 5B).

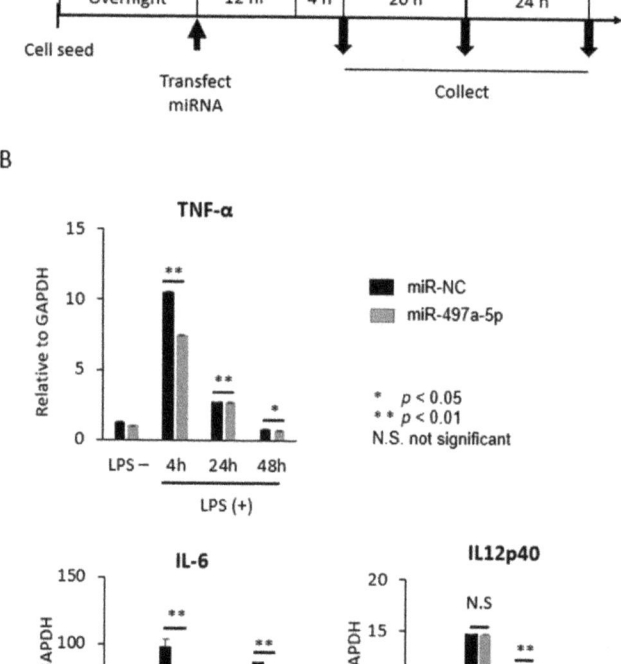

Figure 5. miR-497a-5p suppressed the production of inflammatory cytokine from mouse macrophage cell line J774a.1. (**A**) Time course schedule is shown here. Cells were stimulated by LPS at 100 ng/mL. (**B**) qRT-PCR revealed that miR-497a-5p suppressed the production of inflammatory cytokine, TNF-α, IL-6, and IL-12p40 compared with miR-NC (** $p < 0.01$, * $p < 0.05$. TNF-α: miR-NC vs. miR-497, 4 h $p = 1.45\text{E-}07$, 24 h $p = 0.003$, 48 h $p = 0.033$; IL-6: miR-NC vs. miR-497, 4 h $p = 0.0006$, 24 h $p = 0.003$, 48 h $p = 2.36\text{E-}09$; IL-12p40: miR-NC vs. miR-497, 4 h $p = 0.496$, 24 h $p = 0.006$, 48 h $p = 0.0005$).

2.5. sCA Delivered miRNA to Macrophages in Colonic Mucosa

In our previous study, we showed that sCA incorporating miR-NC tagged with Alexa Fluor 647 was largely co-localized with CD11c$^+$ dendritic cells in the inflamed colon [46]. In this study, we performed in vivo uptake test of miRNA into macrophages. To visualize the extent and localization of miRNA in the normal and inflamed colon, sCA incorporating miR-NC tagged with Alexa Fluor 647 was administered via tail vein, and the colon was excised 4 h after administration. Fluorescence microscopy showed that the red fluorescence of the Alexa 647 conjugate miR-NC was present in the mucosa and submucosa of the colonic epithelium. Immunostaining of macrophages with the anti-F4/80 antibody showed that co-localization of miRNA with the F4/80 positive macrophages was often found (Figure 6A) and the percentage of uptake of miRNA in macrophages was 47.12 ± 8.27 in inflamed colon and 38.23 ± 2.79 in normal mucosa, respectively (Figure 6B). There was no significant difference between the two groups.

Anti-TNF-a antibodies such as infliximab and adalimumab are already used in the treatment of IBD [69]. Because miR-497a-5p was able to suppress IL-6 and IL-12p40 in addition to TNF-α in J774a.1, sCA-miR-497a-5p complex targeting macrophages at inflamed colon may have a clinical benefit.

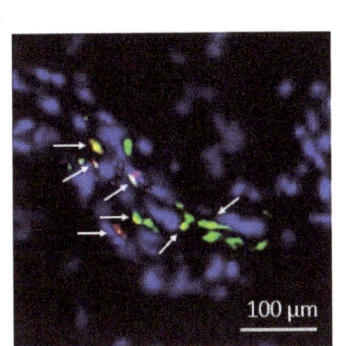

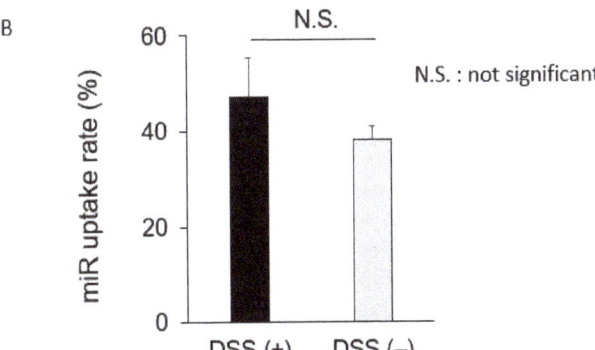

Figure 6. Co-localization of miRNA with macrophages in colonic mucosa. DSS-induced colitis was produced by free drinking of 2% DSS for 7 days in female mice (n = 2). sCA incorporating miR-NC tagged with Alexa Fluor 647 (25 µg) was administered via tail vein, and the colon was excised 4 h after administration. Immunostaining of macrophages with the anti-F4/80 antibody showed that co-localization of miRNA with the F4/80 positive-macrophages was noted 47.12 ± 8.27 in inflamed colon by DSS treatment and 38.23 ± 2.79 in normal mucosa, respectively (n = 6 per mice). Scale bar, 50 µm. Red: miR-NC tagged with Alexa Fluor 647, Green: F4/80 positive-macrophages. Yellow: merged signals, indicated by arrows.

2.6. Therapeutic Efficacy of Systemic Administration of sCA-miR-497a-5p on Mouse DSS-Induced Colitis

Mice were treated with 1.5% DSS in drinking water for 16 days. sCA-miR complexes were injected to tail vein 8 times on days 9, 11, 13, 15, 17, 19, 21, and 23. On day 24, mice were sacrificed (Figure 7A). Here we attempted a long-term experiment to evaluate the therapeutic efficacy of miR-497a-5p; 1.5% DSS for 16 days followed by therapeutic treatments from day 9 to day 23 every two days. Because most studies were performed to assess preventive effect of drugs or gene manipulation in DSS-induced colitis [69–73], we are not aware of any reports that assessed the therapeutic effect of miRNA in DSS-induced colitis especially in such a long-term schedule. As a result, a drastic inflammatory change was noted as early as on day 5 in the inflamed rectum and colon (Supplementary Figure S4). Compared with normal colon epithelium, DSS treatment alone or DSS and sCA-miR-NC destroyed normal epithelial structures, and numerous inflammatory cells infiltrated into the lamina propria of colonic mucosa (Figure 7B). By contrast, DSS and sCA-miR-497a-5p treatment restored epithelial structures of the colonic mucosa and infiltration of inflammatory cells rather decreased (Figure 7B). The colon length was significantly longer in mice treated with DSS and sCA-miR-497a-5p as compared to those treated with DSS alone or DSS and sCA-miR-NC (* $p < 0.05$, Figure 7C). There was no significant difference in body weight loss among the DSS-treated groups (Figure 7D). Significantly worse histological scores in mice treated with DSS alone or DSS and sCA-miR-NC were noted, whereas sCA-miR-497a-5p treatment significantly improved the histological damages (Figure 7E, * $p < 0.05$).

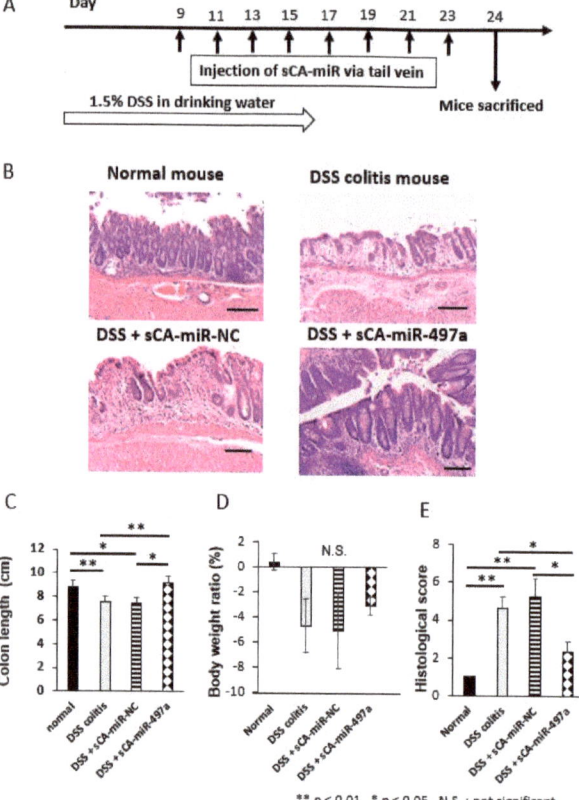

Figure 7. Therapeutic experiment of DSS-induced colitis by intravenous injection of sCA-miR-497a-5p. (**A**) Induction of mouse colitis by 1.5% DSS in drinking water and the therapeutic schedules are shown

here. Normal mice (*n* = 3), DSS-treated mice (*n* = 3), DSS and sCA-miR-NC-treated mice (*n* = 4), DSS and sCA-miR-497a-5p-treated mice (*n* = 3). (**B**) H&E staining of distal colon in each group. The mucosal structure was destroyed and many inflammatory cells were noted in DSS-treated mice or DSS and sCA-miR-NC-treated mice. By contrast, DSS and sCA-miR-497a-5p-treated mice had the notable therapeutic effect. Scale bars, 100 μm for each. (**C**) The colon length was significantly longer in mice treated with DSS and sCA-miR-497a-5p as compared to those treated with DSS alone or DSS and sCA-miR-NC (** $p < 0.01$, * $p < 0.05$, DSS alone vs. DSS and miR-497a-5p, $p = 0.002$; DSS and miR-NC vs DSS and miR-497a-5p, $p = 0.022$). (**D**) There was no significant difference in body weight loss among the DSS-treated groups. (**E**) Significantly worse histological scores in mice treated with DSS alone or DSS and sCA-miR-NC were noted, whereas sCA-miR-497a-5p treatment significantly improved the histological damages (** $p < 0.01$, * $p < 0.05$, DSS alone vs DSS and miR-497a-5p, $p = 0.046$, DSS and miR-NC vs DSS and miR-497a-5p $p = 0.034$).

2.7. Therapeutic Efficacy of Systemic Administration of sCA-miR-186-5p on Mouse DSS-Induced Colitis

Finally, we compared the in vivo efficacy of miR-186-5p and miR-497a-5p loaded on sCA. Studies have shown anti-tumor effect of miR-186-5p in carcinomas of colon, breast, bladder, prostate, and osteosarcoma through maintaining NK cell stability and suppressing epithelial-mesenchymal transition (EMT) [74–79], but its role in IBD has not been investigated. A shorter time course study, where 2% DSS in drinking water was given for 8 days and sCA-miRNAs were injected to tail vein 6 times (Figure 8A), indicated that miR-186-5p had similar therapeutic efficacy to miR-497a-5p in terms of histological score (Figure 8B–E). Our current data with regard to selected three miRNAs acting at activation of TGF-β/Smad signal pathway support the notion that this pathway is an important factor to suppress IBD.

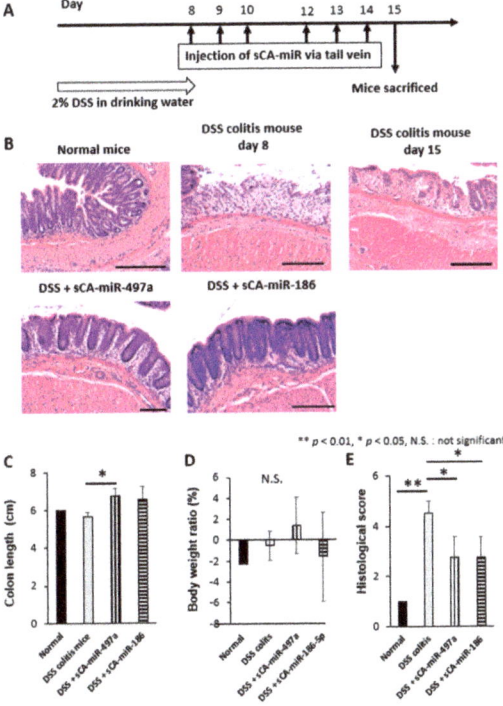

Figure 8. Comparative study on the therapeutic efficacy between sCA-miR-497a-5p and sCA-miR-186-5p. (**A**) The treatment schedule of induction of colitis by DSS and injection of drugs. 2.0% DSS

was administered in drinking water for 8 days. sCA loaded with miRNA (50 µg) was injected on days 8, 9, 10, 12, 13, and 14. Mice were sacrificed on day 15. The mice were divided into four groups as follows: Normal mice ($n = 3$), DSS-treated mice ($n = 3$), DSS and sCA-miR-497a-5p-treated mice ($n = 3$), and DSS and sCA- miR-186-5p-treated mice ($n = 3$). (**B**) H&E staining. The mucosal structure was destroyed in DSS-induced colitis on day 8, only partially regenerated on day 15. On the other hand, the colonic mucosa was largely reconstructed in DSS and sCA-miR-497a-5p and DSS and sCA-miR-186-5p-treated groups. Scale bars, 100 µm. (**C**) Compared with DSS-induced colitis mice, colon length was significantly longer in DSS and sCA-miR-497a-5p or DSS and sCA-miR-186-5p treatment groups compared with DSS-induced colitis mice (* $p < 0.05$, DSS-induced colitis mice vs. DSS and sCA-miR-497a-5p, $p = 0.029$; DSS-induced colitis mice vs. DSS and sCA-miR-186-, $p = 0.196$). (**D**) Changes in body weight. No significant differences were observed among the groups. (**E**) The histological score was significantly improved in DSS and sCA-miR-497a-5p or DSS and sCA-miR-186-5p-treated mice compared with DSS-induced colitis mice (* $p < 0.05$, ** $p < 0.01$, DSS-induced colitis mice vs DSS and sCA-miR-497a-5p $p = 0.026$; DSS-induced colitis mice vs DSS and sCA-miR-186-5p, $p = 0.026$).

2.8. Limitation and Future Perspective

There are several limitations in this study. (i) TGF-β activation and production of cytokines from mouse macrophages had not been examined in the in vivo model yet. (ii) It remains to be clarified how miR-186-5p acts against IBD. (iii) In vivo experiments for miR-186-5p should be repeated although in vivo efficacy of miR-497a-5p was confirmed by two different experiments. During preparation of this manuscript, Zhang M et al. demonstrated a preventive role of miR-497 in DSS-induced colitis using knockout mice and inhibition of Wnt/β-catenin pathway was suggested as one possible mechanism [80]. Collectively it is considered that miR-497 exerts multiple functions such as activation of TGF-β signaling pathway through targeting Smad 7 and inhibition of Wnt/β-catenin pathway. Our study proved therapeutic efficacy of miR-497a-5p using sCA as a delivery tool. Recent review articles introduce sCA nanoparticle as a hopeful non-viral systemic strategy [81–84].

3. Materials and Methods

3.1. Cell Lines and Cell Culture

Human colon cancer cell line HCT116 and human embryonic kidney HEK293 cells were obtained from the American Type Culture Collection (Rockville, MD, USA). Mouse macrophage cell line J774a.1 was purchased from JCRB (Japanese Cancer Research Resources Bank) (Ibaragi, Osaka, Japan). HCT116 and J774a.1 cells were cultured in Dulbecco's modified Eagle medium (Sigma-Aldrich, Cat. No. D6404, St. Louis, MO, USA) supplemented with 10% fetal bovine serum (FBS), 100 U/mL penicillin, and 100 µg/mL streptomycin at 37 °C. HEK293 cells were cultured in DMEM supplemented with 10% FBS, 1% non-essential amino acids (Hyclone, Cat. No. SH30238.01, Tokyo, Japan), 1 mM Na pyruvate (Hyclone, Cat. No. SH30239.01), and 100 U/mL penicillin, and 100 µg/mL streptomycin. Cells were cultured in a humidified incubator at 37 °C in an atmosphere containing 5% CO2.

3.2. miRNAs

The specific miRNAs (mmu miR-125a-5p, mmu miR-148a-3p, mmu miR-148b-3p, mmu miR-152-3p, mmu miR-15a-5p, mmu miR-16-5p, mmu miR-497a-5p, mmu miR-186-5p, mmu miR-195a-5p, mmu miR-19a-3p, mmu miR-19b-3p, mmu miR-196a-5p, and mmu miR-196b-5p), and the two negative control miRNAs (NC-miR-1and NC-miR-2) were used in in vitro experiments.

The specific miRNAs (mmu miR-497a-5p) and the negative control miRNA-1 (NC-miR-1) were used in in vivo experiments. The specific miRNAs and NC-miR-1 were purchased from Gene Design Inc. (Ibaragi, Osaka, Japan) and NC-miR-2 was purchased from Sigma-Aldrich. The sequences of miRNAs used are listed in Supplementary Table S1.

3.3. TGF-β Pathway-Responsive Reporter Assays

The first round screening was performed using HEK293 cells where SBE reporter plasmid was introduced (BPS Bioscience, Cat. No. 60653, Court West, Suite E San Diego, CA, USA). The cells were maintained with 400 μg/mL of Geneticin (Invitrogen, Cat. No. 10131035, Carlsbad, CA, USA). Cells were seeded in 96-well plates at a density of 2.5×10^4 per well and transfected with miR-NC and candidate miRNAs at a final concentration of 50 nM. The second round screening was performed using SBE Reporter Kit (BPS Bioscience, Cat. No. 60654). The kit contains transfection-ready SBE luciferase reporter vector. This reporter contains a firefly luciferase gene under the control of multimerized SBE responsive element located upstream of a minimal promoter. The SBE reporter is premixed with constitutively expressing Renilla-Sea Pansy luciferase vector that serves as internal control for transfection efficiency. Luciferase assay was performed using Dual-Luciferase® Reporter Assay System (Promega, Cat, No. E1910, Madison, WI, USA) and luminescence was measured by a luminometer (TriStar² LB942).

3.4. Transfection

Plasmid DNAs were transfected by Lipofectamine™ 2000 Transfection Reagent (Invitrogen, Cat. No. 11668019) and miRNAs were transfected by Lipofectamine™ RNAiMAX Transfection Reagent (Invitrogen, Cat. No. 13778150). At transfection, Opti-MEM™ I Reduced Serum Medium (Thermo Fisher Scientific, Cat. No. 31985062, Wilmington, DE, USA) was used.

3.5. Western Blotting

Cells were seeded in six-well plates at a density of 1×10^5–2×10^5 per well and transfected with miR-NC, miR-497a-5p and miR-186-5p at a final concentration of 50 nM. After 24 h and 48 h, cell lysates were extracted by lysis buffer (0.05 M Tris-HCl pH8.0, 0.15 M NaCl, 0.5 % Nonidet P-40) with 1% proteinase inhibitor cocktail (Nacalai Tesque, Inc. Kyoto, Kyoto, Japan. Cat. No. 04080-24). The protein samples (30 μg/lane) were electrophoresed by SDS-PAGE using 9% acrylamide gel and transferred to PVDF transfer membranes (Bio-Rad Laboratories, Inc. Hercules, CA, USA. Cat, No. #1620177). The membranes were blocked with 5% non-fat dry milk (Cell Signaling Technology, Inc. Cat, No. #9999, Beverly, MA, USA) in TBS with Tween-20 (TBS-T; 50 mM Tris, 158 mM NaCl, 2.7 mM KCl, pH 7.5, 0.1% Tween-20) or Blocking One (Nacalai Tesque, Inc. Cat, No. 03953-66) or Blocking One-p (Nacalai Tesque, Inc. Cat, No. 05999-84) for 1 h at room temperature and incubated with the following primary antibodies overnight at 4 °C:

Antibodies and dilution used were as follows:

Phospho-Smad 2 (Ser465/467) (138D4) Rabbit mAb (1:1000, Cell Signaling Technology, Cat, No. #3108,), Phospho-Smad 3 (Ser423/425) (C25A9) Rabbit mAb (1:1000, Cell Signaling Technology, Cat, No. #9520), Smad 7 Polyclonal Antibody (1: 500, Invitrogen, Cat, No. 10466413), β-Actin (13E5) Rabbit mAb (1:3000, Cell Signaling Technology, No. #4970), and anti-Rabbit IgG, HRP-Linked Whole Ab Donkey secondary antibody (1: 3000, GE Healthcare, Cat, No. NA934, Chicago, IL, USA). The bands were visualized by the ECL Detection System (GE Healthcare Life Sciences, Cat, No. 89168-782) and analyzed using ImageJ 1.52v software (National Institutes of Health).

3.6. Binding Assay Using pmirGLO Plasmid Vector

RT-PCR was performed to amplify parts of the 3′ UTRs of Smad 7 miRNA. The primer sequences were as follows: insert of Smad 7, forward 5 5′-GCTCGCTAGCCTCGACTGAGC AGGCCACACTTCAAAC-3′, reverse 5′-ATGCCTGCAGGTCGAGGTGTCCTGCCGA TCATACCTG-3′. The amplified product (304 bp) was subcloned and ligated into the multi-cloning site between Sal I and Xho I in the pmirGLO Dual-Luciferase miRNA Target Expression Vector (Promega, Cat, No. E1330) using the In-Fusion HD Cloning Kit (Clontech, Cat, No. 639650, Mountain View, CA, USA).

The sequences of inserts and vectors were confirmed by Sanger sequencing.

Cells were seeded in 96-well plates at a density of 1×10^4 cells per well and were co-transfected with 50 ng pmirGLO plasmid vector containing the insert and either miR-negative control (5 pmol) or miR-497a-5p (5 pmol). At 24 h after transfection, firefly and Renilla luciferase activities were measured using the Dual-Luciferase Reporter Assay System (Promega, Cat. No. E1910). All experiments were conducted in triplicate.

3.7. qRT-PCR

Total RNA was extracted using TRIzol™ Reagent (Invitrogen, Cat. No. 15596018). RNA quality was assessed with a NanoDrop ONE spectrophotometer (Thermo Fisher Scientific, Wilmington, DE, USA). About 2 μg of RNA was reverse transcribed with the high-capacity RNA to cDNA Kit (Applied Biosystems, Cat. No. 4388950, Foster City, CA, USA).

qPCR analysis was performed using THUNDERBIRD SYBR qPCR Mix (TOYOBO LIFE SCIENCE, Cat. No. QPS-201). The qPCR was performed on the LightCycler® 480 real-time PCR system (Roche Diagnostics, Basel, Switzerland). The qPCR conditions were as follows: 95 °C for 30 s; followed by 40 cycles of 95 °C for 10 s, 60 °C for 10 s and 72 °C for 30 s. The expression of the target gene was normalized to endogenous GAPDH expression. Relative expression was quantified by the $2^{-\Delta\Delta Cq}$ method.

The primers used were as follows:

TNF-α: 5′-CGTCAGCCGATTTGCTATCT-3′ (forward) and 5′-CGGACTCCGCAAAGTCTAAG-3′ (reverse).

IL-6: 5′-AGTTGCCTTCTTGGGACTGA-3′ (forward) and 5′-CAGAATTGCCATTGCACAAC-3′ (reverse).

IL-12p40: 5′-AGGTGCGTTCCTCGTAGAGA-3′ (forward) and 5′-AAAGCCAACCAAGCAGAAGA-3′ (reverse).

GAPDH: 5′-AGGTCGGTGTGAACGGATTTG-3′ (forward) and 5′-TGTAGACCATGTAGTTGAGGTCA-3′ (reverse).

3.8. Therapeutic Model for DSS-Induced Mouse Colitis

Eight-week-old BALB/c mice (female) which retain intact immune system were purchased from CLEA (Tokyo, Japan). DSS (MW 36,000–50,000) was purchased from MP Biomedicals (Cat. No. 9011-18-1, Santa Ana, CA, USA). For producing therapeutic model of DSS-induced colitis, drinking water at a concentration of 1.5% DSS was given to mice for 16 days with reference to previous studies [46,81]. MiR-497a-5p loaded on super carbonate apatite nanoparticle was injected eight times on the tail vein from day 9 to day 23 every two days. Mice were sacrificed on day 24. For a comparative therapeutic study between sCA-miR-497a-5p and sCA-miR-186-5p, 2% DSS in drinking water was given to mice for 8 days [82–84]. MiR-497a-5p or miR-186-5p loaded on super carbonate apatite nanoparticle was injected on days 8, 9, 10, 12, 13, and 14. Mice were sacrificed on day 15. The study protocol was in accordance with the Declaration of Helsinki, and the Ethical Guidelines for Medical and Health Research Involving Human Subjects in Osaka University. Animal experiments were approved by the Institutional Animal Care and Use Committee of Osaka University Graduate School of Medicine and by the Committee for the Ethics of Animal Experiments of Osaka University (Permit Number: 30-02-5, 20 June 2018).

3.9. Histological Inflammation Scoring of DSS Colitis Mice

Based on previous reports [46,69], the extent of inflammation in colon and intestinal wall was scored as follows: Mucosal damage: 0, normal; 1, focal damage and 3–10 intraepithelial lymphocytes (IELs)/high power field (HPF); 2, rare crypt abscesses plus >10 IELs /HPF; 3, multiple crypt abscesses and erosion/ulceration plus >10 IELs /HPF. Submucosal damage: 0, normal or widely scattered leukocytes; 1, focal aggregates of leukocytes; 2, diffuse leukocyte infiltration with expansion of the submucosa; 3, diffuse leukocyte infiltration. Muscularis damage: 0, normal or widely scattered leukocytes; 1, widely scattered leukocyte aggregates between muscle layers; 2, leukocyte infiltration with focal effacement of the muscularis; 3, extensive leukocyte infiltration with transmural effacement of the muscularis.

3.10. Production of sCA

sCA was prepared as described previously [44]. Briefly, 50 µg miR-497a-5p or miR-negative control 1 (NC1) was incubated in 25 mL of inorganic solution (44 mM $NaHCO_3$; 0.9 mM NaH_2PO_4; 1.8 mM $CaCl_2$ pH 7.5) at 37 °C for 30 min. The solution was centrifuged at 12,000 rpm for 3 min. The pellets from two tubes were dissolved in 200 µL saline containing 0.5% albumin, and sonicated (38 kHz, 80 W) in a water bath for 10 min. Approximately 50 µg miRNA per one administration was injected into the tail vein.

3.11. Fluorescent Immunostaining of Macrophages at Propria Muscularis of Colon Mucosa

DSS-induced colitis was produced by free drinking of 2% DSS for 7 days in female mice (n = 2). Non-treated mice (n = 2) served as a comparative reference. The Alexia 647-tagged NC-miRNA (25 µg) encapsulated in sCA was injected into the tail vein and the distal colon was collected 4 h later, and frozen in OCT compound. About 8 µm sections were cut and fixed in 4% paraformaldehyde. The frozen sections (n = 6 per mouse) were incubated overnight with rat anti-mouse F4/80 antibody (BIO RAD, Cat, No. MCA497G, Hercules, CA, USA) at a concentration of 1:100. As a secondary antibody, FITC-conjugated goat anti-rat IgG was used (Jackson ImmunoResearch, Cat, No. 112-095-167, West Grove, PA, USA). The nuclei were stained with ProLong Gold anti-fade reagent with DAPI (Invitrogen, Cat, No. #8961). Sections were observed using a fluorescence microscope (BZ-X 700, Keyence Corporation, Osaka, Japan).

3.12. Statistics

F-test was performed to find out if there were equal variances between the two groups. Statistical significance of the difference between two groups was then calculated by Student's t-test or Welch's t-test, and data are presented as means ± standard deviations unless specifically otherwise indicated. When more than two groups were compared, one-way ANOVA was used followed by Bonferroni correction to determine the statistical significance of the differences. Statistical analyses were performed using the JMP13 program (SAS Institute, Cary, NC, USA). Differences with $p < 0.05$ were considered significant (File S1).

4. Conclusions

In conclusion, we have demonstrated that sCA-miR-497a-5p complex exerts a potent anti-inflammatory effect through activation of TGF-β/Smad signal pathway and inhibition of secretion of inflammatory cytokines from macrophages in IBD therapeutic mice model. These results suggest that sCA-miR-497a-5p may potentially have a therapeutic ability against IBD although further investigation is essential.

Supplementary Materials: The following supporting information can be downloaded at: https://www.mdpi.com/article/10.3390/ph16040618/s1, Figure S1: Screening for candidate miRNAs by SBE reporter assays.; Figure S2: Principle of SBE reporter assay; Figure S3: Sequence of mmu-miR-497a-5p and has-miR-497a-5p; Figure S4: HE staining of 1.5% DSS induced colitis mice; Table S1: Sequences of the miRNAs used in this study; File S1: Summary of statistics.

Author Contributions: Conceptualization: H.Y. (Hirofumi Yamamoto); methodology: N.T., T.O., H.H. and H.Y. (Hiroyuki Yamamoto); software: Y.Y.; validation, Y.S., T.H., T.O. and H.T.; formal analysis, N.M., N.T. and H.Y. (Hirofumi Yamamoto); investigation: N.T., T.O., M.U. and T.K.; resources, H.Y. (Hirofumi Yamamoto); data curation: H.Y. (Hirofumi Yamamoto); writing—original draft preparation: N.T., M.H. and H.Y. (Hirofumi Yamamoto); writing—review and editing, T.O., H.E., Y.D., T.M. and H.Y. (Hirofumi Yamamoto); visualization: N.M.; supervision: T.O., H.E., Y.D. and H.Y. (Hirofumi Yamamoto); project administration: H.Y. (Hirofumi Yamamoto); funding acquisition, H.Y. (Hirofumi Yamamoto). All authors have read and agreed to the published version of the manuscript.

Funding: This work was supported by JSPS Grant-in-Aid for Exploratory Research Grant Number 16K15590.

Institutional Review Board Statement: The animal study protocol was approved by the Institutional Review Board of the Institutional Animal Care and Use Committee of Osaka University Graduate School of Medicine and by the Committee for the Ethics of Animal Experiments of Osaka University (Permit Number: 30-02-5, 20 June 2018).

Informed Consent Statement: Not applicable.

Data Availability Statement: Data is contained within the article and Supplementary Materials.

Acknowledgments: We are grateful Kenji Iso and Kazuya Nagata for supporting animal experiments.

Conflicts of Interest: The authors declare no conflict of interest.

References

1. Kaplan, G.G. The global burden of IBD: From 2015 to 2025. *Nat. Rev. Gastroenterol. Hepatol.* **2015**, *12*, 720–727. [CrossRef] [PubMed]
2. Windsor, J.W.; Kaplan, G.G. Evolving Epidemiology of IBD. *Curr. Gastroenterol. Rep.* **2019**, *21*, 40. [CrossRef] [PubMed]
3. Ungaro, R.; Mehandru, S.; Allen, P.; Peyrun-Biroulet, L.; Colombel, J.F. Ulcerative colitis. *Lancet* **2017**, *389*, 1756–1770. [CrossRef] [PubMed]
4. Bouguen, G.; Levesque, B.G.; Feagan, B.G.; Kavanaugh, A.; Peyrin-Biroulet, L.; Jean-Frederic, C.; Hanauer, S.B.; Sandborn, W.J. Treat to target: A proposed new paradigm for the management of Crohnés disease. *Clin. Gastroenterol. Hepatol.* **2015**, *13*, 1042–1050. [CrossRef] [PubMed]
5. Peyrin-Biroulet, L.; Sandborn, W.; Sands, B.E.; Reinisch, W.; Bemelman, W.; Bryant, R.V.; D'Haens, G.; Dotan, I.; Dubinsky, M.; Feagan, B.; et al. Selecting Therapeutic Targets in Inflammatory Bowel Disease (STRIDE): Determining Therapeutic Goals for Treat-to-Target. *Am. J. Gastroenterol.* **2015**, *110*, 1324–1338. [CrossRef] [PubMed]
6. Sandborn, W.J.; Baert, F.; Danese, S.; Krznaric, Z.; Kobayashi, T.; Yao, X.; Chen, J.; Rosario, M.; Bhatia, S.; Kisfalvi, K.; et al. Efficacy and Safety of Vedolizumab Subcutaneous Formulation in a Randomized Trial of Patients With Ulcerative Colitis. *Gastroenterology* **2020**, *158*, 562–572. [CrossRef] [PubMed]
7. Sands, B.E.; Snadborn, W.J.; Panaccione, R.; O'Brien, C.D.; Zhang, H.; Johanns, J.; Adedokun, O.J.; Li, K.; Biroulet, L.; Assche, G.V.; et al. Ustekinumab as Induction and Maintenance Therapy for Ulcerative Colitis. *N. Engl. J. Med.* **2019**, *381*, 1201–1214. [CrossRef] [PubMed]
8. Sandborn, W.J.; Rebuck, R.; Wang, Y.; Zou, B.; Adedokun, O.J.; Gasink, C.; Sands, B.E.; Hanauer, S.B.; Targan, S.; Ghosh, S.; et al. Five-Year Efficacy and Safety of Ustekinumab Treatment in Crohn's Disease: The IM-UNITI Trial. *Clin. Gastroenterol. Hepatol.* **2022**, *20*, 578–590. [CrossRef]
9. Salas, A.; Rocha, C.; Duijvestein, M.; Faubion, W.; McGovern, D.; Vermeire, S.; Vetrano, S.; Casteele, N.V. JAK-STAT pathway targeting for the treatment of inflammatory bowel disease. *Nav. Rev. Gastroenterol. Hepatol.* **2020**, *17*, 323–337. [CrossRef]
10. Mentella, M.C.; Scaldaferii, F.; Pizzoferrato, M.; Gasbarrini, A.; Miggiano, G.A.D. Nutrition, IBD and Gut Microbiota A review. *Nutrients* **2020**, *12*, 944. [CrossRef]
11. Guan, Q. A Comprehensive Review and Update on the Pathogenesis of Inflammatory Bowel Disease. *J. Immunol. Res.* **2019**, *2019*, 7247238. [CrossRef]
12. Glassner, K.L.; Abraham, B.P.; Quigley, E.M.M. The microbiome and inflammatory bowel disease. *J. Allergy Clin. Immunol.* **2020**, *145*, 16–27. [CrossRef]
13. Littman, D.R.; Rudensky, A.Y. Th17 and regulatory T cells in mediating and restraining inflammation. *Cell* **2010**, *140*, 845–858. [CrossRef]
14. Omenetti, S.; Pizarro, T.T. The Treg/Th17 Axis: A Dynamic Balance Regulated by the Gut Microbiome. *Front. Immunol.* **2015**, *6*, 639. [CrossRef] [PubMed]
15. Yan, J.; Luo, M.; Chen, Z.; He, B. The Function and Role of the Th17/Treg Cell Balance in Inflammatory Bowel Disease. *J. Immunol. Res.* **2020**, *2020*, 8813558. [CrossRef] [PubMed]
16. Bai, B.; Li, H.; Han, L.; Mei, Y.; Hu, C.; Mei, Q.; Xu, J.; Liu, X. Molecular mechanism of the TGF-β/Smad7 signaling pathway in ulcerative colitis. *Mol. Med. Rep.* **2022**, *25*, 116. [CrossRef] [PubMed]
17. Monteleone, G.; Kumberova, A.; Croft, N.M.; McKenzie, C.; Steer, H.W.; MacDonald, T.T. Blocking Smad7 restores TGF-beta1 signaling in chronic inflammatory bowel disease. *J. Clin. Investig.* **2001**, *108*, 601–609. [CrossRef] [PubMed]
18. Sedda, S.; Marafini, I.; Dinallo, V.; Fusco, D.D.; Monteleone, G. The TGF-β/Smad System in IBD Pathogenesis. *Inflamm. Bowel Dis.* **2015**, *21*, 2921–2925. [CrossRef] [PubMed]
19. Hill, C.S. Transcriptional Control by the SMADs. *Cold Spring Harb. Perspect. Biol.* **2016**, *8*, a022079. [CrossRef]
20. Hata, A.; Chen, Y.G. TGF-β Signaling from Receptors to Smads. *Cold Spring Harb. Perspect. Biol.* **2016**, *8*, a022061. [CrossRef] [PubMed]

21. Monteleone, G.; Neurath, M.F.; Di Ardizzone, S.; Sabatino, A.; Fantini, M.C.; Castiglione, F.; Scribano, M.L.; Armuzzi, A.; Caprioli, F.; Sturniolo, G.C.; et al. Mongersen, an oral SMAD7 antisense oligonucleotide, and Crohn's disease. *N. Engl. J. Med.* **2015**, *372*, 1104–1113. [CrossRef]
22. Ogino, T.; Takeda, K. Immunoregulation by antigen-presenting cells in human intestinal lamina propria. *Front. Immunol.* **2023**, *14*, 1138971. [CrossRef] [PubMed]
23. Koelink, P.J.; Bloemendaal, F.M.; Li, B.; Westera, L.; Vogels, E.W.M.; Roest, M.; Gloudemans, A.K.; Wout, A.; Korf, H.; Vermerire, S.; et al. Anti-TNF therapy in IBD exerts its therapeutic effect through macrophage IL-10 signaling. *Gut* **2020**, *69*, 1053–1063. [CrossRef] [PubMed]
24. Zhou, X.; Li, E.; Wang, S.; Zhang, P.; Wang, Q.; Xiao, J.; Zhang, C.; Zheng, X.; Xu, X.; Xue, S.; et al. YAP Aggravates Inflammatory Bowel Disease by Regulating M1/M2 Macrophage Polarization and Gut Microbial Homeostasis. *Cell Rep.* **2019**, *27*, 1176–1189. [CrossRef] [PubMed]
25. Ogino, T.; Nishimura, J.; Barman, S.; Kayama, H.; Uematsu, S.; Okuzaki, D.; Osawa, H.; Haraguchi, N.; Uemura, M.; Hata, T.; et al. Increased Th17-inducing activity of CD14+ CD163 low myeloid cells in intestinal lamina propria of patients with Crohn's disease. *Gastroenterology* **2013**, *145*, 1380–1391. [CrossRef] [PubMed]
26. Diag, A.; Schilling, M.; Klironomos, F.; Ayoub, S.; Rajewsky, N. Spatiotemporal m(i)RNA Architecture and 3' UTR Regulation in the *C. elegans* Germline. *Dev. Cell* **2018**, *47*, 785–800. [CrossRef]
27. Kabekkodu, S.; Shakla, V.; Varghese, V.K.; Souza, J.D.; Chakrabarty, S.; Satyamoorthy, K. Clustered miRNAs and their role in biological functions and diseases. *Biol. Rev. Camb. Philos. Soc.* **2018**, *93*, 1955–1986. [CrossRef]
28. Barresi, V.; Musmeci, C.; Rinaldi, A.; Condorelli, D.F. Transcript-Targeted Therapy Based on RNA Interference and Antisense Oligonucleotides: Current Applications and Novel Molecular Targets. *Int. J. Mol. Sci.* **2022**, *23*, 8875. [CrossRef]
29. Fogli, S.; Re, M.D.; Rofi, E.; Posarelli, C.; Figus, M.; Danesi, R. Clinical pharmacology of intravitreal anti-VEGF drugs. *Eye* **2018**, *32*, 1010–1020. [CrossRef]
30. Patel, N.; Hegele, R.A. Mipomersen as a potential adjunctive therapy for hypercholesterolemia. *Expert Opin. Pharmacother.* **2010**, *11*, 2569–2572. [CrossRef]
31. Lim, K.; Maruyama, R.; Yokota, T. Eteplirsen in the treatment of Duchenne muscular dystrophy. *Drug Des. Dev. Ther.* **2017**, *11*, 533–545. [CrossRef] [PubMed]
32. Chiriboga, C.A. Nusinersen for the treatment of spinal muscular atrophy. *Expert Rev. Neurother.* **2017**, *17*, 955–962. [CrossRef]
33. Cooper, C.; Mackie, D. Hepatitis B surface antigen-1018 ISS adjuvant-containing vaccine: A review of HEPLISAV™ safety and efficacy. *Expert Rev. Vaccines* **2011**, *10*, 417–427. [CrossRef]
34. Benson, M.; Dasgupta, N.R.; Monia, B. Inotersen (transthyretin-specific antisense oligonucleotide) for treatment of transthyretin amyloidosis. *Neurodegen. Dis. Manag.* **2019**, *9*, 25–30. [CrossRef]
35. Yang, J. Patisiran for the treatment of hereditary transthyretin-mediated amyloidosis. *Expert Rev. Clin. Pharmacol.* **2019**, *12*, 95–99. [CrossRef]
36. Cai, X.; Zhang, Z.Y.; Yuan, J.T.; Ocansey, D.K.W.; Tu, Q.; Zhang, X.; Qian, H.; Xu, W.R.; Qiu, W.; Mao, F. hucMSC-derived exosomes attenuate colitis by regulating macrophage pyroptosis via the miR-378a-5p/NLRP3 axis. *Stem Cell Res. Ther.* **2021**, *12*, 416. [CrossRef]
37. Feng, Q.; Li, Y.; Zhang, H.; Wang, Z.; Nie, X.; Yao, D.; Han, L.; Chen, W.; Wang, Y. Deficiency of miRNA-149-3p shaped gut microbiota and enhanced dextran sulfate sodium-induced colitis. *Mol. Ther. Nucleic Acids* **2022**, *30*, 208–225. [CrossRef] [PubMed]
38. Zhang, Q.; Wang, S. miR-330 alleviates dextran sodium sulfate-induced ulcerative colitis through targeting IRAK1 in rats. *Kaohsiung J. Med. Sci.* **2021**, *37*, 497–504. [CrossRef]
39. Zhang, J.; Wang, C.; Guo, Z.; Zhu, W.; Li, Q. miR-223 improves intestinal inflammation through inhibiting the IL-6/STAT3 signal pathway in dextran sodium sulfate-induced experimental colitis. *Immune Inflamm. Dis.* **2021**, *9*, 319–327. [CrossRef] [PubMed]
40. Kang, X.; Jiao, Y.; Zhou, Y.; Meng, C.; Zhou, X.; Song, L.; Jiao, X.; Pan, Z. MicroRNA-5112 Targets IKKγ to Dampen the Inflammatory Response and Improve Clinical Symptoms in Both Bacterial Infection and DSS-Induced Colitis. *Front. Immunol.* **2022**, *13*, 779770. [CrossRef]
41. Scalavino, V.; Piccinno, E.; Bianco, G.; Schena, N.; Armentano, R.; Giannelli, G.; Serino, G. The Increase of miR-195-5p Reduces Intestinal Permeability in Ulcerative Colitis, Modulating Tight Junctions' Expression. *Int. J. Mol. Sci.* **2022**, *23*, 5840. [CrossRef]
42. Wang, M.; Guo, J.; Zhao, Y.; Wang, J. IL-21 mediates microRNA-423-5p /claudin-5 signal pathway and intestinal barrier function in inflammatory bowel disease. *Aging* **2020**, *12*, 16099–16110. [CrossRef]
43. Jin, X.; Chen, D.; Zheng, R.; Zhang, H.; Chen, Y.; Xiang, Z. miRNA-133a-UCP2 pathway regulates inflammatory bowel disease progress by influencing inflammation, oxidative stress and energy metabolism. *World J. Gastroenterol.* **2017**, *23*, 76–86. [CrossRef]
44. Wu, X.; Yamamoto, H.; Nakanishi, H.; Yamamoto, Y.; Inoue, A.; Tei, M.; Hirose, H.; Uemura, M.; Nishimura, J.; Hata, T.; et al. Innovative Delivery of siRNA to Solid Tumors by Super Carbonate Apatite. *PLoS ONE* **2015**, *10*, e0116022. [CrossRef]
45. Wang, Y.; Yokoyama, Y.; Hirose, H.; Shimomura, Y.; Bonkobara, S.; Itakura, H.; Kouda, Y.; Morimoto, K.; Minami, K.; Takahashi, H.; et al. Functional assessment of miR-1291 in colon cancer cells. *Int. J. Oncol.* **2022**, *60*, 13. [CrossRef]
46. Fukata, T.; Mizushima, T.; Nishimura, J.; Okuzaki, D.; Wu, X.; Hirose, H.; Yokoyama, Y.; Kubota, Y.; Nagata, K.; Tsujimura, N.; et al. The Supercarbonate Apatite-MicroRNA Complex Inhibits Dextran Sodium Sulfate-Induced Colitis. *Mol. Nucleic Acids* **2018**, *12*, 658–671. [CrossRef] [PubMed]

47. Takeyama, H.; Yamamoto, H.; Yamashita, S.; Wu, X.; Takahashi, H.; Nishimura, J.; Haraguchi, N.; Miyake, Y.; Suzuki, R.; Murata, K.; et al. Decreased miR-340 expression in bone marrow is associated with liver metastasis of colorectal cancer. *Mol. Cancer Ther.* **2014**, *13*, 976–985. [CrossRef] [PubMed]
48. Hiraki, M.; Nishimura, J.; Takahashi, H.; Wu, X.; Takahashi, Y.; Miyo, M.; Nishida, N.; Uemura, M.; Hata, T.; Takemasa, I.; et al. Concurrent Targeting of KRAS and AKT by MiR-4689 Is a Novel Treatment Against Mutant KRAS Colorectal Cancer. *Mol. Nucleic Acids* **2015**, *4*, e231. [CrossRef] [PubMed]
49. Ogawa, Y.; Wu, X.; Kawamoto, K.; Nishida, N.; Konno, M.; Koseki, J.; Matsui, H.; Noguchi, K.; Gotoh, N.; Yamamoto, T.; et al. MicroRNAs Induce Epigenetic Reprogramming and Suppress Malignant Phenotypes of Human Colon Cancer Cells. *PLoS ONE* **2015**, *10*, e0127119. [CrossRef]
50. Takahashi, H.; Nishimura, J.; Kagawa, Y.; Kano, Y.; Takahashi, Y.; Wu, X.; Hiraki, M.; Hamabe, A.; Konno, M.; Haraguchi, N.; et al. Significance of Polypyrimidine Tract-Binding Protein 1 Expression in Colorectal Cancer. *Mol. Cancer Ther.* **2015**, *14*, 1705–1716. [CrossRef]
51. Inoue, A.; Mizushima, T.; Wu, X.; Okuzaki, D.; Kambara, N.; Ishikawa, S.; Wang, J.; Qian, Y.; Hirose, H.; Yokoyama, Y.; et al. A miR-29b Byproduct Sequence Exhibits Potent Tumor-Suppressive Activities via Inhibition of NF-κB Signaling in KRAS-Mutant Colon Cancer Cells. *Mol. Cancer Ther.* **2018**, *17*, 977–987. [CrossRef]
52. Takahashi, H.; Misato, K.; Aoshi, T.; Yamamoto, Y.; Kubota, Y.; Wu, X.; Kuroda, E.; Ishii, K.J.; Yamamoto, H.; Yoshioka, Y. Carbonate Apatite Nanoparticles Act as Potent Vaccine Adjuvant Delivery Vehicles by Enhancing Cytokine Production Induced by Encapsulated Cytosine-Phosphate-Guanine Oligodeoxynucleotides. *Front. Immunol.* **2018**, *9*, 783. [CrossRef] [PubMed]
53. Tamai, K.; Mizushima, T.; Wu, X.; Inoue, A.; Ota, M.; Yokoyama, Y.; Miyoshi, N.; Haraguchi, N.; Takahashi, H.; Nishimura, J.; et al. Photodynamic Therapy Using Indocyanine Green Loaded on Super Carbonate Apatite as Minimally Invasive Cancer Treatment. *Mol. Cancer Ther.* **2018**, *17*, 1613–1622. [CrossRef]
54. Morimoto, Y.; Mizushima, T.; Wu, X.; Okuzaki, D.; Yokoyama, Y.; Inoue, A.; Hata, T.; Hirose, H.; Qian, Y.; Wang, J.; et al. miR-4711-5p regulates cancer stemness and cell cycle progression via KLF5, MDM2 and TFDP1 in colon cancer cells. *Br. J. Cancer* **2020**, *122*, 1037–1049. [CrossRef] [PubMed]
55. Wu, X.; Yokoyama, Y.; Takahashi, H.; Kouda, S.; Yamamoto, H.; Wang, J.; Morimoto, Y.; Minami, K.; Hata, T.; Shamma, A.; et al. Improved In Vivo Delivery of Small RNA Based on the Calcium Phosphate Method. *J. Pers. Med.* **2021**, *11*, 1160. [CrossRef]
56. Monteleone, G.; Stolfi, C.; Marafini, I.; Atreya, R.; Neurath, M.F. Smad7 Antisense Oligonucleotide-Based Therapy in Crohn's Disease: Is it Time to Re-Evaluate? *Mol. Diagn. Ther.* **2022**, *26*, 477–481. [CrossRef]
57. Sands, B.; Feagan, B.; Sandborn, W.; Schreiber, S.; Laurent, P.B.; Colombel, J.; Rossiter, G.; Usiskin, K.; Ather, S.; Zhan, X.; et al. Mongersen (GED-0301) for Active Crohn's Disease: Results of a Phase 3 Study. *Am. J. Gastroenterol.* **2020**, *115*, 738–745. [CrossRef]
58. Marafini, I.; Stolfi, C.; Troncone, E.; Lolli, E.; Onali, S.; Paoluzi, O.; Fantini, M.; Biancone, L.; Calabrese, E.; Grazia, A.; et al. A Pharmacological Batch of Mongersen that Downregulates Smad7 is Effective as Induction Therapy in Active Crohn's Disease: A Phase II, Open-Label Study. *BioDrugs* **2021**, *35*, 325–336. [CrossRef]
59. Bewtra, M.; Lichtenstein, G. Mongersen and SMAD-7 Inhibition, Not a Lucky 7 for Patients With IBD: When Trial Design Is as Important as Disease Therapy. *Am. J. Gastroenterol.* **2020**, *115*, 687–688. [CrossRef] [PubMed]
60. TargetScan. Available online: https://www.targetscan.org/vert_80/ (accessed on 1 July 2017).
61. miRbase. Available online: https://www.mirbase.org (accessed on 1 July 2017).
62. Viviana, S.; Emanuele, P.; Antonio, L.; Angela, T.; Raffaele, A.; Gianluigi, G.; Grazia, S. miR-195-5p Regulates Tight Junctions Expression via Claudin-2 Downregulation in Ulcerative Colitis. *Biomedicines* **2022**, *10*, 919.
63. Chapel, A.; Caligaris, C.; Fenouil, T.; Savary, C.; Aires, S.; Martel, S.; Huchede, P.; Chassot, C.; Chauvet, V.; Ruffino, V.; et al. SMAD2/3 mediate oncogenic effects of TGF-β in the absence of SMAD4. *Commun. Biol.* **2022**, *5*, 1068. [CrossRef] [PubMed]
64. Buwaneka, P.; Ralko, A.; Gorai, S.; Pham, H.; Cho, W. Phosphoinositide-binding activity of Smad2 is essential for its function in TGF-β signaling. *J. Biol. Chem.* **2021**, *297*, 101303. [CrossRef]
65. Mohankumar, K.; Namachivayam, K.; Chapalamadugu, K.C.; Garzon, S.A.; Premkumar, M.H.; Tipparaju, S.M.; Maheshwari, A. Smad7 interrupts TGF-β signaling in intestinal macrophages and promotes inflammatory activation of these cells during necrotizing enterocolitis. *Pediatr. Res.* **2016**, *79*, 951–961. [CrossRef]
66. Chen, X.; Shi, C.; Wang, C.; Liu, W.; Chu, Y.; Xiang, Z.; Hu, K.; Dong, P.; Han, X. The role of miR-497-5p in myofibroblast differentiation of LR-MSCs and pulmonary fibrogenesis. *Sci. Rep.* **2017**, *7*, 40958. [CrossRef]
67. Satsu, H.; Ishimotoa, Y.; Nakanoa, T.; Mochizukia, T.; Iwanaga, T.; Shimizu, M. Induction by activated macrophage-like THP-1 cells of apoptotic and necrotic cell death in intestinal epithelial Caco-2 monolayers via tumor necrosis factor-alpha. *Exp. Cell Res.* **2006**, *312*, 3909–3919. [CrossRef] [PubMed]
68. Petric, Z.; Goncalves, J.; Paixao, P. Under the Umbrella of Clinical Pharmacology: Inflammatory Bowel Disease, Infliximab and Adalimumab, and a Bridge to an Era of Biosimilars. *Pharmaceutics* **2022**, *14*, 1766. [CrossRef] [PubMed]
69. Ozaki, K.; Makino, H.; Aoki, M.; Miyake, T.; Yasumasa, N.; Osako, M.; Nakagami, H.; Rakugi, H.; Morishita, R. Therapeutic effect of ribbon-type nuclear factor-κB decoy oligonucleotides in a rat model of inflammatory bowel disease. *Curr. Gene Ther.* **2012**, *12*, 484–492. [CrossRef]
70. Tahara, K.; Samura, S.; Tsuji, K.; Yamamoto, H.; Tsukada, Y.; Bando, Y.; Tsujimoto, H.; Morishita, R.; Kawashima, K. Oral nuclear factor-κB decoy oligonucleotides delivery system with chitosan modified poly(D,L-lactide-co-glycolide) nanospheres for inflammatory bowel disease. *Biomaterials* **2011**, *32*, 870–878. [CrossRef]

71. Kim, J.J.; Shajib, M.S.; Manocha, M.M.; Khan, W.I. Investigating intestinal inflammation in DSS-induced model of IBD. *J. Vis. Exp.* **2012**, *60*, 3678.
72. Hoffmann, M.; Schwertassek, U.; Seydel, A.; Weber, K.; Falk, W.; Hauschildt, S.; Lehmann, J. A refined and translationally relevant model of chronic DSS colitis in BALB/c mice. *Lab. Anim.* **2018**, *52*, 240–252. [CrossRef]
73. Chassaing, B.; Aitken, J.D.; Malleshappa, M.; Kumar, M. Dextran sulfate sodium (DSS)-induced colitis in mice. *Curr. Protoc. Immunol.* **2014**, *104*, 15.25.1–15.25.14. [CrossRef]
74. Lei, J.; Liu, L.; Zhang, M.; Zhang, Z. METTL3/LINC00662/miR-186-5p feedback loop regulates docetaxel resistance in triple negative breast cancer. *Sci. Rep.* **2022**, *12*, 16715.
75. Ting, H.; Lina, G.; Na, G.; Chaochao, W.; Wuli, G.; Xiaojie, Z.; Qi, L. miR-221-5p and miR-186-5p Are the Critical Bladder Cancer Derived Exosomal miRNAs in Natural Killer Cell Dysfunction. *Int. J. Mol. Sci.* **2022**, *23*, 15177.
76. Rui, W.; Hongbo, B.; Shihua, Z.; Ruiyan, L.; Lijie, C.; Yulan, Z. miR-186-5p Promotes Apoptosis by Targeting IGF-1 in SH-SY5Y OGD/R Model. *Cancer Cell Int.* **2021**, *21*, 114.
77. Zhang, Z.; Wen, Z.; Junsheng, M.; Zheng, X.; Mingyu, F. miR-186-5p Functions as a Tumor Suppressor in Human Osteosarcoma by Targeting FOXK1. *Cell Physiol. Biochem.* **2019**, *52*, 553–564. [PubMed]
78. Ang, L.; Lei, F.; Xiaoya, N.; Qihui, Z.; Bei, L.; Zhen, Y. Downregulation of OIP5-AS1 affects proNGF-induced pancreatic cancer metastasis by inhibiting p75NTR levels. *Aging* **2021**, *13*, 10688–10702.
79. Xian, Z.; Yanli, W.; Rong, D.; Hailong, Z.; Jinzhuo, D.; Haihua, Y.; Guofang, H.; Yuzhang, D.; Qin, C.; Jianxiu, Y. miR186 suppresses prostate cancer progression by targeting Twist1. *Oncotarget* **2016**, *7*, 33136–33151.
80. Zhang, M.; Yang, D.; Yu, H.; Li, Q. MicroRNA-497 inhibits inflammation in DSS-induced IBD model mice and lipopolysaccharide-induced RAW264.7 cells via Wnt/β-catenin pathway. *Int. Immunopharmacol.* **2021**, *101 Pt B*, 108318. [CrossRef]
81. Abd-Aziz, N.; Kamaruzman, N.I.; Poh, C.L. Development of MicroRNAs as Potential Therapeutics against Cancer. *J. Oncol.* **2020**, *2020*, 8029721. [CrossRef] [PubMed]
82. Forterre, A.; Komuro, H.; Aminova, S.; Harada, M. A Comprehensive Review of Cancer MicroRNA Therapeutic Delivery Strategies. *Cancers* **2020**, *12*, 1852. [CrossRef]
83. Merhautova, J.; Demlova, R.; Slaby, O. MicroRNA-Based Therapy in Animal Models of Selected Gastrointestinal Cancers. *Front. Pharmacol.* **2016**, *7*, 329. [CrossRef] [PubMed]
84. Takahashi, R.U.; Prieto-Vila, M.; Kohama, I.; Ochiya, T. Development of miRNA-based therapeutic approaches for cancer patients. *Cancer Sci.* **2019**, *110*, 1140–1147. [CrossRef] [PubMed]

Disclaimer/Publisher's Note: The statements, opinions and data contained in all publications are solely those of the individual author(s) and contributor(s) and not of MDPI and/or the editor(s). MDPI and/or the editor(s) disclaim responsibility for any injury to people or property resulting from any ideas, methods, instructions or products referred to in the content.

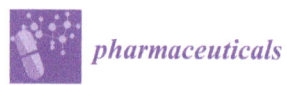

Article

Exploring the Underlying Mechanism of Ren-Shen-Bai-Du Powder for Treating Inflammatory Bowel Disease Based on Network Pharmacology and Molecular Docking

Ni Jin [1], Yao Liu [2], Peiyu Xiong [1], Yiyi Zhang [1], Jingwen Mo [1], Xiushen Huang [1] and Yi Zhou [1,*]

1 School of Basic Medical College, Chengdu University of Traditional Chinese Medicine, Chengdu 611137, China
2 School of Laboratory Medicine, Chengdu Medical College, Chengdu 610500, China
* Correspondence: zhouyi1@cdutcm.edu.cn

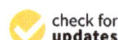

Citation: Jin, N.; Liu, Y.; Xiong, P.; Zhang, Y.; Mo, J.; Huang, X.; Zhou, Y. Exploring the Underlying Mechanism of Ren-Shen-Bai-Du Powder for Treating Inflammatory Bowel Disease Based on Network Pharmacology and Molecular Docking. *Pharmaceuticals* 2022, 15, 1038. https://doi.org/10.3390/ph15091038

Academic Editors: Anderson Luiz-Ferreira and Carmine Stolfi

Received: 27 July 2022
Accepted: 18 August 2022
Published: 23 August 2022

Publisher's Note: MDPI stays neutral with regard to jurisdictional claims in published maps and institutional affiliations.

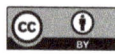

Copyright: © 2022 by the authors. Licensee MDPI, Basel, Switzerland. This article is an open access article distributed under the terms and conditions of the Creative Commons Attribution (CC BY) license (https:// creativecommons.org/licenses/by/ 4.0/).

Abstract: Ren-Shen-Bai-Du Powder (RSBDP) is currently used for inflammatory bowel disease (IBD) therapy in China. However, its potential mechanism against IBD remains unknown. In this study, we initially identified potential targets of RSBDP against IBD through network pharmacology analysis and molecular docking. Afterwards, the DSS-induced colitis mice model was employed to assess the effects of RSBDP. The results of network pharmacology indicated that a total of 39 main active ingredients in RSBDP generated 309 pairs of drug-ingredient and ingredient-target correspondences through 115 highly relevant targets of IBD. The primary ingredients (quercetin, kaempferol, luteolin, naringenin, and sitosterol) exerted functions through multiple targets that include CYP1B1, CA4/7, and ESR1/2, etc. GO functional enrichment analysis revealed that the targets related to IBD were significantly enriched in the oxidation-reduction process, protein binding, and cytosol. Per the KEGG pathway analysis, pathways in cancer, adherens junction, and nitrogen metabolism were pivotal in the RSBDP's treatment of IBD. Additionally, molecular docking demonstrated that a set of active ingredients and their targets displayed good bonding capabilities (e.g., kaempferol and AhR with combined energy < 5 kcal/mol). For the animal experiment, oral RSBDP promoted weight recovery, reduced intestinal inflammation, and decreased serum IL-1, IL-6, and IL-8 concentrations in the DSS + RSBDP group. Meanwhile, oral RSBDP significantly up-regulated the mRNA levels of *CA7*, *CPY1B1*, and *PTPN11*; in particular, the expression level of *CYP1B1* in the DSS + RSBDP group was up-regulated by as high as 9-fold compared to the DSS group. Western blot results indicated that the protein levels of AKR1C1, PI3K, AKT, p-AKT, and Bcl-2 were significantly down-regulated, and Bax was significantly up-regulated in the DSS + RSBDP group. Compared to the DSS and control groups, the Bax/Bcl-2 value in the DSS + RSBDP group increased 4-fold and 8-fold, respectively, which suggested that oral RSBDP promotes apoptosis of intestinal epithelial cells. In short, this study established quercetin, kaempferol, luteolin, naringenin, and sitosterol as the primary key active ingredients of RSBDP that exert synergistic therapeutic effects against IBD through modulating the AhR/CYP1B1 and AKR1C1/PI3K/AKT pathways.

Keywords: Ren-Shen-Bai-Du Powder (RSBDP); inflammatory bowel disease; network pharmacology; molecular docking; underlying mechanism

1. Introduction

Inflammatory bowel disease (IBD) is characterized by an idiopathic chronic inflammatory state of the gastrointestinal tract and encompasses 2 distinct disease states: ulcerative colitis (UC) and Crohn's disease (CD) [1]. Since officially naming the disease in 1875, the number of people subjected with IBD has progressively increased each year. Currently, IBD has become a globalized disease, with five million IBD patients globally and a prevalence of 0.5% in some developed countries [2]. Clinically, it is a heterogeneous disease with numerous phenotypes that commonly characterized by abdominal pain, diarrhea, mucus-like pus, blood in the stool, and damage of the mucosal barrier [3,4]. However, there is no official name for IBD in Chinese medicine. Its clinical features can be classified as "dysentery" and "diarrhea" and are mainly induced by damp-heat and a diet that damages the spleen and stomach.

Drugs used frequently to treat IBD tend to be expensive and have high side effects, rendering their consistent application challenging [5]. Conversely, traditional Chinese medicine (TCM) has fewer toxic side effects and is endowed with a variety of biological activities and pharmacological effects, including anti-inflammatory, antibacterial, and immunomodulatory effects with its multi-targeted action characteristics distinctively superior in the treatment and prevention of IBD [6]. The earliest known use of Ren-Shen-Bai-Du Powder (RSBDP) can be traced back to Qian Yi's "Direct formula for children's drug syndrome" in the Northern Song Dynasty, which consisted of 12 herbs (weight ratio 2:4:2:3:2:2:2:2:2:2:1:1): *Panax ginseng* (Renshen, RS), *Radix bupleuri* (Chaihu, CH), *Radix Peucedani* (Qianhu, QH), *Rhizoma Ligustic Chuanxiong* (Chuanxiong, CX), *Fructus Aurantii* (Zhike, ZK), *Rhizoma et Radix Notopterygii* (Qianghuo, QH), *Radix Angelicae Pubescentis* (Duhuo, DH), *Poria* (Fuling, FL), *Radix Platycodonis* (Jiegeng, JG), *Radix Glycyrrhizae* (Gancao, GC), *Rhizoma Zingiberis Recens* (Shengjiang, SJ), and *Herba Menthae* (Bohe, BH). RSBDP has also shown notable therapeutic properties against infantile diarrhea and has been demonstrated to improve the intestinal mucosal barrier in UC rats [7]. However, the current situation is different from the use of single-target drugs with a specific mechanism, and the potential mechanism of RSBDP for treating IBD is still unclear, which requires further systematic analysis.

The network pharmacology approach includes the use of systems biology, network analysis, connectivity, and multiple effects [8]. It is in line with the holistic and systemic characteristics of TCM and the principles of diagnosis and treatment, which can elucidate the complex network of interactions between disease-specific genes and compounds in TCM herbal medicines. Their association with one another helps reveal the possible molecular mechanism of TCM prescriptions and provides relevant scientific evidence for clinical research [9]. Therefore, the present study aimed to systematically elucidate the mechanism of RSBDP in the treatment of IBD by analyzing the interactional relationships between drug molecules and IBD-related targets through network pharmacology and molecular docking. We also sought to provide a theoretical basis for clinical research. To achieve our objectives, we implemented the technology roadmap in Figure 1.

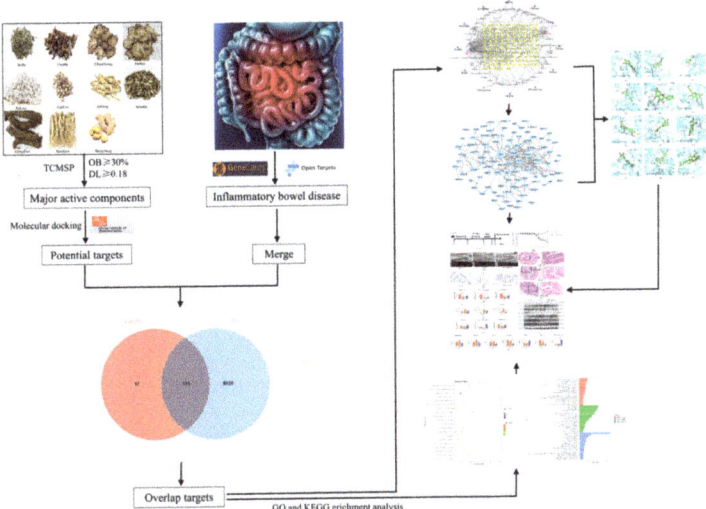

Figure 1. The technology roadmap of network pharmacology in this study.

2. Results

2.1. Screening for Key Active Ingredients of RSBDP and Prediction of Important Targets

Primary bioactive ingredients in RSBDP and corresponding ADME information were extracted from the TCMSP data server. In this study, a total of 39 main bioactive ingredients were identified in RSBDP and obtained the drug targets for the corresponding ingredients utilizing the SwissTargetPrediction database (Table 1). After de-duplication and elimination of invalid gene IDs, we intersected targets with those downloaded from the GeneCards and Open Targets databases to acquire 115 potential targets of RSBDP against IBD. Data collation yielded 309 pairs of drug-ingredient and ingredient-target correspondences.

Table 1. The primary active ingredients of RSBDP.

Drug	Mol ID	Molecule Name	OB (%)	DL
ChaiHu	MOL000354	Isorhamnetin	49.60	0.31
	MOL000422	Kaempferol	41.88	0.24
	MOL000098	Quercetin	46.43	0.28
	MOL000449	Stigmasterol	43.83	0.76
	MOL004718	α-spinasterol	42.98	0.76
ChuanXiong	MOL000359	Sitosterol	36.91	0.75
DuHuo	MOL000358	β-sitosterol	36.91	0.75
FuLing	MOL000287	3β-Hydroxy-24-methylene-8-lanostene-21-oic acid	38.70	0.81
	MOL000282	Ergosta-7,22E-dien-3β-ol	43.51	0.72
	MOL000283	Ergosterol peroxide	40.36	0.81
	MOL000296	Hederagenin	36.91	0.75
	MOL000275	Trametenolic acid	38.71	0.80
GanCao	MOL001792	DFV	32.76	0.18
	MOL004806	Euchrenone	30.29	0.57
	MOL000392	Formononetin	69.67	0.21
	MOL004996	Gadelaidic acid	30.70	0.20
	MOL004910	Glabranin	52.90	0.31
	MOL004828	Glepidotin A	44.72	0.35
	MOL004811	Glyasperin C	45.56	0.40
	MOL004835	Glypallichalcone	61.60	0.19
	MOL004949	Isolicoflavonol	45.17	0.42
	MOL000354	Isorhamnetin	49.60	0.31
	MOL004814	Isotrifoliol	31.94	0.42
	MOL000422	Kaempferol	41.88	0.24
	MOL003656	Lupiwighteone	51.64	0.37
	MOL000211	Mairin	55.38	0.78
	MOL004328	Naringenin	59.29	0.21
	MOL000098	Quercetin	46.43	0.28
	MOL004891	Shinpterocarpin	80.30	0.73
	MOL000359	Sitosterol	36.91	0.75
JieGeng	MOL001689	Acacetin	34.97	0.24
	MOL000006	Luteolin	36.16	0.25
QianHu	MOL005100	5,7-dihydroxy-2-(3-hydroxy-4-methoxyphenyl)chroman-4-one	47.74	0.27
	MOL000358	β-sitosterol	36.91	0.75
	MOL000098	Quercetin	46.43	0.28
	MOL013083	Skimmin (8CI)	38.35	0.32
	MOL007154	tanshinone IIa	49.89	0.40
RenShen	MOL005320	Arachidonate	45.57	0.20
	MOL000358	β-sitosterol	36.91	0.75
	MOL000422	kaempferol	41.88	0.24
	MOL000449	Stigmasterol	43.83	0.76

Table 1. Cont.

Drug	Mol ID	Molecule Name	OB (%)	DL
ZhiKe	MOL000358	β-sitosterol	36.91	0.75
	MOL002341	Hesperetin	70.31	0.27
	MOL004328	Naringenin	61.67	0.52
	MOL005828	Nobiletin	61.67	0.52
BoHe	MOL005190	Eriodictyol	71.79	0.24
ShengJiang	MOL008698	Dihydrocapsaicin	47.07	0.19
	MOL001771	Poriferast-5-en-3β-ol	36.91	0.75

Note: OB: oral bioavailability; DL: drug-likeness.

2.2. The Construction of the Drug-Ingredient-Target Relationship Network

We imported drug–ingredient–target relationships into the Cytoscape (v3.7.2, Paul Shannon, CA, USA) software (containing 12 drugs, 39 active ingredients, and 115 targets) to construct a drug–ingredient–target network diagram for the treatment of IBD with RSBDP (Figure 2). The dark blue color represents the drug composition of RSBDP, the light purple color denotes the main active ingredients of the drug, and the yellow color signifies the common targets of the active ingredients and IBD-related targets. The size of the ingredient node correlates positively with the degrees.

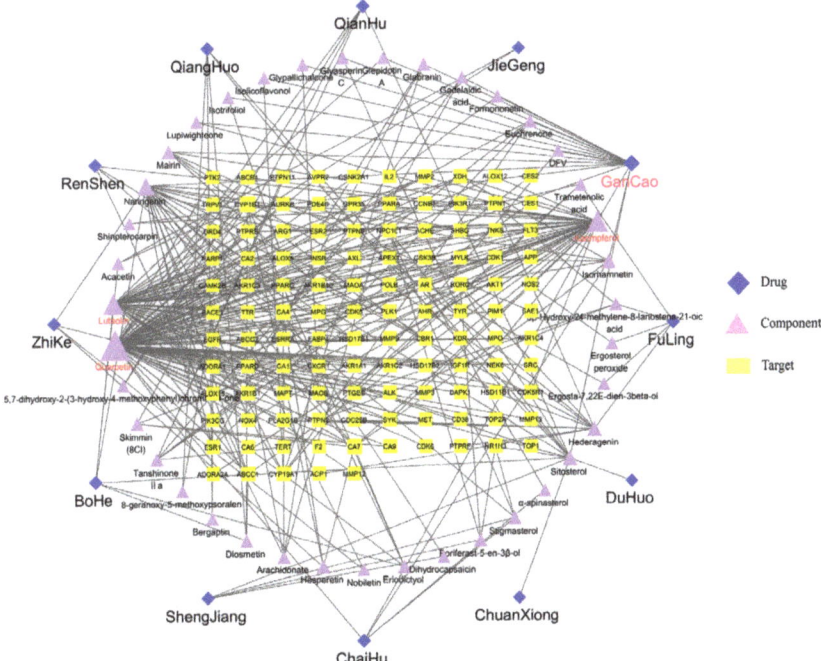

Figure 2. The drug–ingredient–target network for RSBDP in the treatment of IBD. The dark blue diamond the drug; the light purple triangle the pharmaceutical ingredients; the yellow rectangle the potential targets. Node size represents degree value.

We performed topological analyses of the drug-ingredient-target network in the Cytoscape 3.7.2 software using "degree value" as a screening parameter for the active ingredients. Our results suggest that quercetin, kaempferol, luteolin, naringenin, and sitosterol were the potential key molecules for RSBDP's treatment of IBD (Table 2).

Table 2. Key molecules and topological parameters of RSBDP against IBD (Top 5).

Ingredients	Betweenness Centrality	Closeness Centrality	Degree
Quercetin	0.55011787	0.49848943	76
Kaempferol	0.15632436	0.39568345	40
Luteolin	0.1629187	0.3724605	37
Naringenin	0.04758899	0.33199195	23
Sitosterol	0.11861359	0.3674833	13

We also analyzed the core targets of RSBDP for IBD treatment in the same way in the Cytoscape 3.7.2 software. The top 10 targets, namely cytochrome P4501B1 (CYP1B1), carbonic anhydrase 7 (CA7), cytochrome P45019A1 (CYP19A1), carbonic anhydrase 4 (CA4), protein tyrosine phosphatase 1 (PTPN1), estrogen receptor 2 (ESR2), multidrug resistance-associated protein 1 (ABCC1), ATP-binding transporter protein G family member 2 (ABCG2), estrogen receptor 2 (ESR1), and cyclin-dependent kinase 1 (CDK1), are also listed in Table 3.

Table 3. Topological analysis of key targets of RSBDP against IBD (Top 10).

Targets	Betweenness Centrality	Closeness Centrality	Degree
Cytochrome P450 1B1 (CYP1B1)	0.03810726	0.38461538	11
Carbonic anhydrase 7 (CA7)	0.021592	0.37931034	9
Cytochrome P450 19A1 (CYP19A1)	0.01553419	0.35031847	8
Carbonic anhydrase 4 (CA4)	0.01578918	0.37757437	8
Protein-tyrosine phosphatase 1 (PTPN1)	0.03389732	0.264	6
Estrogen receptor 2 (ESR2)	0.00985945	0.35791757	6
Multidrug resistance-associated protein 1 (ABCC1)	0.01345788	0.37585421	6
ATP-binding cassette sub-family G member 2 (ABCG2)	0.01657	0.37078652	5
Estrogen receptor 1 (ESR1)	0.01515971	0.2519084	4
Cyclin-dependent kinase 1 (CDK1)	0.00317045	0.36423841	4

2.3. The Construction and Topological Analysis of the PPI Network

This study imported the 115 obtained common targets into the SRING database to create a PPI network diagram (Figure 3), in which the larger the "degree value", the larger the node. The top 10 targets based on their degree values were retained (Table 4): they included tyrosine kinase Src (SRC), epidermal growth factor receptor (EGFR), serine/threonine-protein kinase AKT (AKT1), phosphoinositide-3-kinase regulatory subunit 1 (PIK3R1), tyrosine-protein phosphatase non-receptor type 11 (PTPN11), estrogen receptor 1 (ESR1), androgen receptor (AR), Aldo-keto reductase 1C3 (AKR1C3), tyrosine-protein phosphatase non-receptor type 1 (PTPN1), and cyclin-dependent kinase 1 (CDK1).

Table 4. Topological analysis of the protein-protein interaction of RSBDP against IBD (Top 10).

Targets	Betweenness Centrality	Closeness Centrality	Degree
Tyrosine kinase Src (SRC)	0.27275215	0.48369565	29
Epidermal growth factor receptor (EGFR)	0.1388039	0.44278607	22
Serine/threonine-protein kinase AKT (AKT1)	0.17437856	0.45641026	21
Phosphoinositide-3-kinase regulatory subunit 1 (PIK3R1)	0.05651908	0.41588785	20
Tyrosine-protein phosphatase non-receptor type 11 (PTPN11)	0.0334887	0.38695652	19
Estrogen receptor α (ESR1)	0.15395677	0.41588785	15
Androgen receptor (AR)	0.2042839	0.41784038	12
Aldo-keto reductase 1C3 (AKR1C3)	0.20965192	0.33584906	11
Tyrosine-protein phosphatase non-receptor type 1 (PTPN1)	0.01003103	0.35742972	11
Cyclin-dependent kinase 1 (CDK1)	0.07792777	0.38864629	11

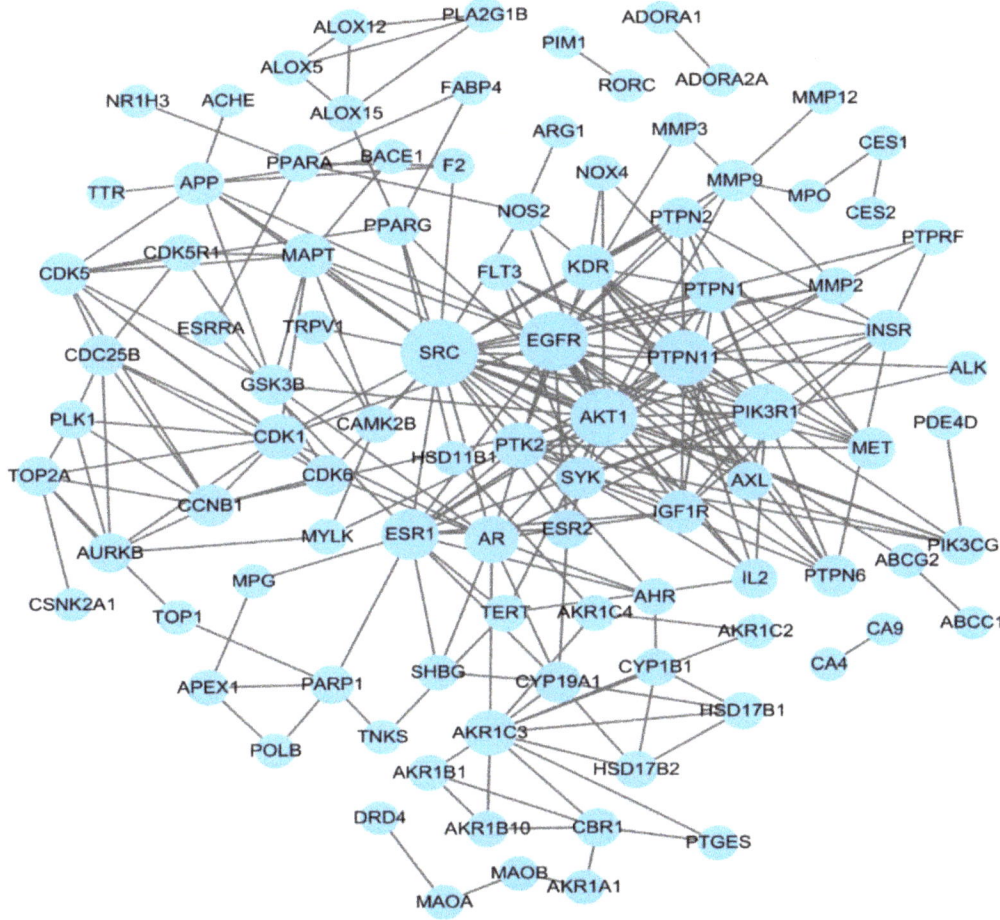

Figure 3. The PPI network of targets. Node size represents degree value.

2.4. GO and KEGG Enrichment Analyses

To further illustrate the biological functions of the 115 intersecting targets, we imported them into the DAVID database for GO and KEGG enrichment analyses. GO examination consisted of three modules: Biological process (BP), Molecular function (MF), and Cellular component (CC). We sorted the top 15 GO items in each module according to the count number (from the largest to the smallest) and then drew the GO function enrichment map (Figure 4). The targets in BP were mainly involved in the oxidation–reduction process, signal transduction, and negative regulation of apoptotic process; the targets in MF mostly took part in protein binding, ATP binding, and zinc ion binding; the targets in CC participated primarily in the cytosol, nucleus, and plasma membrane.

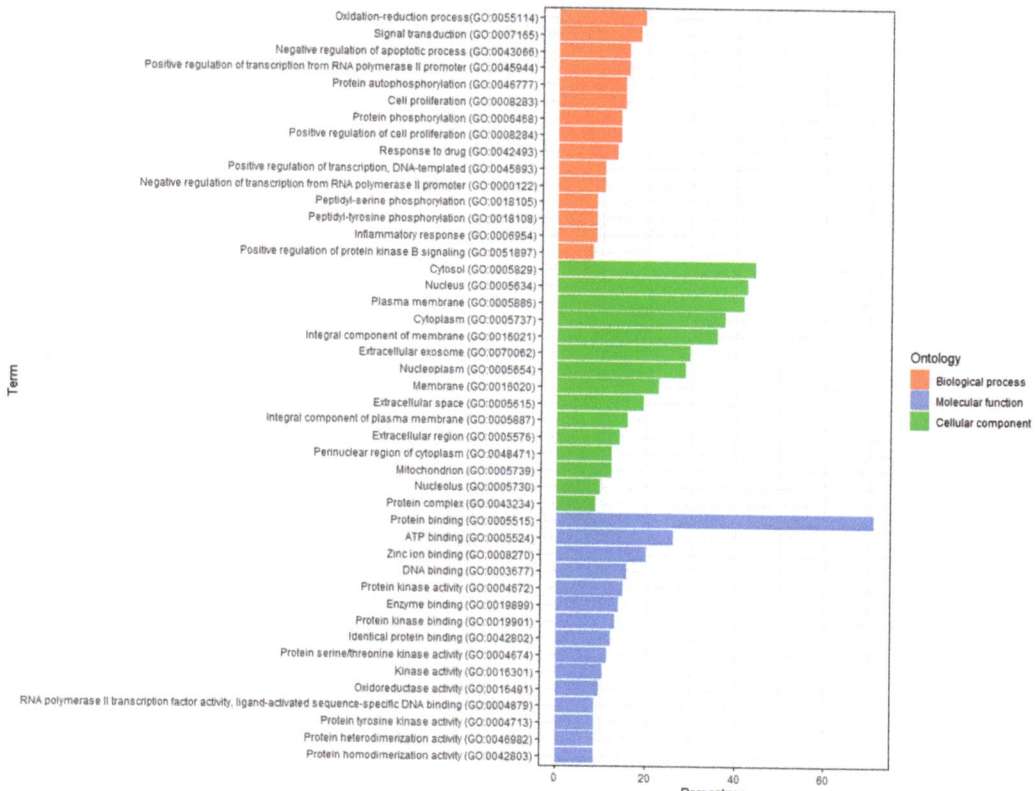

Figure 4. The GO analysis of key targets.

The KEGG pathway analysis returned 74 items, and we selected the top 20 for a visual analysis based on gene count number rank (Figure 5). The analysis revealed that these targets were predominantly enriched in pathways in cancer, proteoglycans in cancer, focal adhesion, insulin resistance, and adherens junction.

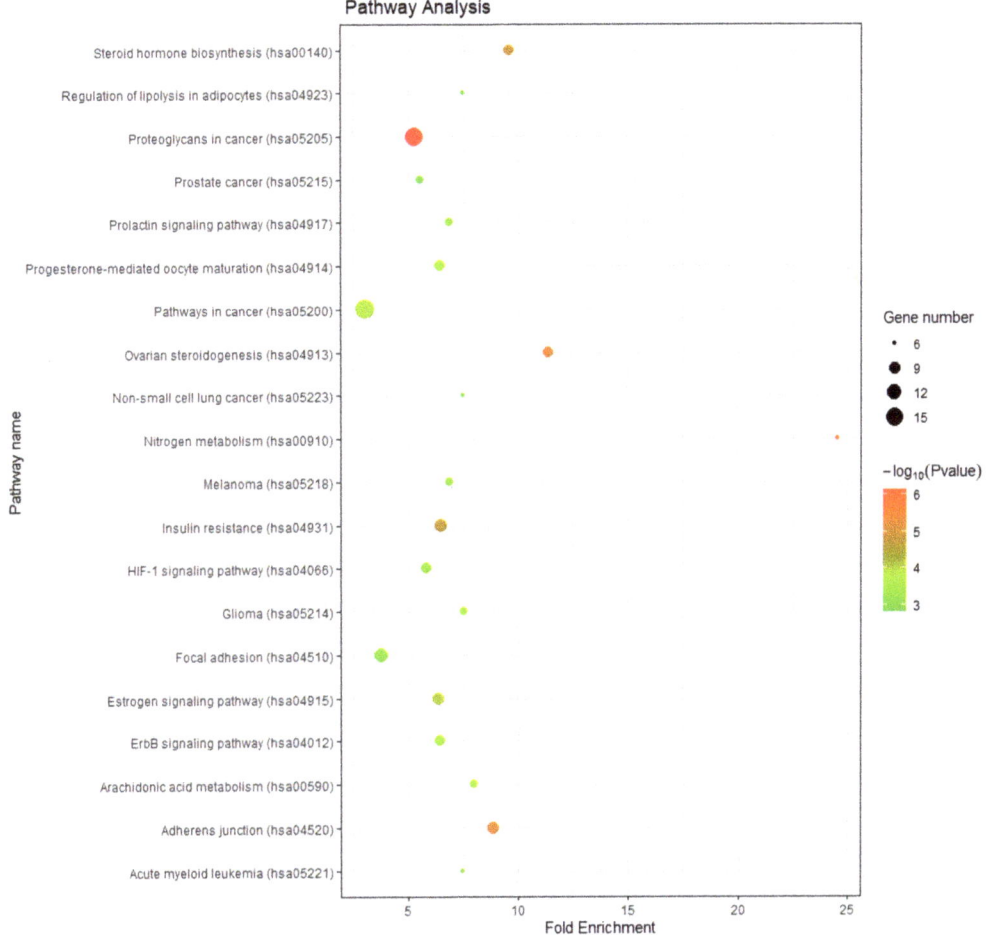

Figure 5. The KEGG pathway analysis of key targets.

2.5. Molecular Docking of Vital Active Ingredients and Core Targets

This study selected a portion of the molecular docking results for display in this study (Figure 6). Five vital active ingredients (quercetin, kaempferol, luteolin, naringenin, and sitosterol) and ingredient-related targets (CYP1B1, SRC, ESR2, ABCG2, CYP19A1, AhR, CA4, ALOX5, ABCC1, ESR1, and NOS2) were designated as ligands and receptors, respectively. A binding energy score of the ligand and receptor less than −5 kcal/mol indicates a strong affinity, as reported previously [10].

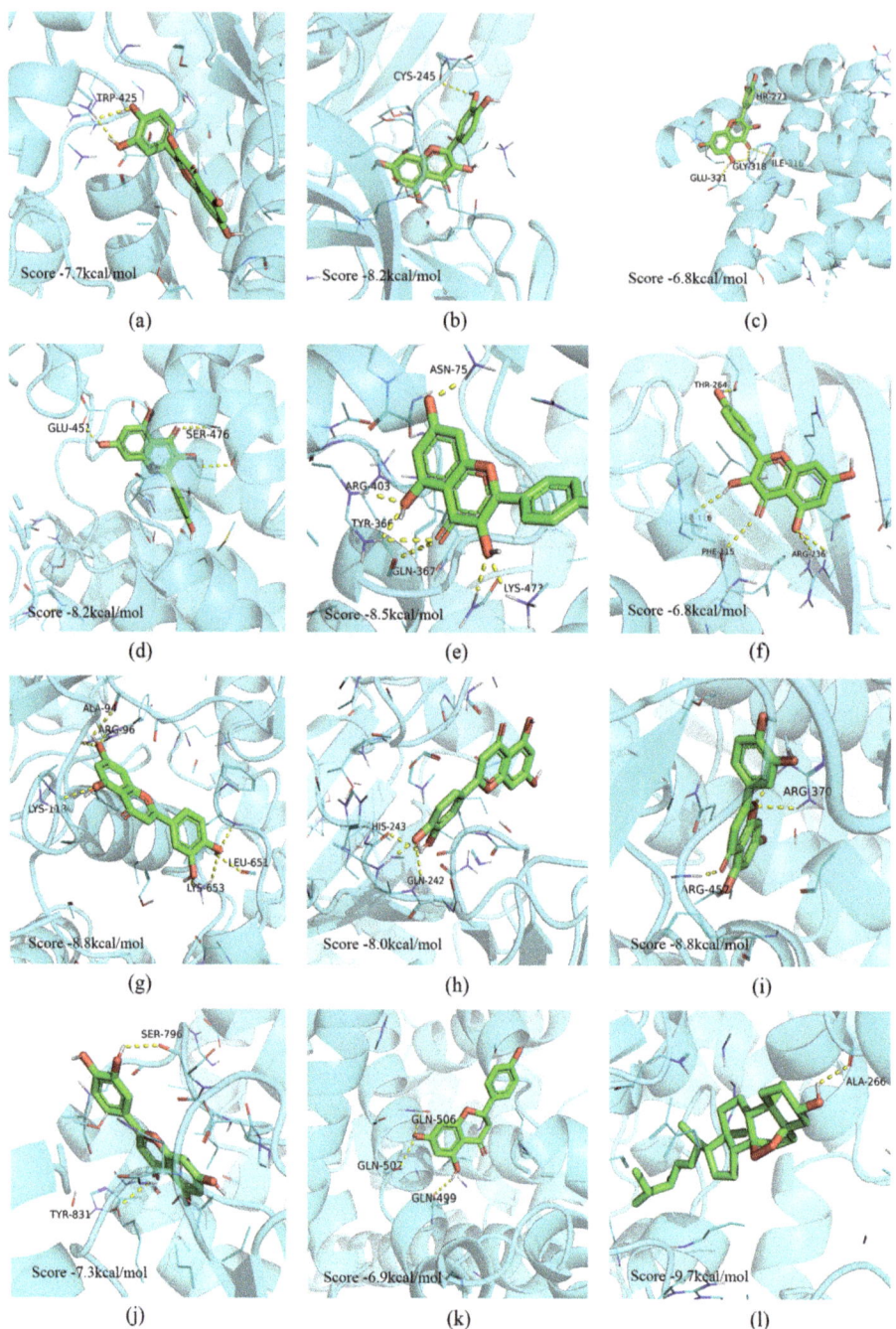

Figure 6. Molecular docking model of vital active ingredients and core targets. (**a**) Quercetin-CYP1B1; (**b**) Quercetin-SRC; (**c**) Quercetin-ESR2; (**d**) Kaempferol-ABCG2; (**e**) Kaempferol-CYP19A1; (**f**) Kaempferol-AhR; (**g**) Luteolin-ABCG2; (**h**) Luteolin-CA4; (**i**) Luteolin-ALOX5; (**j**) Luteolin-ABCC1; (**k**) Naringenin-ESR1; (**l**) Ergosterol peroxide-NOS2.

2.6. Validation of RSBDP Treatment Effectiveness and Targets

To further study the therapeutic effect of RSBDP on treating IBD, we constructed the experimental colitis model using 3% DSS and treated it with RSBDP (Figure 7a). Firstly, we found that the body weight of DSS-induced mice started to decrease from the seventh day. After RSBDP treatment on the ninth day, the body weight of the DSS + RSBDP group gradually recovered, while the body weight of the DSS group still decreased (Figure 7b). Afterward, the intestinal tissues from the mice were removed, and the length of their intestines were measured. The intestines of the DSS group were significantly shorter than the DSS + RSBDP group and still showed signs of congestion and inflammation (Figure 7c). Histological analysis further indicated the remarkable attenuation of inflammatory cell infiltration and mucosal damage in DSS + RSBDP (Figure 7d). Moreover, the ki67 expression level was higher in the DSS + RSBDP group than in the DSS and control groups (Figure 7e). Figure 7f showed that three genes related to the intestinal barrier (*ZO-1*, *Occludin*, and *Claudin-1*) were up-regulated in the DSS + RSBDP group but not statistically different from the DSS group. Serum concentrations of IL-1, IL-6, and IL-8 were lower in the DSS + RSBDP group than in the DSS group, among which the level of IL-8 was significantly lower (Figure 7g). Similarly, the protein level of TNF-α was also declined in DSS + RSBDP group (Figure 7i).

In order to further reveal the underlying mechanism of RSBDP in the treatment of IBD, we performed qRT-PCR to quantify the mRNA abundance of the key targets of RSBDP against IBD in Table 3. As expected, these key targets, such as *CA7*, *CPY1B1*, and *PTPN11*, were significantly up-regulated in the DSS + RSBDP group. In particular, the expression level of *CYP1B1* in the DSS + RSBDP group was up-regulated by as high as 9-fold compared to the DSS group (Figure 7h). Finally, we detected the protein levels of key targets (as shown in Table 4) and their downstream targets. Western blotting results indicated that the protein levels of AKR1C1, PI3K, AKT, p-AKT, Bax, and Bcl-2 were significantly up- and down-regulated in the DSS + RSBDP group. The quantitative analysis of western blot is shown in Figure 7j. Altogether, RSBDP affects the development of IBD by pro-apoptosis and remodeling the intestinal epithelial barrier in the DSS-induced IBD model.

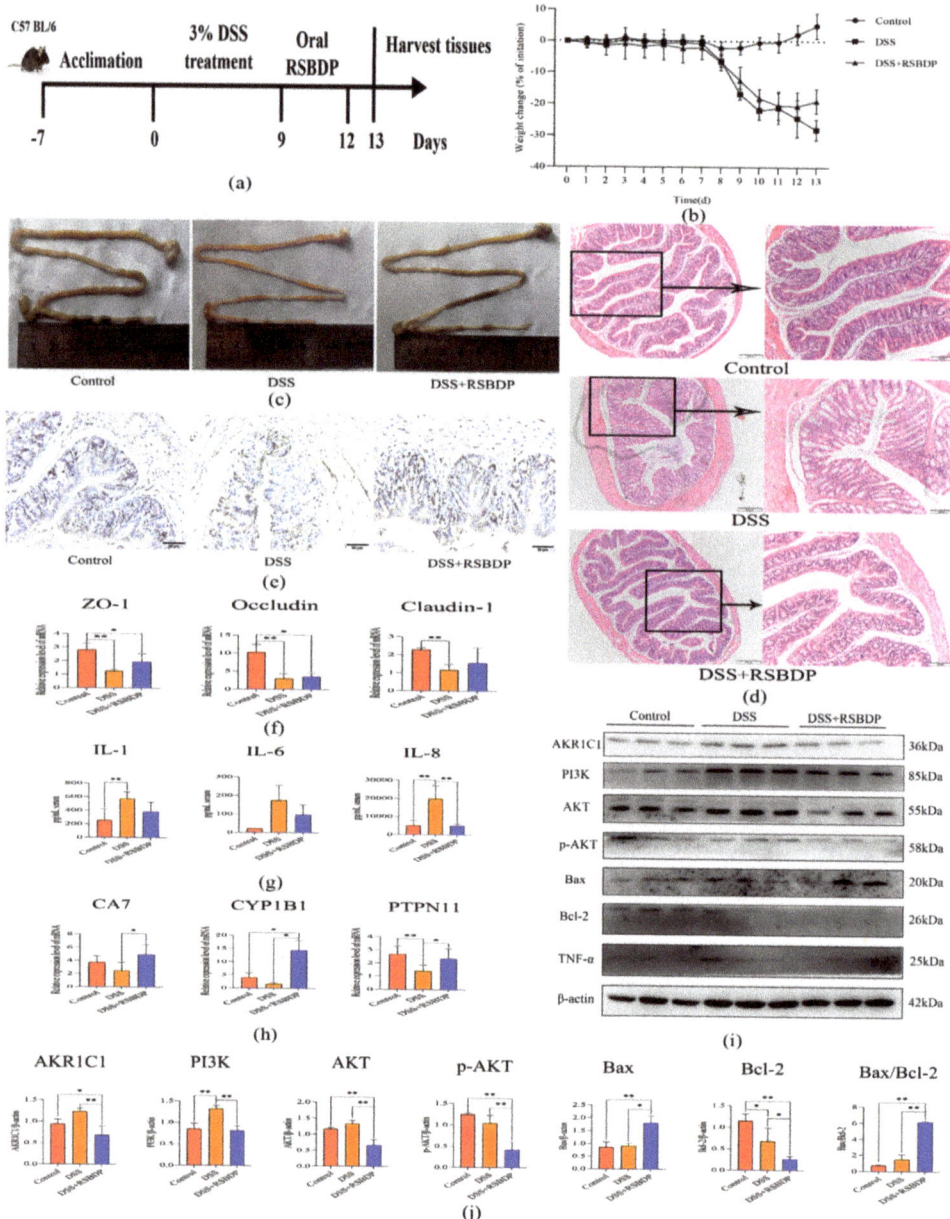

Figure 7. Experimental validation in DSS-induced colitis model. (**a**) An illustration of the mouse model of colitis used in this study. (**b**) Changes in body weight of mice after DSS and RSBDP treatment. (**c**) The intestines from control and IBD mice with RSBDP therapy. (**d**) H&E staining of the colon from control, DSS, and DSS + RSBDP groups. (**e**) The immunohistochemical results of the proliferation-associated maker gene Ki67. (**f**) qRT−PCR results of ZO−1, Occludin, and Claudin−1. (**g**) The concentrations of IL−1, IL−6, and IL−8 in serum. (**h**) qRT−PCR detection of the partial targets in Tables 3 and 4. (**i**) Western blot analysis of AKR1C1, PI3K, AKT, p−AKT, Bax, Bcl−2, and TNF−α. (**j**) The quantitative analysis of western blot. Data were shown as means ± SEM (n = 3–5 per group). * $p < 0.05$, ** $p < 0.01$.

3. Discussion

IBD is a chronic, relapsing, non-specific inflammatory disease of the intestine and is recognizable in two forms, UC and CD. It is persistent and destructive and can cause a variety of complications, including abscesses, fistulas, bleeding, and colitis-related tumors, and cancers [11]. Therefore, finding effective treatments is a high clinical imperative for patients subjected with IBD. While there is no official name for IBD in Chinese medicine, its clinical features are often identified as "dysentery", "diarrhea", and "hemorrhoidal hamorrhage". RSBDP, a well-known formula in Chinese medicine for dysentery therapy, is currently being used to treat IBD and has yielded decent clinical results [12]. To elucidate the potential molecular mechanism of RSBDP's treatment of IBD, we quarried the TCMSP database and screened for the main active ingredients of RSBDP against IBD, obtaining a total of 39 active compounds, comprised predominantly of quercetin, kaempferol, luteolin, naringenin, and sitosterol (Top 5). This is not unexpected, as several studies have demonstrated that these active ingredients (Top 5) relieve symptoms of drug-induced colitis and maintain the integrity of the intestinal epithelium [13–18]. Remarkably, among the 39 main active ingredients, those with similar effects but available in lower quantities, like tanshinone IIa [19], eriodictyol [20], arachidonate [21], acacetin [22], and nobiletin [17], have also displayed acceptable clinical effects in the colitis model. Therefore, RSBDP possibly exerts its therapeutic influence against IBD through the synergy of multiple ingredients.

It is recognized that IBD is a complex immune disease affected by genetic and environmental factors, and a deeper understanding of the unique role of the intestinal epithelium in its pathogenesis appears key to discovering potential targets for drug therapy [23]. Therefore, genes involved in pathways, such as intestinal barrier integrity [24], adaptive immunity [25], inflammation and fibrosis [23], and inflammasome signaling [26], could all be potential therapeutic targets. Therefore, topological, PPI, GO, and KEGG analyses of key targets could provide some insights into RSBDP's actions against IBD.

The aryl hydrocarbon receptor (AhR) is one of the potential targets of RSBDP's treatment of IBD, exerting various regulatory effects through binding to flavonoids or natural drugs and influencing the transduction of downstream signaling pathways [27,28]. Evidence suggests that AhR can induce the regulation of the expression of a series of CYP enzymes [29], pointing to flavonoid-related ingredients of RSBDP's ability to regulate and maintain the homeostasis of the intestinal epithelium by activating the AhR/CYP pathway. Consistent with these reports, our molecular docking results indicated that kaempferol bound well with AhR (Figure 6f). The qRT-PCR results showed that oral administration of RSBDP significantly promoted the expression of *CYP1B1* (Figure 7h). Particularly, members of the CYP family participate in the activation and suppression of inflammation via the synthesis and breakdown of bioactive mediators (e.g., converting fatty acids into pro- or anti-inflammatory factors) [29,30]. The CYP family is also involved in the synthesis and metabolism of various hormones in organisms, and certain hormones (e.g., estrogen and progesterone) promote the wound healing of intestinal epithelium, alleviate the endoplasmic reticulum stress, reduce the pro-inflammatory factors secretion, and improve intestinal epithelial cell barrier [31].

To further reveal the mechanism of RSBDP against IBD, we integrated and analyzed the results of PPI, GO, and KEGG, focusing on the AKR1C1/PI3K/AKT pathway. Although the gene and protein sequences of mouse AKR1C3 were not available in the NCBI database, a previous study analyzed the homology of human AKR1C3 with mouse AKR1C family, and suggested that the mouseAKR1C1 (also known as AKR1C6 in mouse) and human AKR1C3 has higher homology and the similar functions [32]. Interestingly, several studies pointed out that the decreased levels of AKR1C1/AKR1C3 protein can inhibit the phosphorylation of AKT [33,34]. In this study, oral RSBDP decreased the protein concentration of AKR1C1, PI3K, AKT, and p-AKT, which hinted that RSBDP regulates the intestinal epithelial barrier through inhibition of the AKR1C1/PI3K/AKT pathway in the DSS-induced mice. In addition, research shows that PI3K/AKT signaling pathway plays an essential role in cellular processes and apoptosis [35]. Hence, Bax and Bcl-2, two apoptosis-related proteins, were detected in this study. Some evidence suggested that sodium selenite, melatonin, and dapagliflozin alleviate IBD by anti-apoptosis in experimental IBD model [36–38]. Unexpectedly, our study indicated that the protein concentrations of Bax and Bcl-2 were up- and down-regulated after oral RSBDP, respectively. Thus, our results demonstrate that RSBDP displays a unique role in leading to the alleviation of IBD by promoting apoptosis in intestinal epithelial cells. Similarly, several reports suggested that pro-apoptosis may be a new approach to treating colitis [39–41].

In this study, we confirmed the positive effect of RSBDP on DSS-induced mice at the molecular level. However, the ingredients of RSBDP are pretty complex, and it would be fascinating to explore the therapeutic effects of critical ingredients of RSBDP in IBD. As the vital natural flavonoid ingredients of RSBDP, quercetin, kaempferol, luteolin, and naringenin have all been demonstrated to resist IBD through anti-inflammatory and antioxidant pathways [13–17]. Consistent with these studies, our results confirmed that RSBDP exerts its anti-inflammatory effects (significantly reduces serum IL-1, IL-6, and IL-8 concentrations) through these critical ingredients in the IBD model. Remarkably, the natural flavonols are important ligands for AhR, and the activation of AhR plays a pivotal role in the development of IBD [24,42]. Here, the molecule docking results revealed that kaempferol and AhR had an excellent bonding capability (-6.8 kcal/mol), which hints that the major active ingredients of RSBDP might act as ligands of AhR to activate downstream signaling pathways. Moreover, a few studies demonstrated that quercetin cannot alleviate the symptoms of colitis in $AhR^{-/-}$ mice [13]. Hence, the critical ingredients of RSBDP might combat IBD by activating AhR pathway. A recent study indicated that the aromatic compounds in coffee could promote the expression of *CYP1A1* and *CYP1B1* by activating AhR, which alleviates experimental colitis [43]. Our results also demonstrated that RSBDP promotes *CYP1B1* expression through AhR, reducing inflammation in IBD models. RSBDP also promotes the apoptosis of intestinal epithelial cells via AKR1C1/PI3K/AKT and, thus, against IBD. Although there is no direct evidence that the critical ingredients of RSBDP can alleviates the symptoms of IBD by affecting the concentration of *AKR1C1*, indirect evidence suggests that the addition of kaempferol inhibited the mRNA level of *AKR1C1* and induced apoptosis in non-small cell lung cancer cells [44]. Finally, RSBDP alleviation of IBD may function, but is not limited to, through the five major ingredients (quercetin, kaempferol, luteolin, naringenin, and sitosterol).

4. Materials and Methods

4.1. Screening for the Main Active Ingredients of RSBDP

Data on the main active compounds of RSBDP were retrieved from the Traditional Chinese Medicine Systems Pharmacology Database and Analysis Platform (TCMSP, https://lsp.nwu.edu.cn/tcmsp.php, accessed on 4 September 2021) [45]. Oral bioavailability (OB) and drug likeness (DL) indices were used to evaluate drug feasibility. In this study, molecules with OB of $\geq 30\%$ and DL of ≥ 0.18 were considered as the potential active compounds based on screening parameters. The chemical structural formula of ingredients of RSBDP were obtained from the PubChem database (https://pubchem.ncbi.nlm.nih.gov/, accessed on 6 September 2021) by importing the unique IDs of the retrieved compounds [46].

4.2. The Target Prediction of RSBDP Ingredients for IBD Therapy

The collated structural formulae of the main active ingredients were imported into the SwissTargetPrediction database [47] (http://www.swisstargetprediction.ch/, accessed on 15 September 2021) for molecular docking and screened potential targets using a probability threshold ≥ 0.5. Meanwhile, the keywords "inflammatory bowel disease" were input into GeneCards [48] (https://www.genecards.org/, accessed on 15 September 2021) and OpenTargets [49] (https://www.opentargets.org/, accessed on 15 September 2021) databases to search for IBD-related proteins. The IBD targets obtained from both databases were first merged and then overlapped with the potential targets acquired by prediction from the SwissTargetPrediction database for subsequent analysis.

4.3. The Construction and Analysis of a "Drug-Ingredient-Target" Network

We verified the results from Section 2.2, removing ineffective targets and importing effective targets into Cytoscape 3.7.2 to construct a drug-ingredient-target network and perform topological analysis [50].

4.4. The Construction and Analysis of the Protein-Protein Interaction Network

The screened 115 targets were introduced into the STRING database [51] (https://string-db.org/, accessed on 15 September 2021) and set the "minimum required interaction score" for the protein-protein interaction network (PPI) analysis to 0.7 [10]. The PPI network was mapped using the Cytoscape software.

4.5. Gene Ontology and Kyoto Encyclopedia of Genes and Genomes Signal Pathway Enrichment Analysis

We performed the Kyoto Encyclopedia of Genes and Genomes (KEGG) and Gene Ontology (GO) enrichment analyses on the targets from Section 2.3 using the DAVID database. After downloading and collating the relevant data, we visualized them using the ggplot2 package in the R software.

4.6. Molecular Docking Analysis

Molecular docking analyses of the screened key ingredients and their targets were conducted. The 3D molecular structures of the vital active ingredients and their targets were obtained from the Pubchem [46] and PDB [52] databases, respectively, and the Autodock software was employed for the removal of the water molecules of target proteins and generation of PDBQT format files. Molecular docking and importation of the downstream files into the Pymol software to create visual images were carried out using the Autodock Vina program.

4.7. Animal Experiment

4.7.1. Drug

In this study, Panax ginseng, Radix bupleuri, Radix Peucedani, Rhizoma Ligustic Chuanxiong, Fructus Aurantii, Rhizoma et Radix Notopterygii, Radix Angelicae Pubescentis, Poria, Radix Platycodonis, Radix Glycyrrhizae, Rhizoma Zingiberis Recens, and Herba Menthae were purchased from the outpatient department of Chengdu University of traditional Chinese medicine (Chengdu, China), and they were conformed to the quality standards of Chinese Pharmacopoeia (2015 edition). Afterward, these herbs were authenticated by Prof. Jin Pei (Department of Pharmacognosy, Chengdu University of traditional Chinese medicine). Finally, all herbs were crushed separately and mix the above herbs according to the ratio 2:4:2:3:2:2:2:2:2:2:1:1, then added 750 mL (1:10 g/v) of pure water and boiled for 20 min. Subsequently, the drug solution was filtered through a 0.45um filter and concentrated to 75 mL (stored at $-20\ °C$).

4.7.2. Animals and Experimental Design

Six-week-old male C57BL/6 mice were maintained with five to six animals per cage and house in specific pathogen-free facility with a 12-h light and 12-h dark cycle at 22 °C.

All mice were randomly divided into three groups, control group ($n = 5$), DSS group ($n = 6$) and RSBDP+DSS group ($n = 6$). 3% dextran sodium sulfate (DSS, MP Biomedicals) was added to drinking water for 9 days. For the next 5 days, 0.308 mL of saline was gavaged daily in the control and DSS groups, and 0.308 mL of drug solution was gavaged daily in the RSBDP + DSS group. All mice were euthanized at the end of the experiment. Tissues or serum were frozen in liquid nitrogen, and colon specimens were fixed in 4% paraformaldehyde.

4.7.3. Histological Analysis

Hematoxylin and eosin (H&E) was used to measure the degree to which the colon had been damaged and inflamed, and the epithelial proliferation was detected using Ki67 (1:500, Servicebio, Wuhan, China).

4.7.4. Enzyme-Linked Immunosorbent Assay

IL-1, IL-6, and IL-8 were performed on serum using the ELISA Kit according to the manufacturer's instructions (HYCEZMBIO, Wuhan, China).

4.7.5. RNA Extraction and Quantitative Real-Time PCR (qRT-PCR)

RNA extraction was performed using EASYspin Plus Kit (Aidlab, Beijing, China) following the manufacturer's instructions, and the HiScript II qRT SuperMix R223 (Vazyme, Nanjing, China) was used to transcribe total RNA into cDNA. The ChamQ Universal SYBR qPCR Master Mix Q711 (Vazyme, Nanjing, China) was used for qRT-PCR. The primer sequences are listed in Table S1.

4.7.6. Western Blotting

Tissues were lyzed in RIPA buffer (Biosharp, Hefei, China) containing phenylmethylsulfonyl fluoride (PMSF) and phosphatase inhibitors, and the extracts were centrifuged at 14,000 rpm for 10 min at 4 °C. The 10% SDS-PAGE was used to separate total protein, then transferred onto the polyvinylidene fluoride (PVDF) membrane. Primary antibodies include AKR1C1 (A13004), PI3K (A11526), Bax (A19684), Bcl-2 (A20736), TNF-α (A11534), and β-actin (AC028) were purchased from ABclonal (Wuhan, China); AKT (AF6261) was purchased from Affinity (Cincinnati, OH, USA); p-AKT (80455-1-RR) was purchased from Proteintech (Wuhan, China). Anti-rabbit or -mouse IgG conjugated to horseradish peroxidase was applied after secondary antibody incubation for protein detection.

4.7.7. Statistics

The experimental results are presented as means ± SEM for each group with at least three independent experiments. Data analysis using one-way ANOVA followed by LSD test. The $p < 0.05$ was considered statistically significant.

5. Conclusions

In summary, we firstly performed the network pharmacology combined with molecular docking approach to elucidate that the anti-IBD effects and the underlying mechanism of RSBDP, and the key targets of RSBDP against IBD were partially identified by experiments, including CA7, CYP1B1, and PTPN11. In addition, western blotting results revealed multiple functions of RSBDP in the DSS-induced colitis which were exerted by anti-inflammatory and pro-apoptotic activities, relying on the AhR/CYP1B1 and AKR1C1/PI3K/AKT pathways.

Supplementary Materials: The following supporting information can be downloaded at: https://www.mdpi.com/article/10.3390/ph15091038/s1, Table S1: Sequences of primers used for qRT-PCR.

Author Contributions: Conceptualization, N.J., X.H. and Y.Z. (Yi Zhou); methodology, N.J.; software, Y.Z. (Yiyi Zhang); validation, N.J. and Y.L.; formal analysis, N.J., Y.L. and P.X.; investigation, N.J., Y.L., P.X. and J.M.; resources, Y.Z. (Yi Zhou); data curation, N.J.; writing—original draft preparation, N.J.; writing—review and editing, Y.Z. (Yi Zhou) and X.H.; visualization, N.J., J.M. and Y.Z. (Yiyi Zhang); funding acquisition, Y.Z. (Yi Zhou). All authors have read and agreed to the published version of the manuscript.

Funding: This work was supported by the National Facility for Translational Medicine Open Project (TMSK-2021-411).

Institutional Review Board Statement: The animal experimental protocol was approved by the Animal Experimentation Ethics Committee of Chengdu University of Traditional Chinese Medicine (Application Approval No. 2022-03, approved on March 2022).

Informed Consent Statement: Not applicable.

Data Availability Statement: Data is contained within the article and Supplementary Material.

Acknowledgments: Special thanks to Luo Gan from Huazhong Agricultural University for her help with the research.

Conflicts of Interest: The authors declare that there are no conflict of interest.

References

1. Nikolaus, S.; Schulte, B.; Al-Massad, N.; Thieme, F.; Schulte, D.M.; Bethge, J.; Rehman, A.; Tran, F.; Aden, K.; Hasler, R.; et al. Increased Tryptophan Metabolism Is Associated with Activity of Inflammatory Bowel Diseases. *Gastroenterology* **2017**, *153*, 1504–1516.e2. [CrossRef] [PubMed]
2. Zuo, T.; Kamm, M.A.; Colombel, J.F.; Ng, S.C. Urbanization and the gut microbiota in health and inflammatory bowel disease. *Nat. Rev. Gastroenterol. Hepatol.* **2018**, *15*, 440–452. [CrossRef] [PubMed]
3. Olivera, P.; Danese, S.; Jay, N.; Natoli, G.; Peyrin-Biroulet, L. Big data in IBD: A look into the future. *Nat. Rev. Gastroenterol. Hepatol.* **2019**, *16*, 312–321. [CrossRef] [PubMed]
4. Xu, Z.; Zhang, M.; Dou, D.; Kang, T.; Li, F. Effects of Deoxyschisandrin on Visceral Sensitivity of Mice with Inflammatory Bowel Disease. *Evid. Based Complement. Altern. Med.* **2019**, *2019*, 2986097. [CrossRef]
5. Curro, D.; Ianiro, G.; Pecere, S.; Bibbo, S.; Cammarota, G. Probiotics, fibre and herbal medicinal products for functional and inflammatory bowel disorders. *Br. J. Pharmacol.* **2017**, *174*, 1426–1449. [CrossRef]
6. Chen, T.F.; Hsu, J.T.; Wu, K.C.; Hsiao, C.F.; Lin, J.A.; Cheng, Y.H.; Liu, Y.H.; Lee, D.Y.; Chang, H.H.; Cho, D.Y.; et al. A systematic identification of anti-inflammatory active components derived from Mu Dan Pi and their applications in inflammatory bowel disease. *Sci. Rep.* **2020**, *10*, 17238. [CrossRef]
7. Xiong, P.; Chen, L.; Chen, X.; Zhang, P.; Zhong, C.; Liu, X.; Jia, B. Based on "Reverse Flow Carrying Boat" Approach to Explore the Intervention Effect of Renshen Baidu Powder on Intestinal Mucosal Barrier Ulcerative Colitis in Rats. *Mod. Tradit. Chin. Med. Mater. Med. World Sci. Technol.* **2021**, *23*, 2285–2293.
8. Liu, B.; Zheng, X.; Li, J.; Li, X.; Wu, R.; Yang, J.; Liu, W.; Zhao, G. Revealing mechanism of Caulis Sargentodoxae for the treatment of ulcerative colitis based on network pharmacology approach. *Biosci. Rep.* **2021**, *41*, BSR20204005. [CrossRef]
9. Chen, D.; Wu, Y.; Chen, Y.; Chen, Q.; Ye, X.; Xu, S.; Luo, S. Exploration of the molecular targets and mechanisms of suxiao xintong dropping pills for myocardial infarction by network pharmacology method. *Biosci. Rep.* **2021**, *41*, BSR20204211. [CrossRef]
10. Guo, K.; Wang, T.; Luo, E.; Leng, X.; Yao, B. Use of Network Pharmacology and Molecular Docking Technology to Analyze the Mechanism of Action of Velvet Antler in the Treatment of Postmenopausal Osteoporosis. *Evid. Based Complement. Altern. Med.* **2021**, *2021*, 7144529. [CrossRef]
11. Neurath, M.F. Current and emerging therapeutic targets for IBD. *Nat. Rev. Gastroenterol. Hepatol.* **2017**, *14*, 269–278. [CrossRef]
12. Chen, L.; Jia, B.; Deng, H. Treatment of ulcerative colitis based on the Niliu Wanzhou' method. *China J. Tradit. Chin. Med. Pharm.* **2019**, *34*, 527–529.
13. Riemschneider, S.; Hoffmann, M.; Slanina, U.; Weber, K.; Hauschildt, S.; Lehmann, J. Indol-3-Carbinol and Quercetin Ameliorate Chronic DSS-Induced Colitis in C57BL/6 Mice by AhR-Mediated Anti-Inflammatory Mechanisms. *Int. J. Environ. Res. Public Health* **2021**, *18*, 2262. [CrossRef]
14. Ju, S.; Ge, Y.; Li, P.; Tian, X.; Wang, H.; Zheng, X.; Ju, S. Dietary quercetin ameliorates experimental colitis in mouse by remodeling the function of colonic macrophages via a heme oxygenase-1-dependent pathway. *Cell Cycle* **2018**, *17*, 53–63. [CrossRef]
15. Bian, Y.; Dong, Y.; Sun, J.; Sun, M.; Hou, Q.; Lai, Y.; Zhang, B. Protective Effect of Kaempferol on LPS-Induced Inflammation and Barrier Dysfunction in a Coculture Model of Intestinal Epithelial Cells and Intestinal Microvascular Endothelial Cells. *J. Agric. Food Chem.* **2020**, *68*, 160–167. [CrossRef]
16. Lin, T.J.; Yin, S.Y.; Hsiao, P.W.; Yang, N.S.; Wang, I.J. Transcriptomic analysis reveals a controlling mechanism for NLRP3 and IL-17A in dextran sulfate sodium (DSS)-induced colitis. *Sci. Rep.* **2018**, *8*, 14927. [CrossRef]
17. He, W.; Li, Y.; Liu, M.; Yu, H.; Chen, Q.; Chen, Y.; Ruan, J.; Ding, Z.; Zhang, Y.; Wang, T. Citrus aurantium L. and Its Flavonoids Regulate TNBS-Induced Inflammatory Bowel Disease through Anti-Inflammation and Suppressing Isolated Jejunum Contraction. *Int. J. Mol. Sci.* **2018**, *19*, 3057. [CrossRef]
18. Feng, S.; Dai, Z.; Liu, A.; Wang, H.; Chen, J.; Luo, Z.; Yang, C.S. β-Sitosterol and stigmasterol ameliorate dextran sulfate sodium-induced colitis in mice fed a high fat Western-style diet. *Food Funct.* **2017**, *8*, 4179–4186. [CrossRef]
19. Zhang, X.; Wang, Y.; Ma, Z.; Liang, Q.; Tang, X.; Hu, D.; Tan, H.; Xiao, C.; Gao, Y. Tanshinone IIA ameliorates dextran sulfate sodium-induced inflammatory bowel disease via the pregnane X receptor. *Drug Des. Dev. Ther.* **2015**, *9*, 6343–6362. [CrossRef]
20. Wang, R.; Shen, L.; Li, H.; Peng, H. Eriodictyol attenuates dextran sodium sulphate-induced colitis in mice by regulating the sonic hedgehog signalling pathway. *Pharm. Biol.* **2021**, *59*, 974–985. [CrossRef]
21. Gil, A. Polyunsaturated fatty acids and inflammatory diseases. *Biomed. Pharmacother.* **2002**, *56*, 388–396. [CrossRef]
22. Ren, J.; Yue, B.; Wang, H.; Zhang, B.; Luo, X.; Yu, Z.; Zhang, J.; Ren, Y.; Mani, S.; Wang, Z.; et al. Acacetin Ameliorates Experimental Colitis in Mice via Inhibiting Macrophage Inflammatory Response and Regulating the Composition of Gut Microbiota. *Front. Physiol.* **2020**, *11*, 577237. [CrossRef] [PubMed]

23. Graham, D.B.; Xavier, R.J. Pathway paradigms revealed from the genetics of inflammatory bowel disease. *Nature* **2020**, *578*, 527–539. [CrossRef] [PubMed]
24. Yu, M.; Wang, Q.; Ma, Y.; Li, L.; Yu, K.; Zhang, Z.; Chen, G.; Li, X.; Xiao, W.; Xu, P.; et al. Aryl Hydrocarbon Receptor Activation Modulates Intestinal Epithelial Barrier Function by Maintaining Tight Junction Integrity. *Int. J. Biol. Sci.* **2018**, *14*, 69–77. [CrossRef]
25. Geremia, A.; Biancheri, P.; Allan, P.; Corazza, G.R.; Di Sabatino, A. Innate and adaptive immunity in inflammatory bowel disease. *Autoimmun. Rev.* **2014**, *13*, 3–10. [CrossRef]
26. Chen, X.; Liu, G.; Yuan, Y.; Wu, G.; Wang, S.; Yuan, L. NEK7 interacts with NLRP3 to modulate the pyroptosis in inflammatory bowel disease via NF-kappaB signaling. *Cell Death Dis.* **2019**, *10*, 906. [CrossRef]
27. Leclair, H.M.; Tardif, N.; Paris, A.; Galibert, M.D.; Corre, S. Role of Flavonoids in the Prevention of AhR-Dependent Resistance During Treatment with BRAF Inhibitors. *Int. J. Mol. Sci.* **2020**, *21*, 5025. [CrossRef]
28. Yang, T.; Feng, Y.L.; Chen, L.; Vaziri, N.D.; Zhao, Y.Y. Dietary natural flavonoids treating cancer by targeting aryl hydrocarbon receptor. *Crit. Rev. Toxicol.* **2019**, *49*, 445–460. [CrossRef]
29. Vondracek, J.; Umannova, L.; Machala, M. Interactions of the aryl hydrocarbon receptor with inflammatory mediators: Beyond CYP1A regulation. *Curr. Drug Metab.* **2011**, *12*, 89–103. [CrossRef]
30. Christmas, P. Role of Cytochrome P450s in Inflammation. *Adv. Pharmacol.* **2015**, *74*, 163–192. [CrossRef]
31. Van der Giessen, J.; van der Woude, C.J.; Peppelenbosch, M.P.; Fuhler, G.M. A Direct Effect of Sex Hormones on Epithelial Barrier Function in Inflammatory Bowel Disease Models. *Cells* **2019**, *8*, 261. [CrossRef]
32. Velica, P.; Davies, N.J.; Rocha, P.P.; Schrewe, H.; Ride, J.P.; Bunce, C.M. Lack of functional and expression homology between human and mouse aldo-keto reductase 1C enzymes: Implications for modelling human cancers. *Mol. Cancer* **2009**, *8*, 121. [CrossRef]
33. Wei, X.; Wei, Z.H.; Li, Y.Y.; Tan, Z.Q.; Lin, C. AKR1C1 Contributes to Cervical Cancer Progression via Regulating TWIST1 Expression. *Biochem. Genet.* **2021**, *59*, 516–530. [CrossRef]
34. Zheng, J.; Yang, Z.; Li, Y.; Yang, L.; Yao, R. Knockdown of AKR1C3 Promoted Sorafenib Sensitivity Through Inhibiting the Phosphorylation of AKT in Hepatocellular Carcinoma. *Front. Oncol.* **2022**, *12*, 823491. [CrossRef]
35. Fattahi, S.; Amjadi-Moheb, F.; Tabaripour, R.; Ashrafi, G.H.; Akhavan-Niaki, H. PI3K/AKT/mTOR signaling in gastric cancer: Epigenetics and beyond. *Life Sci.* **2020**, *262*, 118513. [CrossRef]
36. Arab, H.H.; Al-Shorbagy, M.Y.; Saad, M.A. Activation of autophagy and suppression of apoptosis by dapagliflozin attenuates experimental inflammatory bowel disease in rats: Targeting AMPK/mTOR, HMGB1/RAGE and Nrf2/HO-1 pathways. *Chem. Biol. Interact.* **2021**, *335*, 109368. [CrossRef]
37. Ala, M.; Jafari, R.M.; Nematian, H.; Shadboorestan, A.; Dehpour, A.R. Sodium Selenite Modulates IDO1/Kynurenine, TLR4, NF-kappaB and Bcl2/Bax Pathway and Mitigates Acetic Acid-Induced Colitis in Rat. *Cell Physiol. Biochem.* **2022**, *56*, 24–35. [CrossRef]
38. Gao, T.; Wang, T.; Wang, Z.; Cao, J.; Dong, Y.; Chen, Y. Melatonin-mediated MT2 attenuates colitis induced by dextran sodium sulfate via PI3K/AKT/Nrf2/SIRT1/RORalpha/NF-kappaB signaling pathways. *Int. Immunopharmacol.* **2021**, *96*, 107779. [CrossRef]
39. Xi, M.; Wang, X.; Ge, J.; Yin, D. N′-[(3-[benzyloxy]benzylidene)-3,4,5-trihydroxybenzohydrazide (1) protects mice against colitis induced by dextran sulfate sodium through inhibiting NFkappaB/IL-6/STAT3 pathway. *Biochem. Biophys. Res. Commun.* **2016**, *477*, 290–296. [CrossRef]
40. Lugering, A.; Lebiedz, P.; Koch, S.; Kucharzik, T. Apoptosis as a therapeutic tool in IBD? *Ann. N. Y. Acad. Sci.* **2006**, *1072*, 62–77. [CrossRef]
41. Saadatdoust, Z.; Pandurangan, A.K.; Ananda Sadagopan, S.K.; Mohd Esa, N.; Ismail, A.; Mustafa, M.R. Dietary cocoa inhibits colitis associated cancer: A crucial involvement of the IL-6/STAT3 pathway. *J. Nutr. Biochem.* **2015**, *26*, 1547–1558. [CrossRef]
42. Bungsu, I.; Kifli, N.; Ahmad, S.R.; Ghani, H.; Cunningham, A.C. Herbal Plants: The Role of AhR in Mediating Immunomodulation. *Front. Immunol.* **2021**, *12*, 697663. [CrossRef]
43. Chapkin, R.S.; Davidson, L.A.; Park, H.; Jin, U.H.; Fan, Y.Y.; Cheng, Y.; Hensel, M.E.; Landrock, K.K.; Allred, C.; Menon, R.; et al. Role of the Aryl Hydrocarbon Receptor (AhR) in Mediating the Effects of Coffee in the Colon. *Mol. Nutr. Food Res.* **2021**, *65*, e2100539. [CrossRef]
44. Fouzder, C.; Mukhuty, A.; Kundu, R. Kaempferol inhibits Nrf2 signalling pathway via downregulation of Nrf2 mRNA and induces apoptosis in NSCLC cells. *Arch. Biochem. Biophys.* **2021**, *697*, 108700. [CrossRef]
45. Ru, J.; Li, P.; Wang, J.; Zhou, W.; Li, B.; Huang, C.; Li, P.; Guo, Z.; Tao, W.; Yang, Y.; et al. TCMSP: A database of systems pharmacology for drug discovery from herbal medicines. *J. Cheminform.* **2014**, *6*, 13. [CrossRef]
46. Wang, Y.; Xiao, J.; Suzek, T.O.; Zhang, J.; Wang, J.; Bryant, S.H. PubChem: A public information system for analyzing bioactivities of small molecules. *Nucleic Acids Res.* **2009**, *37*, W623–W633. [CrossRef]
47. Daina, A.; Michielin, O.; Zoete, V. Swiss Target Prediction: Updated data and new features for efficient prediction of protein targets of small molecules. *Nucleic Acids Res.* **2019**, *47*, W357–W364. [CrossRef]
48. Fishilevich, S.; Nudel, R.; Rappaport, N.; Hadar, R.; Plaschkes, I.; Iny Stein, T.; Rosen, N.; Kohn, A.; Twik, M.; Safran, M.; et al. GeneHancer: Genome-wide integration of enhancers and target genes in GeneCards. *Database* **2017**, *2017*, bax028. [CrossRef]

49. Carvalho-Silva, D.; Pierleoni, A.; Pignatelli, M.; Ong, C.; Fumis, L.; Karamanis, N.; Carmona, M.; Faulconbridge, A.; Hercules, A.; McAuley, E.; et al. Open Targets Platform: New developments and updates two years on. *Nucleic Acids Res.* **2019**, *47*, D1056–D1065. [CrossRef]
50. Shannon, P.; Markiel, A.; Ozier, O.; Baliga, N.S.; Wang, J.T.; Ramage, D.; Amin, N.; Schwikowski, B.; Ideker, T. Cytoscape: A software environment for integrated models of biomolecular interaction networks. *Genome Res.* **2003**, *13*, 2498–2504. [CrossRef]
51. Franceschini, A.; Szklarczyk, D.; Frankild, S.; Kuhn, M.; Simonovic, M.; Roth, A.; Lin, J.; Minguez, P.; Bork, P.; von Mering, C.; et al. STRING v9.1: Protein-protein interaction networks, with increased coverage and integration. *Nucleic Acids Res.* **2013**, *41*, D808–D815. [CrossRef] [PubMed]
52. Sussman, J.L.; Lin, D.; Jiang, J.; Manning, N.O.; Prilusky, J.; Ritter, O.; Abola, E.E. Protein Data Bank (PDB): Database of three-dimensional structural information of biological macromolecules. *Acta Crystallogr. D Biol. Crystallogr.* **1998**, *54*, 1078–1084. [CrossRef] [PubMed]

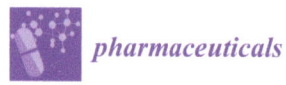

Review

Potential Use of Antioxidant Compounds for the Treatment of Inflammatory Bowel Disease

Alexander V. Blagov [1,*], Varvara A. Orekhova [1,2], Vasily N. Sukhorukov [1,2], Alexandra A. Melnichenko [1] and Alexander N. Orekhov [1,2,*]

[1] Laboratory of Angiopathology, Institute of General Pathology and Pathophysiology, 8 Baltiiskaya Street, Moscow 125315, Russia; v.a.orekhova@yandex.ru (V.A.O.); vnsukhorukov@gmail.com (V.N.S.); sasha.melnichenko@gmail.com (A.A.M.)

[2] Institute for Atherosclerosis Research, Osennyaya Street 4-1-207, Moscow 121609, Russia

* Correspondence: al.blagov2014@gmail.com (A.V.B.); alexandernikolaevichorekhov@gmail.com (A.N.O.)

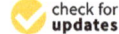

Citation: Blagov, A.V.; Orekhova, V.A.; Sukhorukov, V.N.; Melnichenko, A.A.; Orekhov, A.N. Potential Use of Antioxidant Compounds for the Treatment of Inflammatory Bowel Disease. *Pharmaceuticals* **2023**, *16*, 1150. https://doi.org/10.3390/ph16081150

Academic Editors: Anderson Luiz-Ferreira and Carmine Stolfi

Received: 7 July 2023
Revised: 29 July 2023
Accepted: 11 August 2023
Published: 14 August 2023

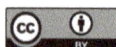

Copyright: © 2023 by the authors. Licensee MDPI, Basel, Switzerland. This article is an open access article distributed under the terms and conditions of the Creative Commons Attribution (CC BY) license (https://creativecommons.org/licenses/by/4.0/).

Abstract: Since inflammatory bowel diseases (IBDs) are chronic, the development of new effective therapeutics to combat them does not lose relevance. Oxidative stress is one of the main pathological processes that determines the progression of IBD. In this regard, antioxidant therapy seems to be a promising approach. The role of oxidative stress in the development and progression of IBD is considered in detail in this review. The main cause of oxidative stress in IBD is an inadequate response of leukocytes to dysbiosis and food components in the intestine. Passage of immune cells through the intestinal barrier leads to increased ROS concentration and the pathological consequences of exposure to oxidative stress based on the development of inflammation and impaired intestinal permeability. To combat oxidative stress in IBD, several promising natural (curcumin, resveratrol, quercetin, and melatonin) and artificial antioxidants (N-acetylcysteine (NAC) and artificial superoxide dismutase (aSOD)) that had been shown to be effective in a number of clinical trials have been proposed. Their mechanisms of action on pathological events in IBD and clinical manifestations from their impact have been determined. The prospects for the use of other antioxidants that have not yet been tested in the treatment of IBD, but have the properties of potential therapeutic candidates, have been also considered.

Keywords: IBD; ulcerative colitis; Crohn's disease; oxidative stress; ROS

1. Introduction

Inflammatory bowel disease (IBD) is characterized by recurrent episodes of inflammation of the gastrointestinal tract caused by an abnormal immune response to the intestinal microflora [1]. Inflammatory bowel disease includes two types of idiopathic bowel disease, which differ in the location and depth of damage to the intestinal wall. Ulcerative colitis (UC) involves diffuse inflammation of the lining of the colon. Ulcerative colitis most commonly affects the rectum (proctitis) but can spread to the sigmoid colon (proctosigmoiditis), and it can also spread out of the sigmoid colon (distal ulcerative colitis) or may cover the entire colon (pancolitis) [2]. Crohn's disease (CD) is characterized by transmural lesions of any part of the gastrointestinal tract (GIT), with the most common pathologies occurring in the ileum and colon [2].

High mortality is typical for patients with Crohn's disease, while the main causes of death are the direct progression of the disease itself, concomitant infections, complications from surgery, and multiple organ failure. IBD is one of the main risk factors for colorectal cancer [3]. At present, the etiology of IBD is not fully understood. Various causes of IBD have been considered, including smoking and diet, but none of them is dominant [4]. It is reliably known that the highest risk of developing IBD is in people who have mutations that determine their predisposition to IBD, the state of dysbacteriosis, and the disruption of the immune tolerance caused by it. Thus, a number of both hereditary and acquired factors are likely to be involved in the occurrence of IBD.

The average incidence of IBD is about 10 cases per 100,000 people in UC and about 7 cases per 100,000 people in CD [5]. The highest incidence of IBD occurs in the United States, Canada, and European countries, while developing countries in Asia and Africa show a lower incidence [5]. On an age scale, young people between the ages of 15 and 30 have the greatest risk of developing IBD. Crohn's disease is somewhat more common to women than in men, but ulcerative colitis is equally present in both sexes [6].

The gut immune system plays a key role in the pathogenesis of IBD. The intestinal epithelium prevents the penetration of bacteria or antigens into the bloodstream due to hermetic intercellular connections. In IBD, these junctions are damaged either due to the disruption of the primary barrier functioning, or as a result of the development of inflammation. Additional defense mechanisms are based on the production of mucus by goblet cells and the production of antimicrobial proteins alpha-defensins by Paneth cells. Increasing inflammation causes even more damage to the structure of the epithelium, which leads to the spread of microbial populations in the intestinal wall, which in turn is a signal for a further increase in inflammation [1].

The basis of IBD treatment is the use of oral drugs based on 5-aminosalicylic acid (5-ASA) with the addition of steroids during an exacerbation of the disease and the transition to tumor necrosis factor inhibitors and immunomodulatory drugs in the absence of remission. Despite tremendous advances in IBD therapy in recent years, approximately 30% of patients do not respond to anti-TNFα therapy in the first place, and even among those who respond, up to 10% lose their response to the drug each year [7]. Additionally, the disadvantage of using current drugs for the treatment of IBD is the risk of developing severe side effects associated with the occurrence of infectious, as well as neoplastic processes [7]. Based on this, it becomes clear that the creation of new effective and safe drugs for the treatment of IBD is an important task for the pharmaceutical industry.

It is known that oxidative stress is a concomitant factor in the pathogenesis of various inflammatory diseases, since reactive oxygen species are direct modulators and initiators of the inflammatory response. Understanding the role of oxidative stress in the pathophysiology of IBD is important for evaluating the relevance of using antioxidants in the treatment of IBD. In most cases, antioxidants are natural compounds and do not cause serious side effects. In addition, the popularity of many of these compounds and methods due to their production from plant materials make the development of therapeutic agents based on them faster and the production less resource-intensive.

Increased oxidative stress with a pronounced weakening of antioxidant protection in IBD was identified in the 1990s [8,9]. This prompted the consideration of antioxidants as potential therapeutic agents in the treatment of CD and UC. Initially, such compounds were investigated in combination with already-registered drugs for the treatment of IBD. Thus, in one study [10], it was demonstrated that combination therapy with sulfasalazine or prednisolone with the addition of one of the antioxidants (allopurinol or dimethyl sulfoxide) led to a greater reduction in relapses among patients with UC than therapy with sulfasalazine or prednisolone alone. Better efficacy of allopurinol in combination with 5-ASA than 5-ASA alone during a 6-month but not a 12-month UC treatment period was shown in a study [11]. Thereby, the primary issues remain the long-term effectiveness of antioxidant therapy against IBD and the possibility of using antioxidants as monotherapy agents in the treatment of CD or UC.

2. The Role of Oxidative Stress in IBD
2.1. Mechanisms of the Formation of Reactive Oxygen Species in the Cell

ROS (reactive oxygen species) are chemical molecules containing one oxygen atom, which, as a result of cellular and extracellular reactions, becomes more reactive than oxygen itself. ROS include both free radical and non-free radical oxygen intermediates (peroxides), such as superoxide radicals (O_2^-), hydrogen peroxide (H_2O_2), hydroxyl radicals (OH), and singlet oxygen (1 O_2) [12].

Oxidative stress is defined as an imbalance between the production of oxidants or ROS and their removal by defense mechanisms or antioxidants. Disruption of this redox balance can result in damage to important cellular components, including proteins, lipids, and DNA, with potential whole-body effects and an increased risk of mutagenesis. ROS are also involved in the initiation and development of pathological processes, including aging, cancer, insulin resistance, diabetes mellitus, cardiovascular disease, Alzheimer's disease, etc. [13].

ROS are formed in two ways. The first is based on the redox reactions occurring in the ETC (electron transport chain) on the mitochondrial membrane during oxidative phosphorylation. ROS generated by this method are the main ROS concentrated in cells [14]. The second is associated with the protective response of immune cells to a bacterial infection or other pathological processes leading to inflammation [15]. These ROS play the role of signaling molecules in the body's immune response.

During respiration, electrons donated from NADH in complex I and FADH2 in complex II pass to complex III through ubiquinone, then through cytochrome C to complex IV, and then the electrons are transferred to molecular oxygen with the formation of water. During oxidative phosphorylation, ETC protein complexes are involved in the process of creating a proton gradient, which is based on an increase in the concentration of protons in the mitochondrial intermembrane space and a decrease in their concentration in the matrix. As a result of the reverse flow of protons into the matrix, ATP is generated [16]. ROS, namely, superoxide, is a by-product of the reaction during electron transfer in the ETC to molecular oxygen [17]. Superoxide is produced by complex I and complex II into the mitochondrial matrix, while complex III additionally directs superoxide into the intermembrane space [18].

As noted, the second way to generate ROS is associated with a protective reaction of immune cells. In this case, ROS are produced by the enzyme nicotinamide adenine dinucleotide phosphate (NADPH) oxidase [15]. NADPH oxidase is associated with the cytoplasmic membrane and is a complex of proteins. The main stimuli that activate the work of NADPH oxidase are foreign microorganisms, increased inflammation, induction of calcium signaling, and an increase in the concentration of growth factors [14]. In addition to the superoxide radical, NADPH oxidase also produces hydrogen peroxide [19].

The tubular network of the endoplasmic reticulum (ER) has a unique oxidative environment, and during stressful conditions, redox signaling mediators are the main initiators of ROS production and directly affect protein folding and secretion [20]. The microsomal cytochrome P450-dependent monooxygenase system, whose role is associated with the metabolism of xenobiotics, is the dominant source of ROS production in hepatocytes [21].

Peroxisomes also contain ROS-producing enzymes, such as xanthine oxidase, which provides the formation of hydrogen peroxide [22]. The catalase enzyme is responsible for the neutralization of peroxide, catalyzing the decomposition of hydrogen peroxide into water and oxygen. The lysosomal electron transport chain, which facilitates the movement of protons to maintain an optimal pH for acid hydrolases, generates OH radicals [16].

2.2. Development of Oxidative Stress in IBD

In the human body, the gastrointestinal tract (GIT) contains a significant number of both stimuli and sources leading to the production of ROS. The epithelial layer, which performs a protective function, cannot provide complete protection against irritants, which include absorbed food components and those coming from outside, as well as microorganisms living in the intestine itself. It can cause an inflammatory reaction leading to the activation of neutrophils and macrophages that produce inflammatory factors, including ROS, which further enhance inflammation [23].

Impaired intestinal barrier function, leading to increased intestinal permeability, is a hallmark of the pathogenesis of IBD. Increased intestinal permeability is determined by the disruption of tight junctions, which leads to the release of pro-inflammatory agents, including ROS, which contribute to the progression of the pathological cascade [24]. As described above, the main ROS producers in IBD are macrophages and neutrophils. With increased inflammation, increased infiltration of these types of immune cells through the intestinal mucosa was noted, accompanied by the release of a large amount of ROS, which in turn play the role of attractants for immune cells [25]. Increased production of ROS in the inflammatory microenvironment of the intestine contributes to enterocyte damage caused by the ability of ROS to cause the destruction of biological macromolecules: proteins, lipids, and DNA. Cell damage leads to the release of cellular components into the extracellular space, where they can act as DAMPs, causing an additional increase in inflammation, including increased production of tumor necrosis factor (TNF)-α and interleukins IL-6 and IL-1β [26]. Dendritic cells play an important role, recognizing the formed DAMPs and then activating naive T-cells, which stimulate their proliferation and maturation and lead to the development of an adaptive immune response [27]. Both main groups of T-lymphocytes take part in IBD, namely, CD8+ T-lymphocytes and CD4+ T-lymphocytes, and the latter can be conditionally divided into two subgroups: effector and regulatory. If effector T-lymphocytes contribute to the further development of inflammation, then regulatory T-cells weaken it. The degree of development of IBD depends, in particular, on the ratio of these cell types [27].

Along with a direct role in the pathogenesis of IBD, oxidative damage to macromolecules, such as DNA damage and actin carbonylation with tubulin nitration, can be initiating factors in the development of colorectal cancer [28]. The relationship of IBD with cancer can also manifest itself when common signaling pathways are activated, including those associated with increased production of the p53 oncogene. Activation of p53 is closely associated with the development of oxidative stress through the expression of the p85 protein, which is a signal molecule in ROS-related p53-dependent apoptosis [29].

A noteworthy fact is the change in the concentration of cellular antioxidant enzymes in the gut mucosa in IBD. The expression of most of the genes of these enzymes, including SOD and CAT, decreases with an increase in inflammation associated with the pathogenesis of IBD, while the expression of the GPx2 gene (a form of GPx specific to the gastrointestinal tract) increases [30]. In studies of tissues of UC patients, it was shown that GPx2 is located in the ER, where it is able to modulate COX-2 activity through the utilization of peroxides and, as a result, reduce the level of prostaglandin E2, which is one of the main mediators of inflammation [31]. Thus, GPx2 is one of the last lines of defense to curb inflammation and carcinogenesis in IBD. Among the pathological effects of ROS, specific for IBD, one can note the effect of nitric oxide (NO•) on chloride anions, which, as a result of such an effect, are released into the intercellular space. It leads to a decrease in the amount of water in the intestinal lumen, and results in the development of osmotic diarrhea [32]. A brief diagram showing the role of oxidative stress in IBD is shown in Figure 1.

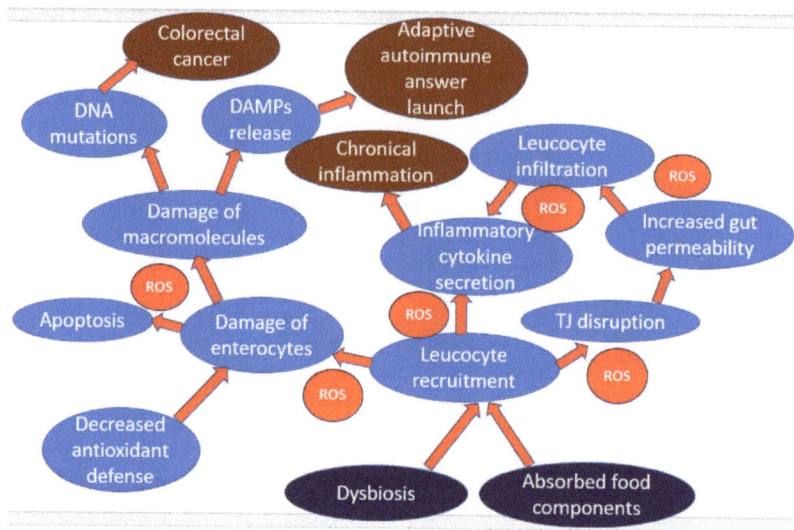

Figure 1. The role of oxidative stress in IBD.

3. Natural Antioxidant Cellular Protection

3.1. Superoxide Dismutase (SOD)

SOD is the most important enzyme protecting against O_2^- radicals. The SOD enzyme family is named after the cofactors used to detoxify excess O_2, such as Cu/Zn-SOD, Fe-SOD, Ni-SOD, and Mn-SOD. SOD is involved in the transformation of the superoxide radical into oxygen and hydrogen peroxide [33]. Thus, SOD can act as an initial defense against ROS as a result of rapid initiation under oxidative stress. Cu/Zn-SOD is presented in a dimeric form and is located in the cytosol, where Cu and Zn are associated with two subunits [34].

It is now well known that mitochondria are the main producers of ROS, as well as the main targets of ROS. Massive accumulation of ROS and free radicals in mitochondria is the reason for the induction of increased expression of Mn-SOD, which suppress oxidative damage in mitochondria. The presence of specific SOD isoforms in different subcellular compartments ensures control of the ROS level in the cell [35].

3.2. Catalase (CAT)

The molecular structure of CAT and its function are based on iron atoms in the composition of the enzyme molecule, which form four heme groups around themselves [33]. The main function of CAT is to clean cells from hydrogen peroxide, which has toxic properties. Peroxisomes are the predominant localization site of CAT in the cell. The rate at which CAT converts hydrogen peroxide into molecular oxygen and water is 6 million hydrogen peroxide molecules per minute. CAT is highly active in hepatocytes, kidney cells, and erythrocytes [36].

3.3. Glutathione Peroxidase (GSH-Px)

The main function of GSH-Px is associated with the protection of the cell under oxidative stress and under normal physiological conditions from hydrogen peroxide, reducing it to water, while simultaneously reducing lipid peroxide. Another extraordinary role of GSH-Px is associated with the inhibition of tumor growth as a result of modulation of the signaling pathways of lipoxygenase and cyclooxygenase [37]. In the human body, there are eight types of GSH-Px, which can be in the form of selenoproteins, which are associated with selenium. Each of the GSH-Px types has a predominant localization in a certain tissue, where it performs its antioxidant function by reducing hydrogen peroxide and other organic peroxides [36].

Thus, GSH-Px1 or cellular GSH-Px (cGSH-Px) is localized in all cell types. GSH-Px2 or gastrointestinal GSH-Px (GSH-Px-GI) is present in human organs such as the stomach, liver, and intestines, but it is not expressed in the heart and lungs [38]. GSH-Px3 or plasma GSH-Px (pGSH-Px) is expressed in the kidney, and more specifically in proximal tubular epithelial cells. GSH-Px4 is a phospholipid localized in various cell types. Its key feature is the ability to reduce phospholipid hydroperoxides to alcohols, thus protecting cell membranes from peroxidation, which is one of the main consequences of oxidative stress leading to cell death [39].

3.4. Glutathione Reductase (GR)

GR promotes an increase in the stores of reduced glutathione, which is the most abundant thiol compound in most cells. Reduced glutathione is directly involved in the control of oxidative stress, being a GSH-Px cofactor. The catalytic function of GR is based on the transformation of glutathione disulfide (GSSG) into reduced GSH via the energy of reduced NADP [40].

3.5. Thioredoxin (Trx)

The Trx antioxidant system, consisting of NADP, thioredoxin reductase (TrxR), and Trx, is very important in combating oxidative stress as an endogenous antioxidant system. Trx antioxidants are involved in DNA and protein repair by reducing ribonucleotide reductase and methionine sulfoxide reductase [41]. Trx systems in cells contribute to the reduction of oxidative stress in the cell due to the presence of thiol and selenol groups. Trx, together with TBP2 and ASK1 proteins, may be involved in the modulation of cell apoptosis, as well as regulate lipid and carbohydrate metabolism. Both the GSH system and the Trx system can protect against oxidative stress by efficiently removing various ROS [42]. Cytosolic Trx1 and mitochondrial Trx2 are major redox proteins that regulate cell proliferation and viability. The reduced/dithiol form of Trxs binds to ASK1 and inhibits its activity, causing blockage of apoptosis. When Trx is oxidized, it dissociates from ASK1, and apoptosis is launched [43].

3.6. Cellular Antioxidant Regulation

The transcription factor nuclear erythroid factor 2 (NRF2) is one of the main modulators of the redox state of the cell, regulating the expression of antioxidant enzymes. The resulting oxidative stress is the reason for the activation of NRF2, which leads to the activation of the expression of heme oxygenase-1, which is an important cytoprotective protein [44]. Normally, NRF2 is associated with Kelch-like ECH-associated protein 1 (KEAP1). ROS at elevated concentrations oxidize cysteine residues on KEAP1 in the NRF2–KEAP1 complex, which facilitates the detachment of KEAP1 from NRF2. Free NRF2 then moves to the nucleus, where it interacts with MAF, resulting in the formation of heterodimers required for binding to antioxidant-responsive elements (ARE) in the regulatory regions of several antioxidant genes that coordinate their expression [45]. The level of mitochondrial ROS is directly related to the likelihood of developing oxidative stress, and, therefore, to ensure adequate cellular homeostasis, a properly functioning system is required to maintain the concentration of ROS within acceptable limits. A sharp increase in the level of ROS as a result of oxidative phosphorylation is the cause of pathological processes in the cell, which lead to oxidative damage to cellular structures and the triggering of apoptosis. With a lack of antioxidant enzymes, namely, SOD2, Trx2, peroxiredoxin, and GPx, the clearance of ROS in the cell is reduced, and the redox balance is disrupted. In addition, the formation of superoxide near NO molecules is a high-risk factor for the appearance of the toxic radical peroxynitrite (ONOO−) [46].

4. Natural Antioxidants in the Treatment of IBD

4.1. Curcumin

Curcumin, isolated from the rhizomes of the *Curcuma longa* plant, has proven antioxidant and anti-inflammatory effects. Curcumin has been shown to be beneficial in animal models of IBD. Thus, it was found that curcumin caused a decrease in the DAI index, which determined the severity of the pathological process. Additionally, it reduces damage caused by inflammation and inhibits neutrophil infiltration. In addition, it causes a decrease in lipid peroxidation [15]. The mechanisms associated with its therapeutic activity are not yet fully understood; however, possible options can be considered, for example, inhibition of the activation of the transcription factors NF-κB and STAT3, and accordingly the subsequent suppression of the expression of proteins that play the role of pro-inflammatory factors, including ROS-producing enzymes such as COX-2 and iNOS [47]. Based on a number of studies, it was shown that the introduction of curcumin reduced the clinical symptoms of IBD and led to the increased proportion of patients who managed to achieve remission [48,49]. Its additional advantage is the absence of serious side effects [1]. A clinical study [50] examined the effect of combination therapy of mesalazine with modified curcumin, which had better hydrophilic properties in patients with mild to moderate UC. According to the results of the study, patients receiving combination therapy demonstrated endoscopic remission, as well as long-term clinical remission, which was assessed at 6 and 12 months, with remission rates of 95% and 84%, respectively.

4.2. Resveratrol

Resveratrol is a polyphenol found in grapes and other fruits. Studies in rat models of IBD have shown that resveratrol reduced the development of lipid peroxidation damage and caused an improvement in cellular antioxidant activity. It could be caused by an increase in glutathione peroxidase activity, as well as an anti-inflammatory effect by inhibiting the expression of pro-inflammatory factors, namely, IL-1β, IL-6, and TGF-β1, and it reduces fibrosis [51,52]. The antioxidant and anti-inflammatory effects of resveratrol have also been demonstrated in several clinical studies. Thus, it was found that resveratrol caused an increase in SOD activity and a decrease in the concentrations of C-reactive protein and TNF-α [52]. Resveratrol, like curcumin, lowers the DAI value [53]. A clinical study [54] demonstrated a significant decrease in the level of inflammatory markers TNF-α and hs-CRP, as well as a decrease in NF-κB activity in patients with mild to moderate UC after 6 weeks of resveratrol supplementation. The disadvantages of resveratrol include its low bioavailability due to rapid absorption in the gastrointestinal tract and liver, as well as poor solubility and low stability [32]. To overcome these shortcomings, a colonic delivery system was developed for resveratrol [55]. This system was made of composite nanoparticles consisting of zinc, pectin, and chitosan, inside which the active substance, resveratrol, was enclosed. Several variants of nanoparticles were obtained by changing a number of parameters, such as cross-linking pH, concentrations of components, cross-linking time, and drug concentration. The nanoparticles obtained at pH 1.5 with 1% chitosan, 2-hour cross-linking time, and a ratio of pectin to resveratrol of 3 to 1 had the best specificity for the colon. Another significant disadvantage of this compound is the possibility of toxicity to normal cells. In high concentrations, resveratrol cannot be used as a drug, as it is considered a toxic compound [56].

4.3. Quercetin

Quercetin has shown beneficial effects in animal models of IBD, including reduced weight loss, rectal bleeding, and bowel injury. In addition, quercetin has an antioxidant effect by initiating a decrease in the activity of the myeloperoxidase enzyme and an increase in the concentration of glutathione, as well as inhibition of lipid peroxidation. Its anti-inflammatory mechanism of action is the inhibition of TNF-α expression [57,58]. An important effect of quercetin regarding the course of IBD is to improve the composition of the intestinal microflora, in particular, by activating macrophage activity against a number of bacteria [57]. It was found using a mice model that 5 weeks of quercetin consumption led to the growth of Bacteroidetes and to a proportional decrease in Gram-negative proteobacteria and Gram-positive actinobacteria concentrations in the colon. Quercetin has also been shown to reduce intestinal permeability by activating tight junction repair [59]. Quercetin can be effectively used in combination with 5-aminosalacylic acid (5-ASA), which allows for a reduction in the dose of 5-ASA, thus minimizing the possibility of side effects [60].

4.4. Melatonin

Melatonin is an organic substance synthesized mainly in the pineal gland, as well as in organs such as the retina and ovaries, which have the ability to produce this natural hormone [61]. Compared to other antioxidants, melatonin has unique properties that prove its uniqueness compared to other antioxidants. First, it is soluble in both water and lipids. Due to this property, melatonin easily penetrates through cell membranes and reaches all cell compartments, but at the same time it is selective towards mitochondria. It is a relatively safe substance, the reported side effects of which are usually harmless [61]. Melatonin can bind heavy metals (for example, iron) and thus prevents the formation of ROS. In addition, melatonin enhances the mechanisms of antioxidant cell defense by activating antioxidant enzymes such as catalase, superoxide dismutase, and others. Another mechanism of melatonin action is based on the anti-inflammatory effect, as a result of which the balance of concentrations of pro-inflammatory and anti-inflammatory cytokines are shifted towards the second [62]. Melatonin has been shown to be effective in the treatment of UC as an adjunct to combination therapy with mesalazine [63]. In a clinical study [63], patients with UC who received adjuvant therapy with melatonin in addition to mesalazine maintained clinical remission for 12 months, and serum CRP levels remained stable. These results were very different from the group receiving mesalazine only: remission was not stable, and CRP levels increased. Another advantage of using melatonin in the treatment of IBD is its ability to modulate intestinal dysbiosis [64]. This study was conducted on two groups of mice with DSS-induced colitis: the first group did not receive any therapy, and the second received melatonin treatment. In the first group, in the plasma of mice, the antioxidant activity, measured by decolorization of ABTS radical cations, was lower than in the second. The proportions of intestinal bacterial communities also differed. In the first group, the percentages of the most common bacteria were as follows: Bacteroidetes (59%), Firmicutes (31%), and Proteobacteria (8%). In the second group, the most common bacterial group was Firmicutes (49%), followed by Bacteroidetes (41%); the amount of Proteobacteria did not change (8%).

5. Artificial Antioxidants in the Treatment of IBD

5.1. N-acetylcysteine

N-acetylcysteine (NAC) is a derivative of L-cysteine, one of the functions of which is associated with the inhibition of the formation of free radicals, the increase in the activity of antioxidant defense enzymes, and the suppression of the production of heat shock proteins, which are considered biomarkers of oxidative stress. NAC can be converted to cysteine, which is a substrate that is involved in the reduction of glutathione in the intestine [65]. NAC also has an anti-inflammatory effect by inhibiting the activation of the NF-kB signaling pathway, thus preventing increased expression of pro-inflammatory cytokines [66]. NAC also increases ATP levels, inhibits apoptosis by acting on caspases, and promotes proliferation, development, and regeneration of intestinal cells [67]. NAC may reduce intestinal barrier permeability by reacting with claudin and occludin proteins [67]. NAC also has a positive effect on the intestinal microflora [68]. In a model of chemically induced colitis in rats, the successful use of NAC in combination with mesalamine was shown, as a result of which the level of inflammatory factors such as iNOS, COX-2, and prostaglandin E2 decreased to a greater extent than when these compounds were administered alone [69]. In a clinical study [70], it was demonstrated that the use of NAC as an adjuvant therapy with simultaneous reduction in the dose of corticosteroids in UC led to an increase in the period of remission. Combination therapy with mesalazine and NAC, evaluated in a clinical trial [71], resulted in better clinical remission, accompanied by a decrease in pro-inflammatory chemokines in UC patients, in contrast to monotherapy with mesalazine.

5.2. Artificial Superoxide Dismutase

One of the enzymes with strong antioxidant properties is superoxide dismutase (SOD), which has been described in detail in the previous paragraphs. However, in diseases associated with high levels of oxidative stress, natural SOD is not effective, as it has a short half-life and is not stable in the gastrointestinal tract. Despite these obstacles, recombinant bacterial strains have been obtained that express human SOD, for example, a strain of *Lactobacillus fermentum*, which has shown an improvement in colitis symptoms and a decrease in mortality in mice [72]. Its antioxidant function is associated with blocking lipid peroxidation and reducing the concentration of MPO in the intestine. The inflammatory response in the gut is reduced as a result of decreased production of pro-inflammatory cytokines caused by activation of the transcription factor NF-κB. Clinical trials of the action of lecithinized superoxide dismutase (PC-SOD) were carried out in patients with ulcerative colitis [73]. This new SOD variant overcomes the shortcomings of the natural version of the enzyme, having a longer half-life, which contributes to its longer action in the intestine. PC-SOD administered intravenously at a dose of 40 or 80 mg per day for four weeks improved the clinical symptoms of IBD and decreased the DAI index. Additionally, according to the results of the study, minor side effects of PC-SOD were revealed, but their occurrence did not depend on the dose of the administered enzyme. Summarizing data on the use of the considered antioxidants for the treatment of IBD are presented in Table 1. Mechanisms of antioxidant action of described antioxidant compounds are shown in Figure 2.

Table 1. Use of antioxidants for the treatment of IBD.

Compound	Chemical Structure	Mechanism of Action	Clinical Manifestation
Curcumin		Inhibition of NF-κB and STAT3 pathways [47]. Inhibition of COX-2 and iNOS expression [47].	Reducing the clinical symptoms of IBD and increasing the achievement of remission [48,49].
Resveratrol		Increase in glutathione peroxidase and SOD activity [51,52]. Inhibition of NF-κB pathway [52].	Lowering the DAI value [53].
Quercetin		Decrease in the activity of myeloperoxidase [57,58]. Increase in the concentration of glutathione [58]. Inhibition of TNF-α expression [57]. Antibacterial activation of macrophages [57].	Reducing the clinical symptoms [60]. Improving the composition of intestinal microflora [57]. Reducing intestinal permeability [59]. Activating tight junction repair [59].

Table 1. Cont.

Compound	Chemical Structure	Mechanism of Action	Clinical Manifestation
Melatonin		Increasing the activity of SOD and catalase [61]. Limiting the production of pro-inflammatory cytokines [62]. Enhancing the production of anti-inflammatory cytokines [62].	Reducing the clinical symptoms [63]. Modulation of intestinal dysbiosis [64].
N-acetylcysteine		Inhibition of NF-κB pathway [66]. Inhibition of apoptosis by acting on caspases [67]. Promotion of intestinal cell proliferation [67]. Modulation claudin and occluding activity [67].	Reducing the clinical symptoms [69,70]. Improving the composition of the intestinal microflora [68]. Reducing intestinal permeability [68].
Artificial superoxide dismutase		Direct inhibition of lipid peroxidation [72]. Decrease in the level of MPO [72]. Inhibition of NF-κB pathway [72].	Reducing the clinical symptoms of IBD [73]. Lowering the DAI value [73].

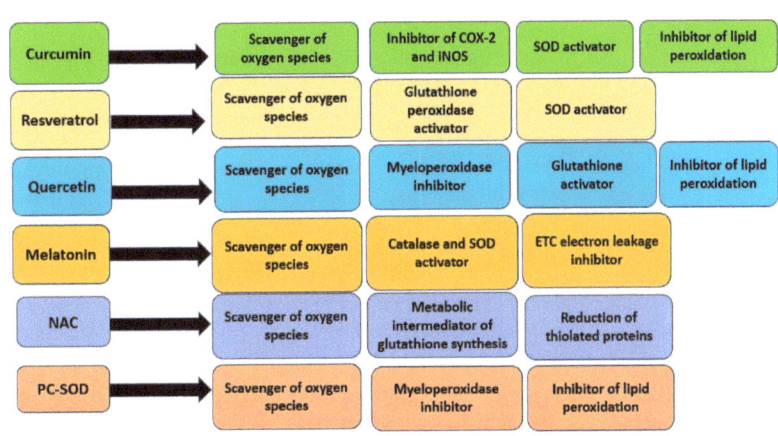

Figure 2. Mechanisms of antioxidant action of described antioxidant compounds.

6. Discussion

Based on the fact that traditional IBD treatment can cause a number of severe side effects, while the aforementioned natural and synthetic antioxidant compounds are well tolerated and have mild side effects in most cases, this therapeutic strategy is a promising avenue for IBD therapy. In addition, the effectiveness of antioxidants in the treatment of IBD also has been shown. The mechanism of antioxidant action is aimed at reducing overall inflammation through an effect on transcription factors, and in some cases, improving the composition of the intestinal microbiota and restoring tight junctions, which shows their high therapeutic specificity with respect to IBD pathogenesis. At the same time, additional larger-scale studies are required to determine the long-term effectiveness of antioxidant-based drugs, as well as to assess the possible risks of chronic toxicity. Determining the best dosage, optimal route of administration, and delivery form that overcome the clinical limitations of the antioxidant substances under consideration are additional tasks, which by solving, the question of the regular use of these compounds in clinical practice can receive a reliable answer. Animal studies are a valuable starting point for clinical trials in humans, but relatively few data have been obtained so far, including in the considered preclinical models of IBD. In view of the fact that IBD is a risk factor for the development of colon cancer, it is interesting to consider the possible antitumor effects of antioxidant compounds. Thus, in a number of studies [74,75], it was demonstrated that PAC ((3,5-bis(4-hydroxy-3-methoxybenzylidene)-N-methyl-4-piperidone)), which is a biological analog of curcumin, could activate apoptosis in cancer cells without being toxic to normal cells.

7. Conclusions

The use of antioxidants is a promising direction in the treatment of IBD, which, first of all, will reduce the frequency of severe side effects arising from the use of traditional therapies. Both natural and artificial antioxidants, in addition to directly affecting oxidative stress, are also able to reduce inflammation by regulating cytokine expression, affect the gut microbiota, and reduce tight junction damage. It has been observed that the most effective clinical use of antioxidants was in combination therapy with an already registered drug for the treatment of IBD, which gave a synergistic effect. However, more research is needed to gain a more complete understanding of the effects of antioxidants.

8. Future Perspectives

We propose that an important future step towards the use of antioxidants for the treatment of IBD is the identification of antioxidants with previously unseen efficacy in the treatment of IBD. Based on the shown therapeutic effects in relation to other inflammatory diseases, the use of such compounds in the therapy of CD and UC may have potential success. In one study [76] it was shown that rosemary extract significantly improved DAI in mice with DDS-induced colitis and helped restore the integrity of the intestinal barrier. The pharmacokinetics of the main components of rosemary extract was determined: carnosic acid (CA) and carnosol (CL). CA had an 11-fold higher serum concentration than carnosine but a shorter half-life: 3.5 h compared to 7.5 h. The revealed pharmacokinetics shows the potential regimens of the isolated compounds. CA should have a fast and powerful therapeutic effect; CL can be used as a drug with a slow but prolonged effect. It was also found that CL inhibits the expression of sestrin-2, the increased concentration of which was previously considered a favorable factor in certain diseases [77]. Thus, these studies also allow scientists to reveal new questions regarding the pathogenesis of IBD that have not been raised before. Another natural compound, anethole, which has shown early antioxidant and anti-inflammatory properties in several disease states, also has the potential to be used in the treatment of IBD. It reduced edema and penetration of immune cells into the focus of inflammation after it was administered to mice with acetic acid-induced colitis [78]. It also reduced malonaldehyde levels and gene expression of inflammatory mediators, including TNF-α, IL-1β, and TLR4.

First of all, researchers should pay attention to antioxidants that exhibit multiple effects and are considered the "strongest" representatives of antioxidants in their class, for example, ergothioneine, whose only antioxidant function has three options: preventing the formation of free radicals, binding ROS, and increasing the activity of natural antioxidants. Ergothioneine is able to inactivate singlet oxygen at a faster rate than other thiols. It has also been shown to be effective in a number of pathological conditions, including those associated with chronic inflammation [79]. Thus, compounds similar to ergothioneine, according to the described criteria, have great potential to become new drugs in the treatment of IBD.

Author Contributions: Writing—original draft preparation, A.V.B., V.N.S. and V.A.O.; writing—review and editing, A.A.M. and A.N.O. All authors have read and agreed to the published version of the manuscript.

Funding: This work was supported by the Russian Science Foundation (Grant #23-65-10014).

Institutional Review Board Statement: Not applicable.

Informed Consent Statement: Not applicable.

Data Availability Statement: Not applicable.

Conflicts of Interest: The authors declare no conflict of interest.

References

1. Maaser, C.; Sturm, A.; Vavricka, S.R.; Kucharzik, T.; Fiorino, G.; Annese, V. ECCO-ESGAR Guideline for Diagnostic Assessment in Inflammatory Bowel Disease. *J. Crohn's Colitis* **2019**, *13*, 144–164. [CrossRef]
2. Dmochowska, N.; Wardill, H. Hughes Advances in Imaging Specific Mediators of Inflammatory Bowel Disease. *Int. J. Mol. Sci.* **2018**, *19*, 2471. [CrossRef]
3. Chung, A.E.; Vu, M.B.; Myers, K.; Burris, J.; Kappelman, M.D. Crohn's and Colitis Foundation of America Partners Patient-Powered Research Network. *Med. Care* **2018**, *56*, S33. [CrossRef]
4. Colombel, J.-F.; Shin, A.; Gibson, R. Functional gastrointestinal symptoms in patients with inflammatory bowel disease: A clinical challenge. *Clin. Gastroenterol. Hepatol.* **2019**, *17*, 380–390. [CrossRef]
5. McDowell, C.; Farooq, U.; Haseeb, M. Inflammatory Bowel Disease. [Updated 2023 April 16]. StatPearls. Available online: https://www.ncbi.nlm.nih.gov/books/NBK470312/ (accessed on 25 July 2023).
6. Su, H.-J.; Chiu, Y.-T.; Chiu, C.-T.; Lin, Y.-C.; Wang, C.-Y.; Hsieh, J.-Y.; Wie, S.-C. Inflammatory bowel disease and its treatment in 2018: Global and Taiwanese status updates. *J. Formos. Med. Assoc.* **2019**, *118*, 1083–1092. [CrossRef]
7. Hazel, K.; O'Connor, A. Emerging treatments for inflammatory bowel disease. *Ther. Adv. Chronic Dis.* **2019**, *11*, 2040622319899297. [CrossRef]
8. McKenzie, S.J.; Baker, M.S.; Buffinton, G.D.; Doe, W.F. Evidence of oxidant-induced injury to epithelial cells during inflammatory bowel disease. *J. Clin. Investig.* **1996**, *98*, 136–141. [CrossRef]
9. Lih-Brody, L.; Powell, S.R.; Collier, K.; Reddy, G.M.; Cerchia, R.; Kahn, E.; Weissman, G.S.; Katz, S.; Floyd, R.A.; McKinley, M.J.; et al. Increased oxidative stress and decreased antioxidant defenses in mucosa of inflammatory bowel disease. *Dig. Dis. Sci.* **1996**, *41*, 2078–2086. [CrossRef]
10. Salim, A.S. Role of oxygen-derived free radical scavengers in the management of recurrent attacks of ulcerative colitis: A new approach. *J. Lab. Clin. Med.* **1992**, *119*, 710–717.
11. Järnerot, G.; Ström, M.; Danielsson, A.; Kilander, A.; Lööf, L.; Hultcrantz, R.; Löfberg, R.; Florén, C.; Nilsson, A.; Broström, O. Allopurinol in addition to 5-aminosalicylic acid based drugs for the maintenance treatment of ulcerative colitis. *Aliment. Pharmacol. Ther.* **2000**, *14*, 1159–1162.
12. Ferreira, C.A.; Ni, D.; Rosenkrans, Z.T.; Cai, W. Scavenging of reactive oxygen and nitrogen species with nanomaterials. *Nano Res.* **2018**, *11*, 4955–4984. [CrossRef]
13. Nogueira, V.; Hay, N. Molecular pathways: Reactive oxygen species homeostasis in cancer cells and implications for cancer therapy. *Clin. Cancer Res. Off. J. Am. Assoc. Cancer Res.* **2013**, *19*, 4309–4314. [CrossRef]
14. Checa, J.; Aran, J.M. Reactive Oxygen Species: Drivers of Physiological and Pathological Processes. *J. Inflamm. Res.* **2020**, *13*, 1057–1073. [CrossRef]
15. Tauffenberger, A.; Magistretti, J. Reactive Oxygen Species: Beyond Their Reactive Behavior. *Neurochem. Res.* **2021**, *46*, 77–87. [CrossRef]
16. Onukwufor, J.O.; Berry, B.J.; Wojtovich, A. Physiologic Implications of Reactive Oxygen Species Production by Mitochondrial Complex I Reverse Electron Transport. *Antioxidants* **2019**, *8*, 285. [CrossRef]
17. Zhao, R.; Jiang, S.; Zhang, L.; Yu, Z. Mitochondrial electron transport chain, ROS generation and uncoupling (Review). *Int. J. Mol. Med.* **2019**, *44*, 3–15. [CrossRef]
18. Nickel, A.; Kohlhaas, M.; Maack, C. Mitochondrial reactive oxygen species production and elimination. *J. Mol. Cell Cardiol.* **2014**, *73*, 26–33. [CrossRef]
19. Cardoso, A.R.; Chausse, B.; da Cunha, F.M.; Luévano-Martínez, L.A.; Marazzi, T.B.M.; Pessoa, S.; Kowaltowski, A.J. Mitochondrial compartmentalization of redox processes. *Free Radic. Biol. Med.* **2012**, *52*, 2201–2208. [CrossRef]
20. Zeeshan, H.; Lee, G.; Kim, H.-R.; Chae, H.-J. Endoplasmic Reticulum Stress and Associated ROS. *Int. J. Mol. Sci.* **2016**, *17*, 327. [CrossRef]
21. Cederbaum, A.I. Cytochrome P450 and Oxidative Stress in the Liver. *Liver* **2017**, 401–419.
22. Del Rio, L.A.; López-Huertas, E. ROS Generation in Peroxisomes and its Role in Cell Signaling. *Plant Cell Physiol.* **2016**, *57*, 1364–1376. [CrossRef] [PubMed]
23. Bhattacharyya, A.; Chattopadhyay, R.; Mitra, S.; Crowe, S.E. Oxidative Stress: An Essential Factor in the Pathogenesis of Gastrointestinal Mucosal Diseases. *Physiol. Rev. Am. Physiol. Soc.* **2014**, *94*, 329. [CrossRef] [PubMed]
24. Lewis, K.; Caldwell, J.; Phan, V.; Prescott, D.; Nazli, A.; Wang, A.; Soderhölm, J.D.; Perdue, M.H.; Sherman, P.M.; McKay, D.M. Decreased epithelial barrier function evoked by exposure to metabolic stress and nonpathogenic E. coli is enhanced by TNF-alpha. *Am. J. Physiol. Gastrointest. Liver Physiol.* **2008**, *294*, 3. [CrossRef] [PubMed]

25. Kashyap, P.; Farrugia, G. Oxidative stress: Key player in gastrointestinal complications of diabetes. *Neurogastroenterol. Motil.* **2011**, *23*, 111–114. [CrossRef] [PubMed]
26. Than, G.; Aytac, E.; Aytekin, H.; Gunduz, F.; Dogusoy, G.; Aydin, S.; Tahan, V.; Uzun, H. Vitamin E has a dual effect of anti-inflammatory and antioxidant activities in acetic acid–induced ulcerative colitis in rats. *Can. J. Surg. Can. Med. Assoc.* **2011**, *54*, 333. [CrossRef] [PubMed]
27. Li, L.; Peng, P.; Ding, N.; Jia, W.; Huang, C.; Tang, Y. Oxidative Stress, Inflammation, Gut Dysbiosis: What Can Polyphenols Do in Inflammatory Bowel Disease? *Antioxidants* **2023**, *12*, 967. [CrossRef] [PubMed]
28. Keshavarzian, A.; Banan, A.; Farhadi, A.; Komanduri, S.; Mutlu, E.; Zhang, Y.; Fields, J.Z. Increases in free radicals and cytoskeletal protein oxidation and nitration in the colon of patients with inflammatory bowel disease. *Gut. BMJ Publ. Group* **2003**, *52*, 720. [CrossRef] [PubMed]
29. Horvath, B.; Liu, G.; Wu, X.; Lai, K.K.; Shen, B.; Liu, X. Overexpression of p53 predicts colorectal neoplasia risk in patients with inflammatory bowel disease and mucosa changes indefinite for dysplasia. *Gastroenterol. Rep.* **2015**, *3*, 344. [CrossRef]
30. Mangerich, A.; Dedon, P.C.; Fox, J.G.; Tannenbaum, S.R.; Wogan, G.N. Chemistry meets biology in colitis-associated carcinogenesis. *Free. Radic. Res.* **2013**, *47*, 958–986. [CrossRef]
31. Banning, A.; Freihaut, B.; Henry, R.; Pierce, S.; Bayer, W.L. GPx2 counteracts PGE2 production by dampening COX-2 and mPGES-1 expression in human colon cancer cells. *Antioxid. Redox Signal.* **2008**, *10*, 1491–1500. [CrossRef]
32. Moura, F.A.; de Andrade, K.Q.; Dos Santos, J.C.F.; Araújo, O.R.P.; Goulart, M.O.F. Antioxidant therapy for treatment of inflammatory bowel disease: Does it work? *Redox Biol.* **2015**, *6*, 617. [CrossRef] [PubMed]
33. He, L.; He, T.; Farrar, S.; Ji, L.; Liu, T.; Ma, X. Antioxidants Maintain Cellular Redox Homeostasis by Elimination of Reactive Oxygen Species. *Cell Physiol. Biochem.* **2017**, *44*, 532–553. [CrossRef] [PubMed]
34. Miller, A.-F. Superoxide dismutases: Ancient enzymes and new insights. *FEBS Lett.* **2011**, *586*, 585–595. [CrossRef] [PubMed]
35. Wang, Y.; Branicky, R.; Noë, A.; Hekimi, S. Superoxide dismutases: Dual roles in controlling ROS damage and regulating ROS signaling. *J. Cell Biol.* **2018**, *217*, 1915–1928. [CrossRef] [PubMed]
36. Unsal, V.; Dalkıran, T.; Çiçek, M.; Kölükçü, E. The Role of Natural Antioxidants Against Reactive Oxygen Species Produced by Cadmium Toxicity: A Review. *Adv. Pharm. Bull.* **2020**, *10*, 184–202. [CrossRef] [PubMed]
37. Unsal, V.; Belge-Kurutaş, E. Experimental Hepatic Carcinogenesis: Oxidative Stress and Natural Antioxidants. *Open Access Maced. J. Med. Sci.* **2017**, *5*, 686. [CrossRef] [PubMed]
38. Unsal, V. Natural Phytotherapeutic Antioxidants in the Treatment of Mercury Intoxication-A Review. *Adv. Pharm. Bull.* **2018**, *8*, 365–376. [CrossRef]
39. Couto, N.; Wood, J.; Barber, J. The role of glutathione reductase and related enzymes on cellular redox homoeostasis network. *Free. Radic. Biol. Med.* **2016**, *95*, 27–42. [CrossRef]
40. Elmallah, M.; Elkhadragy, M.; Al-Olayan, E.; Abdel Moneim, A. Protective Effect of Fragaria ananassa Crude Extract on Cadmium-Induced Lipid Peroxidation, Antioxidant Enzymes Suppression, and Apoptosis in Rat Testes. *Int. J. Mol. Sci.* **2017**, *18*, 957. [CrossRef]
41. Lu, J.; Holmgren, A. The thioredoxin antioxidant system. *Free Radic Biol. Med.* **2014**, *66*, 75–87. [CrossRef]
42. Collins, A.E.; Saleh, T.M.; Kalisch, B.E. Naturally Occurring Antioxidant Therapy in Alzheimer's Disease. *Antioxidants* **2022**, *11*, 213. [CrossRef] [PubMed]
43. Lu, J.; Holmgren, A. Thioredoxin System in Cell Death Progression. *Antioxid. Redox Signal.* **2012**, *17*, 1738–1747. [CrossRef] [PubMed]
44. Niture, S.K.; Khatri, R.; Jaiswal, A.K. Regulation of Nrf2—An update. *Free Radic Biol Med.* **2014**, *66*, 36–44. [CrossRef]
45. Shi, L.; Wu, L.; Chen, Z.; Yang, J.; Chen, X.; Yu, F.; Lin, X. MiR-141 Activates Nrf2-Dependent Antioxidant Pathway via Down-Regulating the Expression of Keap1 Conferring the Resistance of Hepatocellular Carcinoma Cells to 5-Fluorouracil. *Cell Physiol. Biochem.* **2015**, *35*, 2333–2348. [CrossRef] [PubMed]
46. Patel, R.; Rinker, L.; Peng, J.; Chilian, W.M. Reactive Oxygen Species: The Good and the Bad. *React. Oxyg. Species (ROS) Living Cells* **2018**, *7*. [CrossRef]
47. Brumatti, L.V.; Marcuzzi, A.; Tricarico, P.M.; Zanin, V.; Girardelli, M.; Bianco, A.M. Curcumin and Inflammatory Bowel Disease: Potential and Limits of Innovative Treatments. *Molecules* **2014**, *19*, 21127. [CrossRef] [PubMed]
48. Singla, V.; Pratap Mouli, V.; Garg, S.K.; Rai, T.; Choudhury, B.N.; Verma, P.; Deb, R.; Tiwari, V.; Rohatgi, S.; Dhingra, R. Induction with NCB-02 (curcumin) enema for mild-to-moderate distal ulcerative colitis—A randomized, placebo-controlled, pilot study. *J. Crohns. Colitis.* **2014**, *8*, 208–214. [CrossRef]
49. Lang, A.; Salomon, N.; Wu, J.C.; Kopylov, U.; Lahat, A.; Har-Noy, O.; Ching, J.Y.; Cheong, P.K.; Avidan, B.; Gamus, D. Curcumin in Combination with Mesalamine Induces Remission in Patients with Mild-to-Moderate Ulcerative Colitis in a Randomized Controlled Trial. *Clin. Gastroenterol. Hepatol.* **2015**, *13*, 1444–1449.e1. [CrossRef]
50. Banerjee, R.; Pal, P.; Penmetsa, A.; Kathi, P.; Girish, G.; Goren, I.; Reddy, D.N. Novel Bioenhanced Curcumin with Mesalamine for Induction of Clinical and Endoscopic Remission in Mild-to-Moderate Ulcerative Colitis: A Randomized Double-Blind Placebo-controlled Pilot Study. *J. Clin. Gastroenterol.* **2021**, *55*, 702–708. [CrossRef]
51. Rahal, K.; Chmiedlin-Ren, P.; Adler, J.; Dhanani, M.; Sultani, V.; Rittershaus, A.C.; Reingold, L.; Zhu, J.; McKenna, B.J.; Christman, G.M.; et al. Resveratrol has anti-inflammatory and antifibrotic effects in the peptidoglycan-polysaccharide rat model of Crohn's disease. *Inflamm. Bowel Dis.* **2012**, *18*, 613. [CrossRef]

52. Yildiz, G.; Yildiz, Y.; Ulutas, P.A.; Yaylali, A.; Ural, M. Resveratrol Pretreatment Ameliorates TNBS Colitis in Rats. *Recent Pat. Endocr. Metab. Immune Drug Discov.* **2015**, *9*, 134. [CrossRef] [PubMed]
53. Samsamikor, M.; Daryani, N.E.; Asl, P.R.; Hekmatdoost, A. Resveratrol Supplementation and Oxidative/Anti-Oxidative Status in Patients with Ulcerative Colitis: A Randomized, Double-Blind, Placebo-controlled Pilot Study. *Arch. Med. Res.* **2016**, *47*, 304–309. [CrossRef] [PubMed]
54. Samsami-Kor, M.; Daryani, N.E.; Asl, R.; Hekmatdoost, A. Anti-Inflammatory Effects of Resveratrol in Patients with Ulcerative Colitis: A Randomized, Double-Blind, Placebo-controlled Pilot Study. *Arch. Med. Res.* **2015**, *46*, 280–285. [CrossRef] [PubMed]
55. Das, S.; Chaudhury, A.; Ng, K.Y. Preparation and evaluation of zinc-pectin-chitosan composite particles for drug delivery to the colon: Role of chitosan in modifying in vitro and in vivo drug release. *Int. J. Pharm.* **2011**, *406*, 11–20. [CrossRef] [PubMed]
56. Posadino, A.M.; Cossu, A.; Giordo, R.; Zinellu, A.; Sotgia, S.; Vardeu, A.; Hoa, P.T.; Van Nguyen, L.V.; Carru, C.; Pintus, G. Resveratrol alters human endothelial cells redox state and causes mitochondrial-dependent cell death. *Food Chem. Toxicol.* **2015**, *78*, 10–16. [CrossRef] [PubMed]
57. Ju, S.; Ge, Y.; Li, P.; Tian, X.; Wang, H.; Zheng, X.; Ju, S. Dietary quercetin ameliorates experimental colitis in mouse by remodeling the function of colonic macrophages via a heme oxygenase-1-dependent pathway. *Cell Cycle* **2018**, *17*, 53–63. [CrossRef] [PubMed]
58. Dodda, D.; Chhajed, R.; Mishra, J.; Padhy, M. Targeting oxidative stress attenuates trinitrobenzene sulphonic acid induced inflammatory bowel disease like symptoms in rats: Role of quercetin. *Indian J. Pharmacol.* **2014**, *46*, 286. [CrossRef] [PubMed]
59. Suzuki, T.; Hara, H. Role of flavonoids in intestinal tight junction regulation. *J. Nutr. Biochem.* **2011**, *22*, 401–408. [CrossRef]
60. Kamishikiryo, J.; Matsumura, R.; Takamori, T.; Sugihara, N. Effect of quercetin on the transport of N-acetyl 5-aminosalicylic acid. *J. Pharm. Pharmacol.* **2013**, *65*, 1037–1043. [CrossRef]
61. Sánchez, A.; Calpena, A.C.; Clares, B. Evaluating the Oxidative Stress in Inflammation: Role of Melatonin. *Int. J. Mol. Sci.* **2015**, *16*, 16981. [CrossRef]
62. Reiter, R.J.; Mayo, J.C.; Tan, D.X.; Sainz, R.M.; Alatorre-Jimenez, M.; Qin, L. Melatonin as an antioxidant: Under promises but over delivers. *J. Pineal Res.* **2016**, *61*, 253–278. [CrossRef] [PubMed]
63. Chojnacki, C. Evaluation of Melatonin Effectiveness in the Adjuvant Treatment of Ulcerative Colitis. Cochrane Library. Available online: https://www.cochranelibrary.com/central/doi/10.1002/central/CN-00836249/full (accessed on 1 September 2022).
64. Zhu, D.; Ma, Y.; Ding, S.; Jiang, H.; Fang, J. Effects of Melatonin on Intestinal Microbiota and Oxidative Stress in Colitis Mice. *Biomed Res. Int.* **2018**, *2018*, 2607679. [CrossRef] [PubMed]
65. Liu, Y.; Wang, X.; Hu, C.A.A. Therapeutic Potential of Amino Acids in Inflammatory Bowel Disease. *Nutrients* **2017**, *9*, 920. [CrossRef] [PubMed]
66. Elberry, A.A.; Sharkawi, S.M.Z.; Wahba, M.R. Antinociceptive and anti-inflammatory effects of N-acetylcysteine and verapamil in Wistar rats. *Korean J. Pain.* **2019**, *32*, 256–263. [CrossRef] [PubMed]
67. Seril, D.N.; Liao, J.; Ho, K.L.; Yang, C.S.; Yang, G.Y. Inhibition of chronic ulcerative colitis-associated colorectal adenocarcinoma development in a murine model by N-acetylcysteine. *Carcinogenesis* **2002**, *23*, 993–1001. [CrossRef] [PubMed]
68. 68. Zheng, J.; Yuan, X.; Zhang, C.; Jia, P.; Jiao, S.; Zhao, X.; Yin, H.; Du, Y.; Liu, H. N-Acetylcysteine alleviates gut dysbiosis and glucose metabolic disorder in high-fat diet-fed mice. *J. Diabetes* **2019**, *11*, 32–45. [CrossRef] [PubMed]
69. Ancha, H.R.; Kurella, R.R.; McKimmey, C.C.; Lightfoot, S.; Harty, R.F. Effects of N-acetylcysteine plus mesalamine on prostaglandin synthesis and nitric oxide generation in TNBS-induced colitis in rats. *Dig. Dis. Sci.* **2009**, *54*, 758–766. [CrossRef]
70. Masnadi Shirazi, K.; Sotoudeh, S.; Masnadi Shirazi, A.; Moaddab, S.Y.; Nourpanah, Z.; Nikniaz, Z. Effect of N-acetylcysteine on remission maintenance in patients with ulcerative colitis: A randomized, double-blind controlled clinical trial. *Clin. Res. Hepatol. Gastroenterol.* **2021**, *45*, 101532. [CrossRef]
71. Guijarro, L.G.; Mate, J.; Gisbert, J.; Perez-Calle, J.L.; Marin-Jimenez, I.; Arriaza, E.; Olleros, T.; Delgado, M.; Castillejo, M.S.; Prieto-Merino, D.; et al. N-acetyl-L-cysteine combined with mesalamine in the treatment of ulcerative colitis: Randomized, placebo-controlled pilot study. *World J. Gastroenterol.* **2008**, *14*, 2851–2857. [CrossRef]
72. Hou, C.L.; Zhang, J.; Liu, X.T.; Liu, H.; Zeng, X.F.; Qiao, S.Y. Superoxide dismutase recombinant Lactobacillus fermentum ameliorates intestinal oxidative stress through inhibiting NF-κB activation in a trinitrobenzene sulphonic acid-induced colitis mouse model. *J. Appl. Microbiol.* **2014**, *116*, 1621–1631. [CrossRef]
73. Suzuki, Y.; Matsumoto, T.; Okamoto, S.; Hibi, T.A. A lecithinized superoxide dismutase (PC-SOD) improves ulcerative colitis. *Color. Dis.* **2008**, *10*, 931. [CrossRef] [PubMed]
74. Al-Howail, H.A.; Hakami, H.A.; Al-Otaibi, B.; Al-Mazrou, A.; Daghestani, M.H.; Al-Jammaz, I.; Al-Khalaf, H.H.; Aboussekhra, A. PAC down-regulates estrogen receptor alpha and suppresses epithelial-to-mesenchymal transition in breast cancer cells. *BMC Cancer.* **2016**, *16*, 540.
75. Semlali, A.; Contant, C.; Al-Otaibi, B.; Al-Jammaz, I.; Chandad, F. The curcumin analog (PAC) suppressed cell survival and induced apoptosis and autophagy in oral cancer cells. *Sci. Rep.* **2021**, *11*, 11701. [CrossRef] [PubMed]
76. Veenstra, J.; Vemu, B.; Tocmo, R.; Nauman, M.C.; Johnson, J.J. Pharmacokinetic Analysis of Carnosic Acid and Carnosol in Standardized Rosemary Extract and the Effect on the Disease Activity Index of DSS-Induced Colitis. *Nutrients* **2021**, *13*, 773. [CrossRef] [PubMed]
77. Sundararajan, S.; Jayachandran, I.; Subramanian, S.C.; Anjana, R.M.; Balasubramanyam, M.; Mohan, V.; Venkatesan, B.; Manickam, N. Decreased Sestrin levels in patients with type 2 diabetes and dyslipidemia and their association with the severity of atherogenic index. *J. Endocrinol. Investig.* **2021**, *44*, 1395–1405. [CrossRef] [PubMed]

78. Ghasemi-Dehnoo, M.; Safari, A.A.; Rahimi-Madiseh, M.; Lorigooini, Z.; Moradi, M.T.; Amini-Khoei, H. Anethole Ameliorates Acetic Acid-Induced Colitis in Mice: Anti-Inflammatory and Antioxidant Effects. *Evid Based Complement Altern. Med.* **2022**, *2022*, 9057451. [CrossRef]
79. Fu, T.T.; Shen, L. Ergothioneine as a Natural Antioxidant Against Oxidative Stress-Related Diseases. *Front. Pharmacol.* **2022**, *13*, 850813. [CrossRef]

Disclaimer/Publisher's Note: The statements, opinions and data contained in all publications are solely those of the individual author(s) and contributor(s) and not of MDPI and/or the editor(s). MDPI and/or the editor(s) disclaim responsibility for any injury to people or property resulting from any ideas, methods, instructions or products referred to in the content.

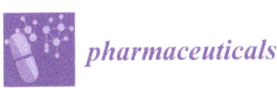

Review

Tackling Inflammatory Bowel Diseases: Targeting Proinflammatory Cytokines and Lymphocyte Homing

Yijie Song [1,†], Man Yuan [1,†], Yu Xu [1,*] and Hongxi Xu [2,*]

1. School of Pharmacy, Shanghai University of Traditional Chinese Medicine, Shanghai 201203, China
2. Shuguang Hospital, Shanghai University of Traditional Chinese Medicine, Shanghai 201203, China
* Correspondence: xyzjh2021@shutcm.edu.cn (Y.X.); hxxu@shutcm.edu.cn (H.X.); Tel.: +86-13601793729 (Y.X.); +86-021-51323089 (H.X.)
† These authors contributed equally to this work.

Abstract: Inflammatory bowel diseases (IBDs) are characterized by chronic inflammatory disorders that are a result of an abnormal immune response mediated by a cytokine storm and immune cell infiltration. Proinflammatory cytokine therapeutic agents, represented by TNF inhibitors, have developed rapidly over recent years and are promising options for treating IBD. Antagonizing interleukins, interferons, and Janus kinases have demonstrated their respective advantages in clinical trials and are candidates for anti-TNF therapeutic failure. Furthermore, the blockade of lymphocyte homing contributes to the excessive immune response in colitis and ameliorates inflammation and tissue damage. Factors such as integrins, selectins, and chemokines jointly coordinate the accumulation of immune cells in inflammatory regions. This review assembles the major targets and agents currently targeting proinflammatory cytokines and lymphatic trafficking to facilitate subsequent drug development.

Keywords: inflammatory bowel disease; cytokines; lymphocyte homing

1. Introduction

Inflammatory bowel diseases (IBDs) are a class of chronic inflammatory disorders including two main clinical entities: Crohn's disease (CD) and ulcerative colitis (UC). The prevalence of IBD is increasing worldwide, imposing a huge socioeconomic burden on society and health care systems [1]. However, a thorough comprehension of IBD pathogenesis remains elusive, and the progression of IBD is widely believed to encompass an intertwining of environmental, genetic, microbial, and immunological factors [2]. Encouragingly, considerable advances in the development of drugs targeting the immune system to block IBD have boosted the efficacy of treatment for IBD in recent decades [3].

Overwhelming cytokine storms and immune cell infiltration impede inflammation regression in IBD and contribute to disease recurrence and tissue damage. As a chronic inflammatory disease, CD has been considered to be correlated with the immune response mediated by type 1 T helper cells (TH1) and TH17, while abnormal TH2 responses are involved in the development of UC, and the eventual imbalance of interactions with other T-cell groups (e.g., Treg and TH9) contributes to the complexity of IBD immunopathogenesis [2]. A variety of cytokines produced by immune cells are uniquely characteristic of patients with IBD, including tumor necrosis factor (TNF), interleukin (IL)-6, and IL-1β, which are critical drivers of inflammatory impairment (Figure 1) [4]. Moderation of such proinflammatory cytokines in IBD appears to be a sound treatment option, evidenced by the successful application of TNF inhibitors, and recognition of cytokines could facilitate IBD therapy. Furthermore, either the innate or adaptive immune response depends primarily on lymphocyte homing to specific tissues, which is mediated by the adhesion of immune cells to vascular endothelial cells [5]. Thus, modulating immune cell trafficking is an efficacious approach to remedy tissue lesions and mucosal inflammation in IBD.

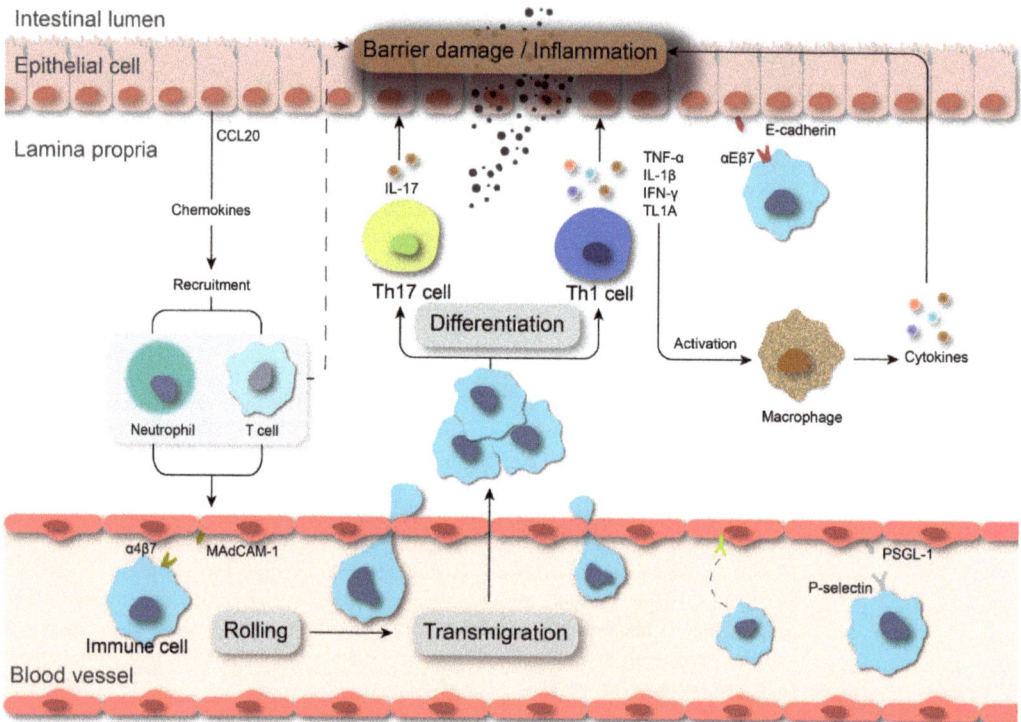

Figure 1. Immune cell homing and cytokine storming drive IBD progression. Lymphocytes roll, adhere, and transmigrate at the site of the lesion through the combined action of integrins, selections, and chemokines, with residence in the lamina propria. Excessive immune responses and external stimulus synergistically lead to a proinflammatory cytokine storm hindering disease recovery.

Given the advanced research on proinflammatory cytokines and lymphatic trafficking associated with IBD in recent years, therapeutic agents for related targets are burgeoning. Therefore, a timely review of targeting cytokines and lymphatic trafficking is needed, and here, the latest relevant studies are collated to facilitate drug developers and clinicians to catch up on research developments and medication choices.

2. Targeting Proinflammatory Cytokines

Cytokines are pivotal influencers of gut homeostasis and perpetual inflammation [6]. The appearance of anti-TNF drugs has drastically altered the therapeutic algorithm for IBD, yet a significant proportion of patients receiving anti-TNF therapy suffer from nonresponse or secondary loss of response. Fortunately, new treatment alternatives have been proactively explored (Figure 2), among which some have entered clinical practice and some have shown good efficacy in preclinical studies [7].

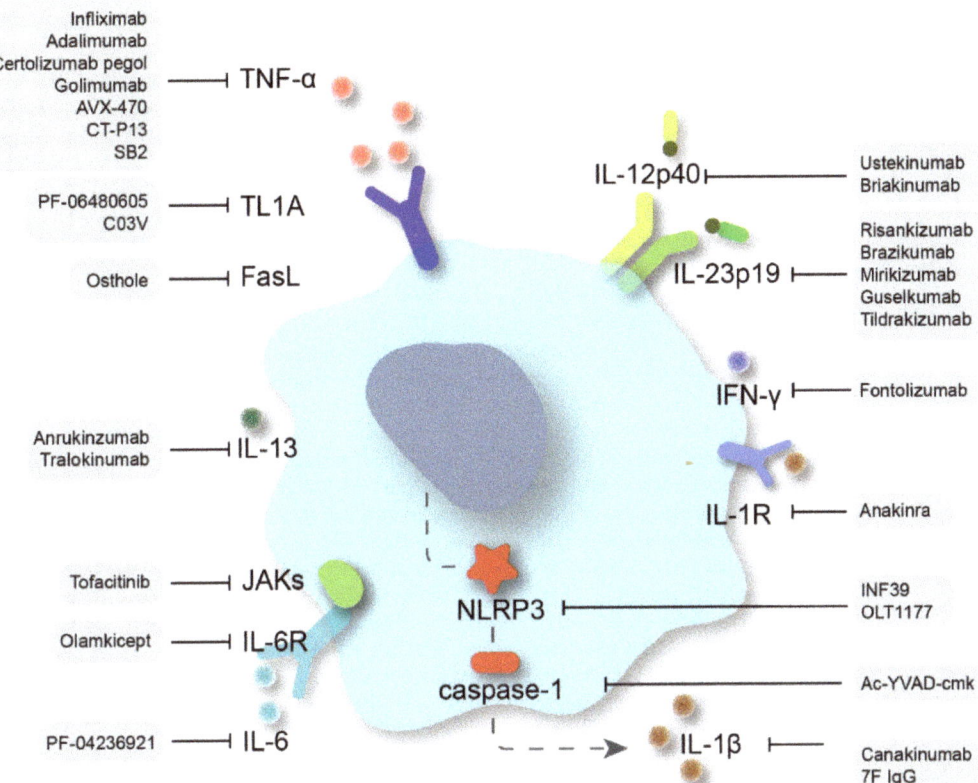

Figure 2. Therapeutic targets of proinflammatory cytokines in IBD treatment and specific therapeutic agents.

2.1. Tumor Necrosis Factor Superfamily

The tumor necrosis factor superfamily (TNFSF) members are molecules with broad-spectrum activity and are well known to have pathological effects on IBD, the best known of which is TNF. The majority of TNFSF members are expressed by immune cells and modulate the homeostasis of T-cell-mediated immune responses [8]. Numerous recent studies have demonstrated that certain TNFSF members, including TNF-α, TL1A, FasL, and others, promote IBD pathogenesis through the enhancement of T-cell proinflammatory function and through the direct disruption of intestinal epithelial integrity [9].

2.1.1. Anti-TNF-α Agents

Infliximab (IFX) is an immunoglobulin G1 monoclonal antibody (mAb) with a high affinity for TNF-α that was initially licensed in 1998 by the FDA for treating patients with refractory active IBD, pioneering the era of biologics for IBD [10,11]. IFX is potent in both attaining and sustaining clinical remission and is also recommended for patients with IBD tha are unresponsive to 5-ASAs or corticosteroid therapy. A multiple-center randomized controlled trial (RCT) of pediatric CD patients [12] showed that first-line IFX intervention outperformed routine treatment in terms of short-term clinical (59% vs. 34%) and endoscopic remission (59% vs. 17%). Sequentially, more anti-TNF mAbs, such as adalimumab, certolizumab pegol, and golimumab, have been developed and licensed, showing promising clinical efficacy [13]. For example, in a multicenter, prospective cohort study of CD patients, approximately two-thirds of patients receiving adalimumab had a good prognosis and long-term maintenance of remission, reducing the incidence of colectomy [14]. In addition to intravenous monotherapy, a new oral polyclonal anti-TNF antibody, AVX-470, prepared from the colostrum of TNF-immune cows, showed efficacy comparable to that of oral prednisolone and parenteral etanercept in murine experimental colitis models and minimized systemic exposure to anti-TNF agents [15]. The first RCT of AVX-470 for UC demonstrated a good safety profile and was beneficial for refractory UC, with clinical, endoscopic, and biomarker (serum CRP and IL-6) improvements [16]. Additionally, TNF-related biosimilars, such as CT-P13 and SB2, have been developed to mitigate the surge in therapeutic costs caused by biological treatments [17], increasing the accessibility of appropriate biologic treatments by patients. Currently, over 20 biosimilars of infliximab and adalimumab are under development and have been described in detail [18].

2.1.2. Anti-TL1A Therapy

TNFSF member 15 gene (TNFSF15, also named TL1A) variants are correlated with the risk of IBD, which impacts the production of multiple cytokines to fuel mucosal inflammation [19]. TL1A is overexpressed in inflamed mucosa and is associated with CD fibrosis [20]. As TL1A is upstream of the proinflammatory process, anti-TL1A regimens may offer an attractive option for individuals unresponsive to TNF-α inhibitors and are a candidate for resolving currently nonreversible intestinal fibrosis. TL1A-overexpressing mice developed idiopathic ileitis with increased proximal colitis-inducing injury and fibrosis, whereas TL1A receptor-deficient mice exhibited resistance to a transmigration model of colitis and had reduced inflammation and intestinal fibrosis [21]. A human immunoglobulin G1 mAb against TL1A, PF-06480605, demonstrated improved endoscopic healing (38.2% at week 14, $p < 0.001$, and 95% CI = 23.82–53.68) and a favorable safety profile among individuals with refractory UC [22], probably in association with inflammatory T cells and fibrosis pathways [23]. C03V, a high affinity and selective human antibody to TL1A that neutralizes the biological activity of TL1A, remarkably attenuated the pathology of colitis triggered by trinitrobenzene sulfonic acid (TNBS) and alleviated fibrosis [24].

2.1.3. Targeting the FasL/FAS System

Mutations in TNFRSF6 (also named FasL) and its receptor FAS cause autoimmune lymphoid tissue proliferation syndrome and are involved in lymphocyte variation in IBD [25]. A marked increase in FasL-containing cells was observed in active UC patients in comparison to either remission or control groups based on immunohistochemistry of the colonic mucosa [26]. Conversely, a study on an acute colitis rat TNBS model discovered that isolated dendritic cells from mesenteric lymph nodes of wild-type rats expressed more FasL than those from colitis rats, and exogenous infusion of DCs genetically engineered to overexpress FasL decreased T-cell IFN-γ production and enhanced T-cell apoptosis, effectively reducing colonic inflammation [27]. Osthole restored the downregulation of Fas and FasL expression in bone marrow mesenchymal stem cells (BMSCs) caused by immune impairment and restored the ability of BMSCs to induce T-cell apoptosis and immunosuppressive function over experimental colitis [28].

2.1.4. Other TNFSF Members with Potential Efficacy

We are gaining insight into the value of other members of TNFSF in the IBD process as research progresses. TNFSF14, also named LIGHT, resides on T cells and participates in their activation, and its transgenic expression on murine T cells drives pathogenic inflammation in several organs, including the intestine [29]. Mice with Tnfsf14 deficiency were found to undergo more serious colitis and have lower survival rates than wild-type mice, suggesting that LIGHT may mediate innate immune activities and the resilience of gut inflammation by transmitting signals through lymphotoxin β receptors in the colon [30]. Furthermore, single-cell analysis of colonic mesenchymal cells in UC patients also revealed a subpopulation of activated mesenchymal populations with TNFSF14 expression, which is assumed to limit colonic epithelial proliferation and impede wound repair responses [31]. TNFSF10, also named TRAIL, mediates autoimmune inflammation and cellular homeostasis by transmitting apoptotic signals to induce apoptosis and was found to suppress autoimmune colitis by inhibiting colonic T-cell activation [32].

It is worth noting that not every patient responds to anti-TNF therapy and many suffer from the underlying opportunistic infections that come with treatment. High-dose administration regimens are recommended by experts to address the insufficient efficacy of anti-TNFs, and individualized dosing strategies are encouraged to be implemented with drug monitoring in clinical practice to avoid inadequate blockade of TNF in serum and tissues [33]. Natural products and herbs have also shown modulation of TNF-α activity in experimental models and clinical trials, which might be an effective intervention to bypass the side effects of specific anti-TNF therapy [34]. Natural polyphenols from plants, such as curcumin [35], mangiferin [36], and catechin [37], have demonstrated anti-inflammatory effects in TNBS/DSS-induced colitis models and reduced TNF-α expression. In addition, complementing anti-TNF therapy with nutritional biocompounds, such as antioxidant-enriched purple corn supplement [38], has exhibited beneficial effects on the induction and maintenance of IBD remission. While studies on natural products are currently mostly preclinical, their potential for the treatment and prevention of IBD deserves constant attention.

2.2. Interleukins

Multiple interleukins secreted by lymphocytes mediate their pro/anti-inflammatory effects, and inhibition of proinflammatory cytokines (IL-6, IL-1β, IL-12, and IL-23) is an effective strategy to ameliorate colitis. Presently, agents targeting interleukins have exhibited some advantages over anti-TNF agents.

2.2.1. Anti-IL-12/IL-23 Agents

IL-12 and IL-23, produced mainly by inflammatory myeloid cells, are highly expressed in colitis patients and induce differentiation and responses in TH1 cells and IL-17-producing T helper cells (TH17), respectively [39]. IL-12 and IL-23, as heterodimeric cytokines, are formed by the homogeneous subunit p40 in conjunction with p35 and p19, respectively. The roles of IL-12 and IL-23 are temporally distinct in the progression of IBD, where IL-12 is engaged in the early stages of colitis by activating TH1 cells and macrophages, while IL-23 shapes the chronic exacerbation of the disease [40].

Antagonizing p40, the cosubunit for IL-12 and IL-23, is a potent blockade of disease development. Ustekinumab (UST), a mAb against the p40 subunit, has already been licensed for CD treatment. In two 8-week RCTs of intravenous induction therapy for intermediate-to-severe active CD patients (UNITI-1 and UNITI-2), patients undergoing either primary or secondary nonresponse to TNF antagonists achieved significantly higher remission rates in patients receiving intravenous UST than those receiving placebo (in UNITI-1, 34.3% vs. 21.5%; in UNITI-2, 51.7% vs. 28.7%). A double-blind, active comparative phase 3b RCT (SEAVUE) involving multiple countries showed that 124 (65%) moderate-to-severe CD patients (n = 191) without biologic therapy remained in clinical remission after UST treatment at week 52 [41]. Moreover, patients taking maintenance doses of UST injections every 8 or 12 weeks achieved prolonged disease remission, and the occurrence of undesirable events was comparable to the placebo [42]. UST is equally effective in inducing and sustaining remission for patients with moderate-to-severe UC compared with placebo [43], and future studies are expected to compare the effectiveness of UST with existing biologics in treating UC [44]. Briakinumab, an anti-IL-12p40 mAb, has been terminated from production and follow-up studies due to uncertainty and low confidence in its actual role in the induction and maintenance of clinical remission in CD patients [45].

IL-23 is a pivotal promoter for chronic intestinal inflammation, and targeting IL-23-specific p19 subunits has proven to be effective in phase 2 studies of IBD [46], which may facilitate selective blockade of intestinal lymphatic trafficking without compromising systemic immune defense [47]. There are four mAbs (risankizumab, brazikumab, mirikizumab, and guselkumab) currently applied in clinical trials for either CD or UC [48]. Risankizumab showed curative efficacy and an admissible safety profile in patients suffering moderate-to-severe CD [49], and subcutaneous risankizumab demonstrated maintenance efficacy (including >71% clinical relief and >42% endoscopic remission) in a phase 2 study with good treatment tolerability [50]. Additionally, IL-23/IL-17 axis-related genes were differentially expressed in the transcriptome profile of the ileum and colon of patients after risankizumab treatment [51]. Brazikumab treatment was correlated with clinical improvement in patients with moderate-to-severe CD at 8 and 24 weeks [52]. Mirikizumab exhibited an effective induction of a positive clinical response following 12 weeks of treatment in UC patients (22.6% in the 200 mg group vs. 4.8% in the placebo group) and showed lasting benefits during the entire maintenance period, while it should be noted that the treatment effect of mirikizumab did not seem to proceed in a dose-dependent manner, and further studies are required to determine the optimal dose [53]. Comparatively, approximately 50% of patients initially unresponsive to mirikizumab achieved a clinical response after receiving a prolonged induction period at an increased dose (600 or 1000 mg [54]). Different doses of guselkumab had a good safety profile compared to placebo, achieving better clinical and endoscopic remission (200 mg: 57.4%, 500 mg: 55.6%, and 1200 mg: 45.9% vs. placebo: 16.4%) in a phase 2 clinical trial (GLAXI-1). Additionally, tildrakizumab, a high affinity humanized IgG1κ antibody targeting IL23p19, has proven efficacy in chronic plaque psoriasis and is expected to be implemented into IBD management [55].

Since the effect of IL-23 blockers in the management of chronic inflammatory diseases was first confirmed in psoriasis and subsequently revalidated in other inflammatory diseases, such as IBD, learning from the long-term experience of their applications in other diseases may help to accelerate the optimization of IL-12/23 dosing regimens for IBD patients by gastroenterologists and avoid drug adverse events [56].

2.2.2. IL-6/IL-6R Inhibitors

The engagement of IL-6 in IBD and colorectal cancer pathogenesis has been well explored [57], and some anti-IL-6 mAbs have been tested in RCTs against autoimmune diseases. IL-6 is rapidly produced in response to tissue injury and infection and promotes host immunity by stimulating acute phase responses and immune reactivity, while imbalanced IL-6 synthesis contributes to the pathological effects on chronic inflammation and immune action [58]. IL-6 mediates the proliferation of TH17 cells in concert with TGF-β by affecting signal transducers and activators of transcription (STAT3), which is essential for TH17 cell maintenance and function [59].

PF-04236921, an antibody against IL-6, was investigated among adult CD patients (ANDANTE I and II), with an increased remission rate after a 12-week treatment period (27.4% in PF-04236921 vs. 10.9% in placebo) [60]. PF-04236921 has the potential to induce clinical responses and palliations for refractory CD patients not responding to anti-TNF regimens, but its possible side effects (gastrointestinal abscesses and abdominal pain) warrant attention during subsequent development. Clone MP5-20F3 (an IL-6 mAb) neutralized DSS-induced elevated IL-6 concentrations and inhibited Claudin-2 expression in mice, improving intestinal inflammation and permeability, and its therapeutic effects were further amplified upon coadministration with an anti-TNF-α mAb [61]. An intriguing study on diet and colon cancer demonstrated that a high-calorie diet elevated IL-6 expression in porcine colonic mucosa and changed the expression of IL-6-associated proteins such as PI3KR4, IL-1α, and Map2k1, while a whole food diet inhibited HCD-induced alterations in IL-6-related proteins and modulation of IL-6 signaling was strongly associated with diet-related colitis/cancer [62]. Notably, IL-6 is involved in conditioning critical pharmacokinetic enzymes, such as cytochrome P450s (CYPs), and receiving anti-IL-6 management may restrict the AUCs of drugs with CYP substrates [63], which would impair drug management of many diseases.

Blocking IL-6R also effectively restricts IL-6 complex formation and modulates IL-6-mediated chronic inflammation. Tocilizumab, a humanized IL-6R blocker, is currently approved as a treatment for rheumatoid arthritis and has proven effective in other recalcitrant autoimmune diseases, and its therapeutic applications in IBD are promising [64]. Furthermore, since the chronic proinflammatory activity of IL-6 depends on the gp130 coreceptor for trans-signaling, the decoy protein sgp130Fc (olamkicept) was developed to specifically block IL-6 trans-signaling. Olamkicept resulted in a clinical response by 44% of patients with active IBD in a prospective 2a trial, and its clinical effectiveness was consistent with transcriptional changes in target inhibition [65].

Overall, IL-6 inhibition is a viable treatment option for IBD, but the benefit of completely blocking IL-6 or related receptors is restricted by its strong immunosuppression [65].

2.2.3. IL-1β/IL-1R Antagonists

IL-1β is the main proinflammatory mediator of inflammation. Its secretion is triggered predominantly by macrophages in response to injurious stimuli and it has high expression in IBD patients. The analysis of intestinal biopsy specimens and circulating cytokine profiles from 30 UC patients showed that nearly three-quarters of primary nonresponders to anti-TNF therapy were characterized by hyperexpression of IL-1β in serum and gut tissue [66]. Despite the fact that IL-1β is considered to be as crucial a cytokine as TNF-α in the onset of IBD, there are currently few specific antibodies against IL-1β, excluding canakinumab [67]. The absence of binding to murine-derived IL-1β hindered preclinical studies of canakinumab [68].

A novel chimeric anti-IL-1β-specific mAb, 7F IgG, with high affinity for various mammalian IL-1βs, blocked IL-1β to regulate proinflammatory cytokines and showed anticolitis activity in a TNBS-induced murine model [68]. Antagonism of the IL-1 receptor (IL-1R) is a therapeutic alternative to reduce the IL-1β stimulatory response. Endogenous IL-1R antagonists have been discovered to be important in host defense against overwhelming endotoxin-induced injury, and they are generated in experimental animal models of multiple diseases and in human autoimmune inflammatory diseases and are essential natural anti-inflammatory proteins in colitis [69]. Anakinra (an IL-1R antagonist) treatment ameliorated dinitrobenzene sulfonate (DNBS)-induced colitis in terms of macroscopic and histological changes, inflammatory cell infiltration, and oxidative stress [70]. Two IL10R-deficient patients with severe refractory IBD had significant clinical, endoscopic, and histological responses following 4–7 weeks of anakinra therapy [71]. A phase 2, multicenter RCT (IASO) of short-term anakinra treatment in patients with acute severe ulcerative colitis (ASUC) has been approved by the Cambridge Central Ethics Committee, a clinical trial has been authorized [72], and the prognostic outcome of using anakinra to intervene in IL-1 signaling in patients with ASUC is of ongoing interest. A proportion of de-N-acetylated oligomers ($13 < dp < 20$) were reported to rescue inflammatory impairments via an IL-1Ra-dependent pathway, and water-soluble galactosaminogalactan oligosaccharides might be therapeutically applicable as new anti-inflammatory glycosides in IL-1-mediated hyperinflammatory diseases [73].

Indeed, the release of IL-1β is driven by the activated NOD-like receptor family pyrin domain containing 3 (NLRP3) inflammasome, which is harmful in colitis [74]. In a comparative preclinical study of NLRP3 inflammasome signaling inhibitors, it was found that administration of INF39 (an NLRP3 inflammasome irreversible direct blocker), Ac-YVAD-cmk (a caspase-1 inhibitor), and anakinra to rats with DNBS-induced colitis resulted in colitis relief and that INF39 was more effective in reducing organizational increments of myeloperoxidase, TNF, and IL-1β, and attenuating intestinal inflammation [75]. OLT1177, a selective inhibitor of NLRP3 inflammasomes, was administered during the induction period of DSS-induced mice to alleviate the disease phenotype, and OLT1177 was effective in preventing the onset of DSS colitis. However, the administration of OLT1177 during the recovery phase of colitis did not promote the recovery course or tissue remission [75]. Curcumin potently inhibited NLRP3 inflammasome activation to alleviate colitis in a DSS-induced murine model, and the therapeutic outcome was partially limited following the use of MCC950 (a specific NLRP3 blocker) [76].

2.2.4. Other Interleukin Neutralizers with Potential Efficacy

Experimental animal studies and human genetic studies are gradually revealing the importance of the interleukin superfamily in regulating inflammation and tissue damage in the intestinal mucosa [77]. More members of the interleukin family are being noticed in colitis, and targeted therapies are being explored.

IL-18 is a proinflammatory interleukin matured by NLRP3 inflammasome activation, and IL-18 equilibrium in the epithelium has been implicated in barrier function in colitis, where IL-18 coordinates goblet cell maturation transcriptional programs [78]. Mokry conducted a Mendelian randomization study of 12,882 cases and 21,770 controls to examine the effect of elevated IL-18 on IBD susceptibility, and the results revealed that each genetically predicted SNP change (rs385076, rs17229943, and rs71478720) in IL-18 was associated with elevated susceptibility to IBD [79]. GSK1070806, a neo-IgG1 mAb that neutralizes IL-18, has been tested in a pilot trial in type 2 diabetes and kidney transplantation [80], and a corresponding RCT based on genomic detection of IL-18 in IBD is warranted.

Overproduction of IL-13 in active UC causes disturbances in the intestinal epithelium and may promote fibrosis. Anrukinzumab is a humanized IgG1 antibody conjugated to IL-13 that impedes the binding of IL-13 and IL-4Rα without affecting the attachment of IL-13 to IL-13α1/α2. After receiving anrukinzumab intravenously, the total serum level of IL-13 increased (free IL-13 binds to anrukinzumab) in patients with active UC, while changes in fecal calprotectin at 14 weeks posttreatment were not significantly different compared to placebo, and the treatment effect did not have a statistically significant difference [81]. Tralokinumab, an IL-13 neutralizing antibody, failed to induce a clinical response when used as an add-on therapy randomized to ambulatory adult UC patients, whereas tralokinumab had higher rates of clinical remission (18% vs. 6%) and mucosal healing (32% vs. 20%) than placebo, suggesting that it may benefit some UC patients and be well tolerated [82]. Likewise, although IL-17A is an active cytokine in gut inflammation, the clinical outcome of anti-IL-17A therapy (secukinumab and ixekizumab, anti-IL-17A mAbs) in CD patients is not favorable [83], and a study based on IL-17a-/- mice found that blockade of IL-17A may cause IL-6 upregulation and RORγt+ ILC recruitment during chronic colitis, leading to elevated IL-22 and even worsened disease [84].

Apart from the interleukins mentioned above, the role played by other interleukins, such as IL-5 [85], IL-21 [86], and IL-33 [87], in IBD development is being uncovered as the disease mechanism comes to be better understood, and subsequent drug development for them is anticipated. The network of interleukin family actions is intertwined, and a complete blockade of a singular interleukin may lead to systemic involvement. This may explain the involvement of some interleukin family members in mediating IBD and the lack of efficacy in targeted antagonistic therapy [88]. Long-term follow-up after anti-interleukin control and regular monitoring of relevant therapeutic indicators are necessary to avoid potential adverse drug effects.

2.3. Anti-Interferon Agents

Interferons (IFNs) are an essential family of immunostimulatory cytokines, classified broadly into three subtypes: type I (IFN-α, β, ε, κ and ω), type II (IFN-γ), and the recently defined type III (IFN-λ) [89], among which INF-γ has been extensively studied in IBD. IFN-γ upregulation is common in IBD, and IFN-γ is vital for mucosal barrier defense function and stimulates immunomodulatory signaling. Increased populations of INF-γ-secreting cells in the lamina propria were identified as correlating with a higher disease activity index in CD [90], and a population-based screening cohort study of plasma samples identified IFN-γ as a potential key regulator of UC [91]. The pathogenic effect of IFN-γ on IBD may not only involve its immunomodulatory effects but also depend on its participation in the disruption of the vascular barrier [92]. The profile of serum type I and type II IFN in IBD patients receiving anti-TNF therapy correlated significantly with the treatment response in IBD patients and could be regarded as a clinical biomarker [93]. Excess type I interferon signaling in the intestinal epithelium is involved in intestinal panniculocyte dysfunction, and the Western diet is one of the environmental triggers leading to this process and ultimately to the pathogenesis of CD [94]. Recently, IFN-λ has also been proven to be involved in IBD, disrupting colonic epithelial healing and inducing small intestinal epithelial death, although associated studies are at a preliminary stage with complex and "paradoxical" effects of IFN-λ [95].

Fontolizumab, an anti-IFN-γ antibody, demonstrated efficacy in individuals with refractory CD, in which patients received two doses of fontolizumab intravenously followed by increased treatment response rates and remission on day 56, whereas clinical remission on day 28 after a single dose of fontolizumab was not significant [96]. Unfortunately, there have been no subsequent reports of fontolizumab for the treatment of colitis in recent years. Although quite a few biologics with activity against type I and II interferons are currently available, such as sifalumumab, rontalizumab, and anifrolumab (some of which have been approved for treating other immune diseases) [97], very few studies have been performed for the treatment of colitis. This is inextricably bound up with the double-sided action of IFN for colitis, and IFN profiling and other biomarkers in the serum of clinical patients could help to find suitable recipients for such therapies. Alternatively, small molecules of plant origin could be a potential breakthrough, offering a more "moderate" inhibitory activity against interferon than monoclonal antibodies. For example, feeding berberine inhibits IFN-γ and IL-17A in SCID mice administered with CD4+CD45RB high T cells, reduces lamina propria lymphocyte infiltration, and improves colitis [98].

2.4. Janus Kinase Inhibitors

Activation of Janus kinases (JAKs) is required for cytokine signaling and mediates the binding of cytokines and receptors. Consequently, blocking JAKs may be an efficient way to simultaneously modulate the activity of multiple proinflammatory cytokines to improve colitis [99].

Tofacitinib, a small-molecule JAK suppressor, is currently a promising medication for IBD and is approved for UC management [99]. Tofacitinib was superior to placebo for both inducing and maintaining treatment in three phase 3 clinical trials (OCTAVE) for UC. Clinical remission occurred in 18.5% of patients treated with 10 mg tofacitinib for 8 weeks and 8.2% of the placebo group, and similar improvements in treatment outcomes were reached in the other parallel trials. At 52 weeks, the maintenance effect of tofacitinib was apparent, as the remission rates in the 5 mg tofacitinib, 10 mg tofacitinib, and placebo groups were 34.3%, 40.6%, and 11.1%, respectively [100]. However, the risk of infection and cardiovascular events emerging from this study are of ongoing concern for follow-up. Tofacitinib is a rescue option for TNF inhibitor treatment failures, and an additional 10 mg of tofacitinib treatment usually leads to positive clinical responses for most patients [101]. In addition, recent studies have provided evidence of endoscopic and tissue remissions with tofacitinib for patients with refractory UC [102]. Nevertheless, the therapeutic benefit of tofacitinib on CD was not as pronounced as that on UC, and the results of several CD-related studies [103,104] demonstrated that the primary efficacy endpoint of tofacitinib was fundamentally similar to that of a placebo.

3. Targeting Leukocyte Trafficking

Leukocyte trafficking in the gut is strictly coordinated and engaged in maintaining intestinal immune equilibrium, mediating immune responses, and modulating inflammation, while in cases of colitis, large numbers of leukocytes migrate through the lymphatic and blood circulation into the gut and are activated, which is considered a vital step for a flare-up of IBD [105]. With the success of the anti-α4β7 antibody vedolizumab, the concept of addressing leukocyte homing for IBD management has been highlighted, which has become an exciting pillar of IBD therapy [106]. Leukocyte recruitment in inflammation is a complicated and sophisticated process requiring the binding of chemoattractants and receptors, the recognition of integrins, and the fastening of adhesion molecules. Thus, this section presents an overview of IBD agents targeting leukocyte trafficking (Figure 3), mainly including integrins, cell adhesion molecules (CAMs), chemokines, selectins, and sphingosine 1-phosphate (S1P) signaling.

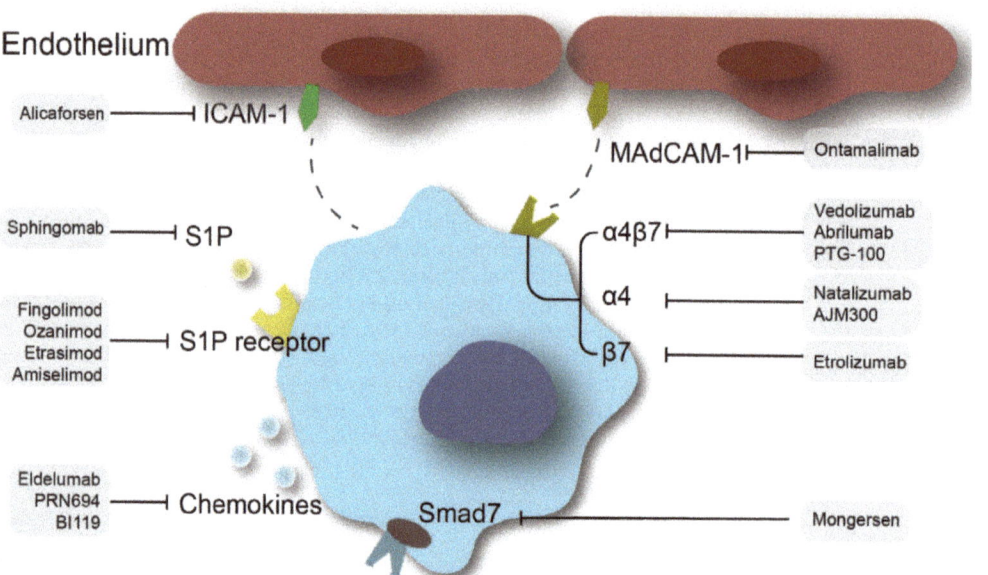

Figure 3. Therapeutic targets of leukocyte trafficking in IBD treatment and specific therapeutic agents.

3.1. Integrins

The integrin family is of particular importance in lymphatic homing, and various integrins expressed on endothelial cells are fundamental to this process. Integrins expressed on specific lymphocyte subpopulations are implicated in the onset of IBD [107]. Briefly, integrins are glycoprotein receptors present on the cell surface and are comprised of heterodimeric α and β subunits, to which CAMs and extracellular matrix bind [108]. Morphological alterations of integrins sparked by external stimuli (e.g., cytokines) boost their avidity for their corresponding ligands and guide the migration of lymphocytes. As an example, the integrins α4β1 and α4β7 enhance the translation of proinflammatory T lymphocytes into the lamina propria. Subsequently, cytotoxic T lymphocytes are preserved by the interaction between αEβ7 and E-cadherin once they have entered the lamina propria [109].

3.1.1. Anti-α4 Antibody

α4 was the first integrin explored as a potential target for the management of UC and CD, and as a common subunit of α4β1 and α4β7, HP1/2 (an anti-α4 mAb) significantly alleviated acute colitis in a cotton-top tamarin spontaneous colitis model [110]. Consequently, blocking leukocyte–vascular adhesion and other integrin-mediated IBD management options have been acknowledged and developed rapidly over the past three decades.

Natalizumab (a humanized α4 antibody) induced and maintained remission in refractory CD patients in a phase 3 trial, but its increased risk of progressive multifocal leukoencephalopathy was unacceptable; therefore, it has basically been withdrawn from clinical use [111]. Nonintestinal selective anti-α4 mAb impairs leukocyte recycling of the central nervous system, and the oral small-molecule α4 inhibitor AJM300 is currently the most promising agent. After receiving oral AJM300, 102 patients with moderately active UC presented with significantly higher clinical response rates (62.7% vs. 25.5%), clinical remission rates (23.5% vs. 3.9%), and mucosal healing rates (58.8% vs. 29.4%) at week 8 compared to the placebo and were free of serious adverse events [112]. The effectiveness and safety of AJM300 were recently reaffirmed in a double-blind phase 3 study, in which 45% of UC patients who did not respond to mesalazine intervention achieved clinical remission after AJM300 intervention (compared to 21% in the placebo), while the frequency of adverse incidents was comparable to placebo [113].

3.1.2. Anti-α4β7 Antibody

α4β7 integrin conjugates with its ligand MAdCAM-1 to accomplish intercellular anchoring, and since MAdCAM-1 is expressed mostly within the intestine, anti-α4β7 antagonism is deemed to be gut-selective, circumventing the potential risk of systemic inhibition by anti-α4 therapies.

Vedolizumab, a selective anti-α4β7 integrin mAb, achieved improved and durable clinical responses in refractory UC patients in a phase 3 double-dummy trial with both subcutaneous and intravenous administration [114]. In a phase 3b head-to-head clinical trial, vedolizumab was preferable to adalimumab in terms of attaining clinical remission and endoscopic improvement [115]. Additionally, vedolizumab had the best safety profile according to a network meta-analysis of small-molecule drugs and biologics for UC [116]. The efficacy of vedolizumab in CD patients is also remarkable, given that in a prospective trial, approximately one-third of active CD patients reached endoscopic remission at week 52 after treatment with vedolizumab, and two-thirds of patients attained histological remission at week 26 [116]. In a phase 3 RCT (VISIBLE 2), a new subcutaneous formulation of vedolizumab was reported to be active and safe in the maintenance treatment of adults with active CD [117]. Abrilumab, a fully human anti-α4β7 mAb, was investigated in a phase 2 trial in Japanese refractory UC patients (receiving conventional therapy) and exhibited superior clinical remission outcomes relative to placebo at week 8 [118]. PTG-100, an oral α4β7 antagonist peptide, has shown potential for IBD treatment in both preclinical models and phase 2a trials in UC patients, effectively inhibiting memory T-cell trafficking with a good safety profile [119].

3.1.3. Anti-β7 Antibody

Selective antagonism of the cosubunit β7 in α4β7 and αEβ7 integrins is another anti-integrin strategy being investigated. Etrolizumab, an anti-β7 integrin mAb, markedly induced clinical remission among patients suffering active UC in an early phase 2 study, while in a recent phase 3 trial (HICKORY), etrolizumab significantly increased the remission proportion at week 14 in refractory UC patients who had already received anti-TNF therapy [120]. A double-dummy phase 3 RCT (GARDENIA) involving 397 active UC patients demonstrated that etrolizumab had similar activity as infliximab in terms of improving clinical remission from a clinical perspective [121]. The efficacy of etrolizumab in CD patients was assessed in an RCT (BERGAMOT) and the open-label extension trial JUNIPER. A higher rate of clinical endoscopic remission was achieved with etrolizumab compared to placebo, suggesting that blocking α4β7 and αEβ7 may be beneficial in the refractory CD population [122].

3.2. Inhibitors of Cell Adhesion Molecules

Cell adhesion molecules are overexpressed in inflamed mucosa, and their binding to integrins is responsible for leukocyte recruitment, making targeting of CAMs attractive [123].

MAdCAM, a member of the immunoglobulin superfamily, influences the adhesion of circulating leukocytes to inflamed areas and regulates lymphocyte infiltration [124]. Immunohistochemical analysis of colonic biopsies from UC patients showed that MAdCAM-1 expression persisted after venous inflammation had subsided and then it increased in subsequent episodes, possibly as a trigger for disease recurrence and as a chronic therapeutic target [125]. The efficacy and safety of ontamalimab for UC, a fully human mAb against MAdCAM-1, was preliminarily confirmed, and ontamalimab was well tolerated by patients in the long term (144 weeks) with acceptable adverse events [126].

Intercellular adhesion molecule 1 (ICAM-1), as a hyperglycosylated transmembrane protein, is expressed on nonhematopoietic cells and is rapidly upregulated upon exposure to inflammatory stimuli [127], whereas the expression pattern of ICAM-1 in IBD implies a relevant pathological role [128]. Alicaforsen, an anti-ICAM-1 antisense oligonucleotide, shows only mild efficacy in IBD by inhibiting the translation of ICAM-1 mRNA [128]. Although alicaforsen did not appear therapeutically effective in phase II trials for parenteral application, its efficacy in distal UC as a topical enema was improved [129]. In addition, increased expression of multiple CAMs (PECAM-1, ICAM-3, and VCAM-1) in colon biopsies from quiescent IBD patients is suspected to be associated with subsequent disease onset.

Collectively, although CAMs have been progressively confirmed to participate in IBD pathogenesis, current treatment options for CAMs are limited and do not achieve the desired results.

3.3. Regulation of Chemokines

Chemokines, namely, chemotactic cytokines, regulate the movement and localization of peripheral immune cells in tissues, directing activated cells to drain lymph nodes to initiate and imprint adaptive immune responses [130]. A range of chemokines is distinctly increased in IBD patients compared with normal healthy donors [131], and chemokines and related receptors are potential targets for IBD treatment.

CCL20 is a member of the CC chemokine superfamily, constitutively expressed by intestinal epithelial cells, whose production is markedly increased in CD patients [132]. CCL20 inhibits TGF-β1-induced Treg (iTreg) differentiation and predisposes cells toward the pathogenic TH17 lineage in a CCR6-dependent manner [133]. The subtle equilibrium between TH17 and Treg cells maintained by the CCL20/CCR6 axis is disrupted under inflammatory states, violating mucosal tolerance. Genome-wide association studies in IBD patients have indicated a robust correlation between CCR6 expression and disease severity, and blockade of CCR6 or CCL20 with antagonists provides relief by preventing the trafficking of CCR6-expressing lymphocytes at sites of inflammation [134]. *Taraxacum officinale* extract significantly reduced the expression of CCL20, CCR6, and CXCL1/5 in DSS-induced mice and alleviated colitis by modulating fatty acid metabolism and microorganisms [135]. After two weeks of treatment with mongersen (an anti-Smad7 oligonucleotide), a proportion of active CD patients responded with reduced serum levels of CCL20, which may be a potential treatment modality [132]. PRN694 significantly hindered the development of T-cell-driven adoptive transfer model colitis and T-cell infiltration in tissues, which may be associated with impaired CXCL11 and CCL20 migration [136]. BI119, a novel oral RORγt antagonist, downregulated the expression of CXCL1, CXCL8, and CCL20 in intestinal crypt cultures in vitro, and BI119 exhibited the same regulatory effect in a T-cell transfer animal model [137].

CXCL10 promotes the recruitment of neutrophils, T-cell activation, and secretion of downstream cytokines. Eldelumab, a fully human anti-CXCL10 mAb, showed a higher clinical remission and response rate in anti-TNF-primed UC patients, despite not meeting the primary induction treatment endpoint in a placebo-controlled phase 2b study [138]. Induction therapy with eldelumab in active CD exhibited clinical and endoscopic efficacy trends, without an observed exposure–remission relationship for eldelumab [139].

Serum CCL11 is significantly increased in IBD patients, considered to be associated with increased colonic eosinophils, and Ccl11-/- mice were found to be tolerant to DSS-induced colitis and to reduce the colonic tumor load induced by azomethine (AOM)-DSS, suggesting that CCL11 antibodies might be valuable for IBD treatment and cancer prevention [140]. As research progresses, a growing list of chemokines are being identified as relevant to IBD progression or as disease-monitoring indicators, but the development of anti-chemotactic agents still needs further optimization. For instance, the poor pharmacokinetics of vercirnon (a prototype CCR9 antagonist) might cause invalid clinical trial results, and oral CCR antagonists based on the 1,3-dioxoindoline backbone could offer a possible direction for optimization [141].

3.4. Selectins

Selectins are an adhesion molecule family comprising L-, E-, and P-selectins that primarily bridge the interactions between leukocytes and the endothelium [142]. L-selectin is widely represented by leukocytes, whereas E-selectin and P-selectin are mainly expressed on the surface of endothelial cells exposed to inflammatory stimuli. Selectin deficiency or dysfunction contributes to inflammatory diseases, and targeting selectins in IBD has been proven to be feasible. P-selectin exerts its physiological function by binding to P-selectin glycoprotein ligands (PSGL-1). The serum concentration of soluble PSGL-1 in UC patients is significantly increased compared with that in controls, and the anti-PSGL-1 antibody resulted in a short-term blockade of neutrophil trafficking and reduced UC activity [143]. L-selectin is a promising independent predictor of anti-TNF management based on a 5-year clinical follow-up of IBD, aiding patients in personalizing treatment and reducing the risk of adverse events [144].

3.5. Modulation of Sphingosine 1-Phosphate Signaling

Sphingosine-1-phosphate (S1P) signaling is a promising target for immune cell homing, which regulates lymphocyte efflux into recirculation and the accumulation of lymphocytes in inflamed intestinal segments [145]. Although anti-S1P mAb (Sphingomab) has shown encouraging therapeutic results in maintaining inflammatory endothelial barrier function, no study has been conducted for IBD.

Antagonizing S1P receptors is the prevailing research direction for interrupting S1P signaling. Fingolimod, the first FDA-approved S1P receptor immunomodulator for multiple sclerosis treatment, has shown symptomatic relief in multiple experimental murine colitis models [145]. However, fingolimod has been proven to cause lymphopenia and has potential cardiac and vascular side effects. Currently, of greater interest is a novel class of oral small-molecule S1P receptor modulators.

Ozanimod, as a selective S1P receptor subtype 1 and 5 modulator, offers great induction and the maintenance of therapeutic efficacy in IBD treatment. In a multicenter phase 3 study of patients with moderate-to-severe active UC, the proportion of patients achieving clinical remission with ozanimod treatment in the induction phase was 16% compared to 6% for placebo, and 37% of patients achieved clinical remission with ozanimod treatment in the maintenance phase compared to 18.5% for placebo [146]. Meanwhile, during the 52-week trial, the incidence of infection with ozanimod was similar to placebo, with serious infections occurring in extremely few patients. A 4-year follow-up of the phase 2 TOUCHSTONE trial showed that the tolerability and long-term benefit rates of ozanimod administration were substantial, with 93.3% and 82.7% clinical response and remission rates at week 200, respectively, based on Mayo measurements, and no new safety risks were observed during the follow-up period [147]. Ozanimod has also contributed to treating refractory CD. Endoscopic improvement was observed in 23.2% of patients, clinical remission in 39.1%, and treatment response in 56.5% of patients at 12 weeks after receiving ozanimod. In addition, relevant phase 3 placebo-controlled trials are under investigation [148].

Etrasimod, a selective S1P1 receptor modulator, is being evaluated for immune-mediated inflammatory diseases. Patients with refractory UC met the primary and all secondary endpoints of the trial when given a daily oral dose of 2 mg of etrasimod at week 12. Endoscopic improvement was reported in 41.8% of patients receiving etrasimod versus 17.8% of patients receiving placebo [149]. A long-term efficacy study on etrasimod for UC treatment (OASIS) described the favorable therapeutic effect and safety of etrasimod in UC patients, approximately half of whom had a clinical response and endoscopic remission over 12 weeks of continuous treatment [150]. Although the vast majority of adverse events occurring during 52 weeks of etrasimod treatment were acceptably mild/moderate, such as anemia and exacerbation of UC, appropriate caution could not be exercised regarding drug safety monitoring.

Amiselimod, an oral S1P1 receptor modulator, may have a better safety profile than other S1P receptor modulators, given its lower EC50 value. After 3 days of continuous amiselimod administration, the expression of the S1P1 receptor on mesenteric lymph node T cells in mice was almost completely eliminated, and amiseimod inhibited disease progression and T-cell infiltration in the lamina propria in the T-cell adoptive transfer colitis model [151]. However, amiselimod did not show a marked advantage over the placebo group in terms of induction of a clinical response in a recent phase 2a trial on refractory CD patients [152].

4. Discussion

Cytokines secreted by activated lymphocytes lead to damage to the mucosal barrier and increased inflammation, participating in the pathogenesis of IBD [4]. Targeting proinflammatory cytokines and lymphocyte trafficking in IBD is a comparatively flawless therapeutic strategy [5]. Since more biological and small-molecule medications are available, both patients and clinicians are challenged to choose the "right" drug. Therefore, in this review, the recent targets and agents aimed at cytokines and immune cell homing in IBD are summarized to assist in understanding the current status of drug development.

New treatment strategies offer extended options for IBD treatment. Steroid-free remission is one of the main goals of IBD treatment due to the adverse effects of corticosteroids, and prolonged usage of corticosteroids is a sign of unsatisfactory care [153]. The annual use of corticosteroids has indeed declined yearly with the emergence of new biological therapies [154]. Over the past few decades, anti-TNF agents and vedolizumab have been adopted for clinical IBD treatment, and facilitate the reduction of corticosteroid use and improve the response and remission rates [155]. However, no guidance is currently available on the most suitable second-line treatment after the failure of anti-TNF therapy [156]. The novel therapeutic agents listed herein combined with the monitoring of disease-related biomarkers during treatment will enlarge our existing therapeutic armamentarium to achieve deep remission of IBD [157]. Cytokines and cell trafficking blockers have yielded promising results facilitating individualized treatment of IBD. Head-to-head comparative trials are now required to supply proof for choosing appropriate medications. Moreover, a more proactive attitude is needed toward emerging agents. The preference of patients and providers for "relatively safe and effective" standard therapies has led to a dilemma in the usage of new medications. The proportion of patients receiving first-line combination therapy (any biologic therapy with any immunomodulator) was less than 1% [158]. With the drugs available, there are more opportunities to greatly improve the quality of life of patients [159].

Overall, selective inhibition of proinflammatory cytokines provides expanded options for achieving clinical remission in IBD [160], while blockade of lymphocyte homing may be a more effective option for modulating proinflammatory mediators. Treatment follow-up and drug safety evaluation will facilitate the subsequent development and clinical application of these agents.

Author Contributions: Conceptualization, H.X. and Y.X.; methodology, Y.S.; software, Y.S. and M.Y.; validation, Y.X.; formal analysis, Y.S.; investigation, M.Y.; resources, H.X.; data curation, Y.S.; writing—original draft preparation, Y.S.; writing—review and editing, Y.X.; visualization, M.Y.; supervision, H.X. and Y.X.; project administration, H.X.; funding acquisition, H.X. and M.Y. All authors have read and agreed to the published version of the manuscript.

Funding: This research received no external funding.

Institutional Review Board Statement: Not applicable.

Informed Consent Statement: Not applicable.

Data Availability Statement: Not applicable.

Conflicts of Interest: The authors declare no conflict of interest.

References

1. The global, regional, and national burden of inflammatory bowel disease in 195 countries and territories, 1990–2017: A systematic analysis for the Global Burden of Disease Study 2017. *Lancet Gastroenterol. Hepatol.* **2020**, *5*, 17–30. [CrossRef]
2. de Souza, H.S.; Fiocchi, C. Immunopathogenesis of IBD: Current state of the art. *Nat. Rev. Gastroenterol. Hepatol.* **2016**, *13*, 13–27. [CrossRef] [PubMed]
3. Zhao, M.; Gönczi, L.; Lakatos, P.L.; Burisch, J. The Burden of Inflammatory Bowel Disease in Europe in 2020. *J. Crohn's Colitis* **2021**, *15*, 1573–1587. [CrossRef]
4. Neurath, M.F. Cytokines in inflammatory bowel disease. *Nat. Rev. Immunol.* **2014**, *14*, 329–342. [CrossRef] [PubMed]
5. Neurath, M.F. Targeting immune cell circuits and trafficking in inflammatory bowel disease. *Nat. Immunol.* **2019**, *20*, 970–979. [CrossRef]
6. Chen, M.L.; Sundrud, M.S. Cytokine Networks and T-Cell Subsets in Inflammatory Bowel Diseases. *Inflamm. Bowel Dis.* **2016**, *22*, 1157–1167. [CrossRef]
7. Verstockt, B.; Ferrante, M.; Vermeire, S.; Van Assche, G. New treatment options for inflammatory bowel diseases. *J. Gastroenterol.* **2018**, *53*, 585–590. [CrossRef]
8. Croft, M.; Siegel, R.M. Beyond TNF: TNF superfamily cytokines as targets for the treatment of rheumatic diseases. *Nat. Rev. Rheumatol.* **2017**, *13*, 217–233. [CrossRef]
9. Lebioda, T.J.; Kmieć, Z. Tumour necrosis factor superfamily members in the pathogenesis of inflammatory bowel disease. *Mediat. Inflamm.* **2014**, *2014*, 325129. [CrossRef]
10. Koelink, P.J.; Bloemendaal, F.M.; Li, B.; Westera, L.; Vogels, E.W.M.; Van Roest, M.; Gloudemans, A.K.; Wout, A.V.; Korf, H.; Vermeire, S.; et al. Anti-TNF therapy in IBD exerts its therapeutic effect through macrophage IL-10 signalling. *Gut* **2019**, *69*, 1053–1063. [CrossRef]
11. Knight, D.M.; Trinh, H.A.N.; Le, J.; Siegel, S.; Shealy, D.; McDonough, M.; Scallon, B.; Moore, M.A.; Vilcek, J.A.N.; Daddona, P.; et al. Construction and initial characterization of a mouse-human chimeric anti-TNF antibody. *Mol. Immunol.* **1993**, *30*, 1443–1453. [CrossRef]
12. Jongsma, M.M.; Aardoom, M.A.; Cozijnsen, M.A.; van Pieterson, M.; de Meij, T.; Groeneweg, M.; Norbruis, O.F.; Wolters, V.M.; van Wering, H.M.; Hojsak, I.; et al. First-line treatment with infliximab versus conventional treatment in children with newly diagnosed moderate-to-severe Crohn's disease: An open-label multicentre randomised controlled trial. *Gut* **2022**, *71*, 34–42. [CrossRef] [PubMed]
13. Gerriets, V.; Goyal, A.; Khaddour, K. Tumor Necrosis Factor Inhibitors. In *StatPearls*; StatPearls Publishing: St. Petersburg, FL, USA, 2022.
14. Bouhnik, Y.; Carbonnel, F.; Laharie, D.; Stefanescu, C.; Hébuterne, X.; Abitbol, V.; Nachury, M.; Brixi, H.; Bourreille, A.; Picon, L.; et al. Efficacy of adalimumab in patients with Crohn's disease and symptomatic small bowel stricture: A multicentre, prospective, observational cohort (CREOLE) study. *Gut* **2018**, *67*, 53–60. [CrossRef] [PubMed]
15. Bhol, K.C.; Tracey, D.E.; Lemos, B.R.; Lyng, G.D.; Erlich, E.C.; Keane, D.M.; Quesenberry, M.S.; Holdorf, A.D.; Schlehuber, L.D.; Clark, S.A.; et al. AVX-470: A novel oral anti-TNF antibody with therapeutic potential in inflammatory bowel disease. *Inflamm. Bowel Dis.* **2013**, *19*, 2273–2281. [CrossRef] [PubMed]
16. Harris, M.S.; Hartman, D.; Lemos, B.R.; Erlich, E.C.; Spence, S.; Kennedy, S.; Ptak, T.; Pruitt, R.; Vermeire, S.; Fox, B.S. AVX-470, an Orally Delivered Anti-Tumour Necrosis Factor Antibody for Treatment of Active Ulcerative Colitis: Results of a First-in-Human Trial. *J. Crohn's Colitis* **2016**, *10*, 631–640. [CrossRef]
17. Zheng, M.K.; Shih, D.Q.; Chen, G.C. Insights on the use of biosimilars in the treatment of inflammatory bowel disease. *World J. Gastroenterol.* **2017**, *23*, 1932–1943. [CrossRef]
18. Danese, S.; Bonovas, S.D.S.; Peyrin-Biroulet, L. Biosimilars in IBD: From theory to practice. *Nat. Rev. Gastroenterol. Hepatol.* **2017**, *14*, 22–31. [CrossRef]
19. Gonsky, R.; Fleshner, P.; Deem, R.L.; Biener-Ramanujan, E.; Li, D.; Potdar, A.A.; Bilsborough, J.; Yang, S.; McGovern, D.P.; Targan, S.R. Association of Ribonuclease T2 Gene Polymorphisms With Decreased Expression and Clinical Characteristics of Severity in Crohn's Disease. *Gastroenterology* **2017**, *153*, 219–232. [CrossRef]
20. Furfaro, F.; Alfarone, L.; Gilardi, D.; Correale, C.; Allocca, M.; Fiorino, G.; Argollo, M.; Zilli, A.; Zacharopoulou, E.; Loy, L.; et al. TL1A: A New Potential Target in the Treatment of Inflammatory Bowel Disease. *Curr. Drug Targets* **2021**, *22*, 760–769. [CrossRef]
21. Jacob, N.; Kumagai, K.; Abraham, J.P.; Shimodaira, Y.; Ye, Y.; Luu, J.; Blackwood, A.Y.; Castanon, S.L.; Stamps, D.T.; Thomas, L.S.; et al. Direct signaling of TL1A-DR3 on fibroblasts induces intestinal fibrosis in vivo. *Sci. Rep.* **2020**, *10*, 18189. [CrossRef]
22. Danese, S.; Klopocka, M.; Scherl, E.J.; Romatowski, J.; Allegretti, J.R.; Peeva, E.; Vincent, M.S.; Schoenbeck, U.; Ye, Z.; Hassan-Zahraee, M.; et al. Anti-TL1A Antibody PF-06480605 Safety and Efficacy for Ulcerative Colitis: A Phase 2a Single-Arm Study. *Clin. Gastroenterol. Hepatol.* **2021**, *19*, 2324–2332.e6. [CrossRef] [PubMed]
23. Hassan-Zahraee, M.; Ye, Z.; Xi, L.; Baniecki, M.L.; Li, X.; Hyde, C.L.; Zhang, J.; Raha, N.; Karlsson, F.; Quan, J.; et al. Antitumor Necrosis Factor-like Ligand 1A Therapy Targets Tissue Inflammation and Fibrosis Pathways and Reduces Gut Pathobionts in Ulcerative Colitis. *Inflamm. Bowel Dis.* **2022**, *28*, 434–446. [CrossRef] [PubMed]

24. Clarke, A.W.; Poulton, L.; Shim, D.; Mabon, D.; Butt, D.; Pollard, M.; Pande, V.; Husten, J.; Lyons, J.; Tian, C.; et al. An anti-TL1A antibody for the treatment of asthma and inflammatory bowel disease. *MAbs* **2018**, *10*, 664–677. [CrossRef]
25. Gitlin, A.D.; Heger, K.; Schubert, A.F.; Reja, R.; Yan, D.; Pham, V.C.; Suto, E.; Zhang, J.; Kwon, Y.C.; Freund, E.C.; et al. Integration of innate immune signalling by caspase-8 cleavage of N4BP1. *Nature* **2020**, *587*, 275–280. [CrossRef] [PubMed]
26. Yukawa, M.; Iizuka, M.; Horie, Y.; Yoneyama, K.; Shirasaka, T.; Itou, H.; Komatsu, M.; Fukushima, T.; Watanabe, S. Systemic and local evidence of increased Fas-mediated apoptosis in ulcerative colitis. *Int. J. Color. Dis.* **2002**, *17*, 70–76. [CrossRef] [PubMed]
27. De Jesus, E.R.; Isidro, R.A.; Cruz, M.L.; Marty, H.; Appleyard, C.B. Adoptive Transfer of Dendritic Cells Expressing Fas Ligand Modulates Intestinal Inflammation in a Model of Inflammatory Bowel Disease. *J. Clin. Cell. Immunol.* **2016**, *7*, 411. [CrossRef]
28. Yu, Y.; Chen, M.; Yang, S.; Shao, B.; Chen, L.; Dou, L.; Gao, J.; Yang, D. Osthole enhances the immunosuppressive effects of bone marrow—Derived mesenchymal stem cells by promoting the Fas/FasL system. *J. Cell. Mol. Med.* **2021**, *25*, 4835–4845. [CrossRef]
29. Shaikh, R.B.; Santee, S.; Granger, S.W.; Butrovich, K.; Cheung, T.; Kronenberg, M.; Cheroutre, H.; Ware, C.F. Constitutive Expression of LIGHT on T Cells Leads to Lymphocyte Activation, Inflammation, and Tissue Destruction. *J. Immunol.* **2001**, *167*, 6330–6337. [CrossRef]
30. Krause, P.; Zahner, S.P.; Kim, G.; Shaikh, R.B.; Steinberg, M.W.; Kronenberg, M. The Tumor Necrosis Factor Family Member TNFSF14 (LIGHT) Is Required for Resolution of Intestinal Inflammation in Mice. *Gastroenterology* **2014**, *146*, 1752–1762.e4. [CrossRef]
31. Kinchen, J.; Chen, H.H.; Parikh, K.; Antanaviciute, A.; Jagielowicz, M.; Fawkner-Corbett, D.; Ashley, N.; Cubitt, L.; Mellado-Gomez, E.; Attar, M.; et al. Structural Remodeling of the Human Colonic Mesenchyme in Inflammatory Bowel Disease. *Cell* **2018**, *175*, 372–386.e17. [CrossRef]
32. Chyuan, I.T.; Tsai, H.F.; Wu, C.S.; Hsu, P.N. TRAIL suppresses gut inflammation and inhibits colitogeic T-cell activation in experimental colitis via an apoptosis-independent pathway. *Mucosal Immunol.* **2019**, *12*, 980–989. [CrossRef]
33. Roblin, X.; Williet, N.; Boschetti, G.; Phelip, J.-M.; Del Tedesco, E.; Berger, A.-E.; Vedrines, P.; Duru, G.; Peyrin-Biroulet, L.; Nancey, S.; et al. Addition of azathioprine to the switch of anti-TNF in patients with IBD in clinical relapse with undetectable anti-TNF trough levels and antidrug antibodies: A prospective randomised trial. *Gut* **2020**, *69*, 1206–1212. [CrossRef]
34. Guo, B.-J.; Bian, Z.-X.; Qiu, H.-C.; Wang, Y.-T.; Wang, Y. Biological and clinical implications of herbal medicine and natural products for the treatment of inflammatory bowel disease. *Ann. N. Y. Acad. Sci.* **2017**, *1401*, 37–48. [CrossRef] [PubMed]
35. Goulart, R.A.; Barbalho, S.M.; Lima, V.M.; Souza, G.A.; Matias, J.N.; Araújo, A.C.; Rubira, C.J.; Buchaim, R.L.; Buchaim, D.V.; Carvalho, A.; et al. Effects of the Use of Curcumin on Ulcerative Colitis and Crohn's Disease: A Systematic Review. *J. Med. Food* **2021**, *24*, 675–685. [CrossRef]
36. Szandruk, M.; Merwid-Ląd, A.; Szeląg, A. The impact of mangiferin from Belamcanda chinensis on experimental colitis in rats. *Inflammopharmacology* **2018**, *26*, 571–581. [CrossRef]
37. Du, Y.; Ding, H.; Vanarsa, K.; Soomro, S.; Baig, S.; Hicks, J.; Mohan, C. Low Dose Epigallocatechin Gallate Alleviates Experimental Colitis by Subduing Inflammatory Cells and Cytokines, and Improving Intestinal Permeability. *Nutrients* **2019**, *11*, 1743. [CrossRef]
38. Liso, M.; Sila, A.; Verna, G.; Scarano, A.; Donghia, R.; Castellana, F.; Cavalcanti, E.; Pesole, P.L.; Sommella, E.M.; Lippolis, A.; et al. Nutritional Regimes Enriched with Antioxidants as an Efficient Adjuvant for IBD Patients under Infliximab Administration, a Pilot Study. *Antioxidants* **2022**, *11*, 138. [CrossRef]
39. Teng, M.W.L.; Bowman, E.P.; McElwee, J.J.; Smyth, M.; Casanova, J.-L.; Cooper, A.; Cua, D.J. IL-12 and IL-23 cytokines: From discovery to targeted therapies for immune-mediated inflammatory diseases. *Nat. Med.* **2015**, *21*, 719–729. [CrossRef]
40. Eftychi, C.; Schwarzer, R.; Vlantis, K.; Wachsmuth, L.; Basic, M.; Wagle, P.; Neurath, M.F.; Becker, C.; Bleich, A.; Pasparakis, M. Temporally Distinct Functions of the Cytokines IL-12 and IL-23 Drive Chronic Colon Inflammation in Response to Intestinal Barrier Impairment. *Immunity* **2019**, *51*, 367–380.e4. [CrossRef]
41. Sands, B.E.; Irving, P.M.; Hoops, T.; Izanec, J.L.; Gao, L.L.; Gasink, C.; Greenspan, A.; Allez, M.; Danese, S.; Hanauer, S.B.; et al. Ustekinumab versus adalimumab for induction and maintenance therapy in biologic-naive patients with moderately to severely active Crohn's disease: A multicentre, randomised, double-blind, parallel-group, phase 3b trial. *Lancet* **2022**, *399*, 2200–2211. [CrossRef]
42. Feagan, B.G.; Sandborn, W.J.; Gasink, C.; Jacobstein, D.; Lang, Y.; Friedman, J.R.; Blank, M.A.; Johanns, J.; Gao, L.-L.; Miao, Y.; et al. Ustekinumab as Induction and Maintenance Therapy for Crohn's Disease. *N. Engl. J. Med.* **2016**, *375*, 1946–1960. [CrossRef]
43. Sands, B.E.; Sandborn, W.J.; Panaccione, R.; O'Brien, C.D.; Zhang, H.; Johanns, J.; Adedokun, O.J.; Li, K.; Peyrin-Biroulet, L.; Van Assche, G.; et al. Ustekinumab as Induction and Maintenance Therapy for Ulcerative Colitis. *N. Engl. J. Med.* **2019**, *381*, 1201–1214. [CrossRef]
44. Biancone, L.; Ardizzone, S.; Armuzzi, A.; Castiglione, F.; D'Incà, R.; Danese, S.; Daperno, M.; Gionchetti, P.; Rizzello, F.; Scribano, M.L.; et al. Ustekinumab for treating ulcerative colitis: An expert opinion. *Expert Opin. Biol. Ther.* **2020**, *20*, 1321–1329. [CrossRef]
45. Davies, S.C.; Nguyen, T.M.; Parker, C.E.; MacDonald, J.K.; Jairath, V.; Khanna, R. Anti-IL-12/23p40 antibodies for maintenance of remission in Crohn's disease. *Cochrane Database Syst. Rev.* **2019**, *12*, Cd012804. [CrossRef]
46. Sewell, G.W.; Kaser, A. Interleukin-23 in the Pathogenesis of Inflammatory Bowel Disease and Implications for Therapeutic Intervention. *J. Crohn's Colitis* **2022**, *16*, ii3–ii19. [CrossRef]
47. Ma, C.; Panaccione, R.; Khanna, R.; Feagan, B.G.; Jairath, V. IL12/23 or selective IL23 inhibition for the management of moderate-to-severe Crohn's disease? *Best Pract. Res. Clin. Gastroenterol.* **2019**, *38–39*, 101604. [CrossRef]

48. Gottlieb, Z.S.; Sands, B.E. Personalised Medicine with IL-23 Blockers: Myth or Reality? *J. Crohn's Colitis* **2022**, *16* (Suppl. S2), ii73–ii94. [CrossRef]
49. Feagan, B.G.; Sandborn, W.J.; D'Haens, G.; Panés, J.; Kaser, A.; Ferrante, M.; Louis, E.; Franchimont, D.; Dewit, O.; Seidler, U.; et al. Induction therapy with the selective interleukin-23 inhibitor risankizumab in patients with moderate-to-severe Crohn's disease: A randomised, double-blind, placebo-controlled phase 2 study. *Lancet* **2017**, *389*, 1699–1709. [CrossRef]
50. Ferrante, M.; Feagan, B.G.; Panés, J.; Baert, F.; Louis, E.; Dewit, O.; Kaser, A.; Duan, W.R.; Pang, Y.; Lee, W.-J.; et al. Long-Term Safety and Efficacy of Risankizumab Treatment in Patients with Crohn's Disease: Results from the Phase 2 Open-Label Extension Study. *J. Crohn's Colitis* **2021**, *15*, 2001–2010. [CrossRef]
51. Visvanathan, S.; Baum, P.; Salas, A.; Vinisko, R.; Schmid, R.; Grebe, K.M.; Davis, J.W.; Wallace, K.; Böcher, W.O.; Padula, S.J.; et al. Selective IL-23 Inhibition by Risankizumab Modulates the Molecular Profile in the Colon and Ileum of Patients With Active Crohn's Disease: Results From a Randomised Phase II Biopsy Sub-study. *J. Crohn's Colitis* **2018**, *12*, 1170–1179. [CrossRef]
52. Sands, B.E.; Chen, J.; Feagan, B.G.; Penney, M.; Rees, W.A.; Danese, S.; Higgins, P.; Newbold, P.; Faggioni, R.; Patra, K.; et al. Efficacy and Safety of MEDI2070, an Antibody Against Interleukin 23, in Patients With Moderate to Severe Crohn's Disease: A Phase 2a Study. *Gastroenterology* **2017**, *153*, 77–86.e6. [CrossRef]
53. Sandborn, W.J.; Ferrante, M.; Bhandari, B.R.; Berliba, E.; Feagan, B.G.; Hibi, T.; Tuttle, J.L.; Klekotka, P.; Friedrich, S.; Durante, M.; et al. Efficacy and Safety of Mirikizumab in a Randomized Phase 2 Study of Patients With Ulcerative Colitis. *Gastroenterology* **2020**, *158*, 537–549.e10. [CrossRef]
54. Sandborn, W.J.; Ferrante, M.; Bhandari, B.R.; Berliba, E.; Hibi, T.; D'Haens, G.R.; Tuttle, J.L.; Krueger, K.; Friedrich, S.; Durante, M.; et al. Efficacy and Safety of Continued Treatment With Mirikizumab in a Phase 2 Trial of Patients With Ulcerative Colitis. *Clin. Gastroenterol. Hepatol.* **2022**, *20*, 105–115.e14. [CrossRef]
55. Reich, K.; Papp, K.A.; Blauvelt, A.; Tyring, S.K.; Sinclair, R.; Thaçi, D.; Nograles, K.; Mehta, A.; Cichanowitz, N.; Li, Q.; et al. Tildrakizumab versus placebo or etanercept for chronic plaque psoriasis (reSURFACE 1 and reSURFACE 2): Results from two randomised controlled, phase 3 trials. *Lancet* **2017**, *390*, 276–288. [CrossRef]
56. Valenti, M.; Narcisi, A.; Pavia, G.; Gargiulo, L.; Costanzo, A. What Can IBD Specialists Learn from IL-23 Trials in Dermatology? *J. Crohn's Colitis* **2022**, *16* (Suppl. S2), ii20–ii29.
57. Atreya, R.; Mudter, J.; Finotto, S.; Müllberg, J.; Jostock, T.; Wirtz, S.; Schütz, M.; Bartsch, B.; Holtmann, M.; Becker, C.; et al. Blockade of interleukin 6 trans signaling suppresses T-cell resistance against apoptosis in chronic intestinal inflammation: Evidence in Crohn disease and experimental colitis in vivo. *Nat. Med.* **2000**, *6*, 583–588. [CrossRef]
58. Tanaka, T.; Narazaki, M.; Kishimoto, T. IL-6 in inflammation, immunity, and disease. *Cold Spring Harb. Perspect. Biol.* **2014**, *6*, a016295. [CrossRef]
59. Harbour, S.N.; DiToro, D.F.; Witte, S.J.; Zindl, C.L.; Gao, M.; Schoeb, T.R.; Jones, G.W.; Jones, S.A.; Hatton, R.D.; Weaver, C.T. T H 17 cells require ongoing classic IL-6 receptor signaling to retain transcriptional and functional identity. *Sci. Immunol.* **2020**, *5*, eaaw2262. [CrossRef]
60. Danese, S.; Vermeire, S.; Hellstern, P.; Panaccione, R.; Rogler, G.; Fraser, G.; Kohn, A.; Desreumaux, P.; Leong, R.W.; Comer, G.M.; et al. Randomised trial and open-label extension study of an anti-interleukin-6 antibody in Crohn's disease (ANDANTE I and II). *Gut* **2019**, *68*, 40–48. [CrossRef]
61. Xiao, Y.-T.; Yan, W.-H.; Cao, Y.; Yan, J.-K.; Cai, W. Neutralization of IL-6 and TNF-α ameliorates intestinal permeability in DSS-induced colitis. *Cytokine* **2016**, *83*, 189–192. [CrossRef]
62. Sido, A.; Radhakrishnan, S.; Kim, S.W.; Eriksson, E.; Shen, F.; Li, Q.; Bhat, V.; Reddivari, L.; Vanamala, J.K. A food-based approach that targets interleukin-6, a key regulator of chronic intestinal inflammation and colon carcinogenesis. *J. Nutr. Biochem.* **2017**, *43*, 11–17. [CrossRef]
63. Wang, L.; Chen, Y.; Zhou, W.; Miao, X.; Zhou, H. Utilization of physiologically-based pharmacokinetic model to assess disease-mediated therapeutic protein-disease-drug interaction in immune-mediated inflammatory diseases. *Clin. Transl. Sci.* **2022**, *15*, 464–476. [CrossRef]
64. Jena, A.; Mishra, S.; Deepak, P.; Kumar-M, P.; Sharma, A.; Patel, Y.I.; Kennedy, N.A.; Kim, A.; Sharma, V.; Sebastian, S. Response to SARS-CoV-2 vaccination in immune mediated inflammatory diseases: Systematic review and meta-analysis. *Autoimmun. Rev.* **2022**, *21*, 102927. [CrossRef]
65. Schreiber, S.; Aden, K.; Bernardes, J.P.; Conrad, C.; Tran, F.; Höper, H.; Volk, V.; Mishra, N.; Blase, J.I.; Nikolaus, S.; et al. Therapeutic Interleukin-6 Trans-signaling Inhibition by Olamkicept (sgp130Fc) in Patients With Active Inflammatory Bowel Disease. *Gastroenterology* **2021**, *160*, 2354–2366.e11. [CrossRef]
66. Liso, M.; Verna, G.; Cavalcanti, E.; De Santis, S.; Armentano, R.; Tafaro, A.; Lippolis, A.; Campiglia, P.; Gasbarrini, A.; Mastronardi, M.; et al. Interleukin 1β Blockade Reduces Intestinal Inflammation in a Murine Model of Tumor Necrosis Factor–Independent Ulcerative Colitis. *Cell. Mol. Gastroenterol. Hepatol.* **2022**, *14*, 151–171. [CrossRef]
67. De Benedetti, F.; Gattorno, M.; Anton, J.; Ben-Chetrit, E.; Frenkel, J.; Hoffman, H.M.; Koné-Paut, I.; Lachmann, H.J.; Ozen, S.; Simon, A.; et al. Canakinumab for the Treatment of Autoinflammatory Recurrent Fever Syndromes. *N. Engl. J. Med.* **2018**, *378*, 1908–1919. [CrossRef]
68. Oh, Y.S.; Kwak, M.-K.; Kim, K.; Cho, E.-H.; Jang, S.-E. Development and application of an antibody that binds to interleukin-1β of various mammalian species for the treatment of inflammatory diseases. *Biochem. Biophys. Res. Commun.* **2020**, *527*, 751–756. [CrossRef]

69. Arend, W.P.; Malyak, M.; Guthridge, C.J.; Gabay, C. Interleukin-1 Receptor Antagonist: Role in Biology. *Annu. Rev. Immunol.* **1998**, *16*, 27–55. [CrossRef]
70. Impellizzeri, D.; Siracusa, R.; Cordaro, M.; Peritore, A.F.; Gugliandolo, E.; Mancuso, G.; Midiri, A.; Di Paola, R.; Cuzzocrea, S. Therapeutic potential of dinitrobenzene sulfonic acid (DNBS)-induced colitis in mice by targeting IL-1β and IL-18. *Biochem. Pharmacol.* **2018**, *155*, 150–161. [CrossRef]
71. Shouval, D.S.; Biswas, A.; Kang, Y.H.; Griffith, A.E.; Konnikova, L.; Mascanfroni, I.D.; Redhu, N.S.; Frei, S.M.; Field, M.; Doty, A.L.; et al. Interleukin 1β Mediates Intestinal Inflammation in Mice and Patients With Interleukin 10 Receptor Deficiency. *Gastroenterology* **2016**, *151*, 1100–1104. [CrossRef]
72. Thomas, M.G.; Bayliss, C.; Bond, S.; Dowling, F.; Galea, J.; Jairath, V.; Lamb, C.; Probert, C.; Timperley-Preece, E.; Watson, A.; et al. Trial summary and protocol for a phase II randomised placebo-controlled double-blinded trial of Interleukin 1 blockade in Acute Severe Colitis: The IASO trial. *BMJ Open* **2019**, *9*, e023765. [CrossRef] [PubMed]
73. Gressler, M.; Heddergott, C.; N'Go, I.C.; Renga, G.; Oikonomou, V.; Moretti, S.; Coddeville, B.; Gaifem, J.; Silvestre, R.; Romani, L.; et al. Definition of the Anti-inflammatory Oligosaccharides Derived From the Galactosaminogalactan (GAG) From Aspergillus fumigatus. *Front. Cell. Infect. Microbiol.* **2019**, *9*, 365. [CrossRef]
74. Corcoran, S.E.; Halai, R.; Cooper, M.A. Pharmacological Inhibition of the Nod-Like Receptor Family Pyrin Domain Containing 3 Inflammasome with MCC950. *Pharmacol. Rev.* **2021**, *73*, 968–1000. [CrossRef] [PubMed]
75. Pellegrini, C.; Fornai, M.; Colucci, R.; Benvenuti, L.; D'Antongiovanni, V.; Natale, G.; Fulceri, F.; Giorgis, M.; Marini, E.; Gastaldi, S.; et al. A Comparative Study on the Efficacy of NLRP3 Inflammasome Signaling Inhibitors in a Pre-clinical Model of Bowel Inflammation. *Front. Pharmacol.* **2018**, *9*, 1405. [CrossRef] [PubMed]
76. Gong, Z.; Zhao, S.; Zhou, J.; Yan, J.; Wang, L.; Du, X.; Li, H.; Chen, Y.; Cai, W.; Wu, J. Curcumin alleviates DSS-induced colitis via inhibiting NLRP3 inflammsome activation and IL-1β production. *Mol. Immunol.* **2018**, *104*, 11–19. [CrossRef]
77. Moschen, A.R.; Tilg, H.; Raine, T. IL-12, IL-23 and IL-17 in IBD: Immunobiology and therapeutic targeting. *Nat. Rev. Gastroenterol. Hepatol.* **2019**, *16*, 185–196. [CrossRef]
78. Nowarski, R.; Jackson, R.; Gagliani, N.; De Zoete, M.R.; Palm, N.W.; Bailis, W.; Low, J.S.; Harman, C.C.D.; Graham, M.; Elinav, E.; et al. Epithelial IL-18 Equilibrium Controls Barrier Function in Colitis. *Cell* **2015**, *163*, 1444–1456. [CrossRef]
79. Mokry, L.E.; Zhou, S.; Guo, C.; Scott, R.A.; Devey, L.; Langenberg, C.; Wareham, N.; Waterworth, D.; Cardon, L.; Sanseau, P.; et al. Interleukin-18 as a drug repositioning opportunity for inflammatory bowel disease: A Mendelian randomization study. *Sci. Rep.* **2019**, *9*, 9386. [CrossRef]
80. Wlodek, E.; Kirkpatrick, R.B.; Andrews, S.; Noble, R.; Schroyer, R.; Scott, J.; Watson, C.J.E.; Clatworthy, M.; Harrison, E.M.; Wigmore, S.J.; et al. A pilot study evaluating GSK1070806 inhibition of interleukin-18 in renal transplant delayed graft function. *PLoS ONE* **2021**, *16*, e0247972. [CrossRef]
81. Reinisch, W.; Panes, J.; Khurana, S.; Toth, G.; Hua, F.; Comer, G.M.; Hinz, M.; Page, K.; O'Toole, M.; Moorehead, T.M.; et al. Anrukinzumab, an anti-interleukin 13 monoclonal antibody, in active UC: Efficacy and safety from a phase IIa randomised multicentre study. *Gut* **2015**, *64*, 894–900. [CrossRef]
82. Danese, S.; Rudziński, J.; Brandt, W.; Dupas, J.-L.; Peyrin-Biroulet, L.; Bouhnik, Y.; Kleczkowski, D.; Uebel, P.; Lukas, M.; Knutsson, M.; et al. Tralokinumab for moderate-to-severe UC: A randomised, double-blind, placebo-controlled, phase IIa study. *Gut* **2015**, *64*, 243–249. [CrossRef] [PubMed]
83. Fauny, M.; Moulin, D.; D'Amico, F.; Netter, P.; Petitpain, N.; Arnone, D.; Jouzeau, J.-Y.; Loeuille, D.; Peyrin-Biroulet, L. Paradoxical gastrointestinal effects of interleukin-17 blockers. *Ann. Rheum. Dis.* **2020**, *79*, 1132–1138. [CrossRef] [PubMed]
84. Park, C.H.; Lee, A.-R.; Ahn, S.B.; Eun, C.S.; Han, D.S. Role of innate lymphoid cells in chronic colitis during anti-IL-17A therapy. *Sci. Rep.* **2020**, *10*, 297. [CrossRef] [PubMed]
85. Abo, H.; Flannigan, K.L.; Geem, D.; Ngo, V.L.; Harusato, A.; Denning, T.L. Combined IL-2 Immunocomplex and Anti-IL-5 mAb Treatment Expands Foxp3+ Treg Cells in the Absence of Eosinophilia and Ameliorates Experimental Colitis. *Front. Immunol.* **2019**, *10*, 459. [CrossRef] [PubMed]
86. Di Fusco, D.; Izzo, R.; Figliuzzi, M.; Pallone, F.; Monteleone, G. IL-21 as a therapeutic target in inflammatory disorders. *Expert Opin. Ther. Targets* **2014**, *18*, 1329–1338. [CrossRef]
87. Phuong, N.N.T.; Palmieri, V.; Adamczyk, A.; Klopfleisch, R.; Langhorst, J.; Hansen, W.; Westendorf, A.M.; Pastille, E. IL-33 Drives Expansion of Type 2 Innate Lymphoid Cells and Regulatory T Cells and Protects Mice From Severe, Acute Colitis. *Front. Immunol.* **2021**, *12*, 2764. [CrossRef]
88. Tong, X.; Zheng, Y.; Li, Y.; Xiong, Y.; Chen, D. Soluble ligands as drug targets for treatment of inflammatory bowel disease. *Pharmacol. Ther.* **2021**, *226*, 107859. [CrossRef]
89. Schneider, W.M.; Chevillotte, M.D.; Rice, C.M. Interferon-Stimulated Genes: A Complex Web of Host Defenses. *Annu. Rev. Immunol.* **2014**, *32*, 513–545. [CrossRef]
90. Tindemans, I.; Joosse, M.E.; Samsom, J.N. Dissecting the Heterogeneity in T-Cell Mediated Inflammation in IBD. *Cells* **2020**, *9*, 110. [CrossRef]
91. Bergemalm, D.; Andersson, E.; Hultdin, J.; Eriksson, C.; Rush, S.T.; Kalla, R.; Adams, A.T.; Keita, A.V.; D'Amato, M.; Gomollon, F.; et al. Systemic Inflammation in Preclinical Ulcerative Colitis. *Gastroenterology* **2021**, *161*, 1526–1539.e9. [CrossRef]

92. Langer, V.; Vivi, E.; Regensburger, D.; Winkler, T.H.; Waldner, M.J.; Rath, T.; Schmid, B.; Skottke, L.; Lee, S.; Jeon, N.L.; et al. IFN-γ drives inflammatory bowel disease pathogenesis through VE-cadherin–directed vascular barrier disruption. *J. Clin. Investig.* **2019**, *129*, 4691–4707. [CrossRef] [PubMed]
93. Mavragani, C.P.; Nezos, A.; Dovrolis, N.; Andreou, N.-P.; Legaki, E.; Sechi, L.A.; Bamias, G.; Gazouli, M. Type I and II Interferon Signatures Can Predict the Response to Anti-TNF Agents in Inflammatory Bowel Disease Patients: Involvement of the Microbiota. *Inflamm. Bowel Dis.* **2020**, *26*, 1543–1553. [CrossRef]
94. Liu, T.-C.; Kern, J.T.; Jain, U.; Sonnek, N.M.; Xiong, S.; Simpson, K.F.; VanDussen, K.L.; Winkler, E.S.; Haritunians, T.; Malique, A.; et al. Western diet induces Paneth cell defects through microbiome alterations and farnesoid X receptor and type I interferon activation. *Cell Host Microbe* **2021**, *29*, 988–1001.e6. [CrossRef] [PubMed]
95. Wallace, J.W.; Constant, D.A.; Nice, T.J. Interferon Lambda in the Pathogenesis of Inflammatory Bowel Diseases. *Front. Immunol.* **2021**, *12*, 4234. [CrossRef] [PubMed]
96. Hommes, D.W.; Mikhajlova, T.L.; Stoinov, S.; Stimac, D.; Vucelic, B.; Lonovics, J.; Zákuciová, M.; D'Haens, G.; Van Assche, G.; Ba, S. Fontolizumab, a humanised anti-interferon gamma antibody, demonstrates safety and clinical activity in patients with moderate to severe Crohn's disease. *Gut* **2006**, *55*, 1131–1137. [CrossRef]
97. Baker, K.; Isaacs, J. Novel therapies for immune-mediated inflammatory diseases: What can we learn from their use in rheumatoid arthritis, spondyloarthritis, systemic lupus erythematosus, psoriasis, Crohn's disease and ulcerative colitis? *Ann. Rheum. Dis.* **2018**, *77*, 175–187. [CrossRef]
98. Takahara, M.; Takaki, A.; Hiraoka, S.; Adachi, T.; Shimomura, Y.; Matsushita, H.; Nguyen, T.T.T.; Koike, K.; Ikeda, A.; Takashima, S.; et al. Berberine improved experimental chronic colitis by regulating interferon-γ- and IL-17A-producing lamina propria CD4+ T cells through AMPK activation. *Sci. Rep.* **2019**, *9*, 11934. [CrossRef]
99. Salas, A.; Hernandez-Rocha, C.; Duijvestein, M.; Faubion, W.; McGovern, D.; Vermeire, S.; Vetrano, S.; Casteele, N.V. JAK–STAT pathway targeting for the treatment of inflammatory bowel disease. *Nat. Rev. Gastroenterol. Hepatol.* **2020**, *17*, 323–337. [CrossRef]
100. Sandborn, W.J.; Su, C.; Sands, B.E.; D'Haens, G.R.; Vermeire, S.; Schreiber, S.; Danese, S.; Feagan, B.G.; Reinisch, W.; Niezychowski, W.; et al. Tofacitinib as Induction and Maintenance Therapy for Ulcerative Colitis. *N. Engl. J. Med.* **2017**, *376*, 1723–1736. [CrossRef]
101. Sandborn, W.J.; Peyrin-Biroulet, L.; Sharara, A.I.; Su, C.; Modesto, I.; Mundayat, R.; Gunay, L.M.; Salese, L.; Sands, B.E. Efficacy and Safety of Tofacitinib in Ulcerative Colitis Based on Prior Tumor Necrosis Factor Inhibitor Failure Status. *Clin. Gastroenterol. Hepatol.* **2022**, *20*, 591–601.e8. [CrossRef]
102. Verstockt, B.; Volk, V.; Jaeckel, C.; Alsoud, D.; Sabino, J.; Nikolaus, S.; Outtier, A.; Krönke, N.; Feuerhake, F.; De Hertogh, G.; et al. Longitudinal monitoring of STAT3 phosphorylation and histologic outcome of tofacitinib therapy in patients with ulcerative colitis. *Aliment. Pharmacol. Ther.* **2022**, *56*, 282–291. [CrossRef] [PubMed]
103. Panés, J.; Sandborn, W.J.; Schreiber, S.; Sands, B.E.; Vermeire, S.; D'Haens, G.; Panaccione, R.; Higgins, P.; Colombel, J.F.; Feagan, B.G. Tofacitinib for induction and maintenance therapy of Crohn's disease: Results of two phase IIb randomised placebo-controlled trials. *Gut* **2017**, *66*, 1049–1059. [CrossRef] [PubMed]
104. Fenster, M.; Alayo, Q.A.; Khatiwada, A.; Wang, W.; Dimopoulos, C.; Gutierrez, A.; Ciorba, M.A.; Christophi, G.P.; Hirten, R.P.; Ha, C.; et al. Real-World Effectiveness and Safety of Tofacitinib in Crohn's Disease and IBD-U: A Multicenter Study From the TROPIC Consortium. *Clin. Gastroenterol. Hepatol.* **2020**, *19*, 2207–2209.e3. [CrossRef] [PubMed]
105. Habtezion, A.; Nguyen, L.P.; Hadeiba, H.; Butcher, E.C. Leukocyte Trafficking to the Small Intestine and Colon. *Gastroenterology* **2016**, *150*, 340–354. [CrossRef]
106. Wiendl, M.; Becker, E.; Müller, T.M.; Voskens, C.J.; Neurath, M.F.; Zundler, S. Targeting Immune Cell Trafficking—Insights from Research Models and Implications for Future IBD Therapy. *Front. Immunol.* **2021**, *12*, 1546. [CrossRef]
107. Dotan, I.; Allez, M.; Danese, S.; Keir, M.; Tole, S.; McBride, J. The role of integrins in the pathogenesis of inflammatory bowel disease: Approved and investigational anti—Integrin therapies. *Med. Res. Rev.* **2020**, *40*, 245–262. [CrossRef]
108. Shattil, S.J.; Kim, C.; Ginsberg, M.H. The final steps of integrin activation: The end game. *Nat. Rev. Mol. Cell Biol.* **2010**, *11*, 288–300. [CrossRef]
109. Fischer, A.; Zundler, S.; Atreya, R.; Rath, T.; Bosch-Voskens, C.; Hirschmann, S.; López-Posadas, R.; Watson, A.; Becker, C.; Schuler, G.; et al. Differential effects of α4β7 and GPR15 on homing of effector and regulatory T cells from patients with UC to the inflamed gut in vivo. *Gut* **2016**, *65*, 1642–1664. [CrossRef]
110. Podolsky, D.K.; Lobb, R.; King, N.; Benjamin, C.D.; Pepinsky, B.; Sehgal, P.; Debeaumont, M. Attenuation of colitis in the cotton-top tamarin by anti-alpha 4 integrin monoclonal antibody. *J. Clin. Investig.* **1993**, *92*, 372–380. [CrossRef]
111. Lamb, C.; O'Byrne, S.; Keir, M.E.; Butcher, E.C. Gut-Selective Integrin-Targeted Therapies for Inflammatory Bowel Disease. *J. Crohn's Colitis* **2018**, *12*, S653–S668. [CrossRef]
112. Yoshimura, N.; Watanabe, M.; Motoya, S.; Tominaga, K.; Matsuoka, K.; Iwakiri, R.; Watanabe, K.; Hibi, T. Safety and Efficacy of AJM300, an Oral Antagonist of α4 Integrin, in Induction Therapy for Patients With Active Ulcerative Colitis. *Gastroenterology* **2015**, *149*, 1775–1783.e2. [CrossRef]
113. Matsuoka, K.; Watanabe, M.; Ohmori, T.; Nakajima, K.; Ishida, T.; Ishiguro, Y.; Kanke, K.; Kobayashi, K.; Hirai, F.; Watanabe, K.; et al. AJM300 (carotegrast methyl), an oral antagonist of α4-integrin, as induction therapy for patients with moderately active ulcerative colitis: A multicentre, randomised, double-blind, placebo-controlled, phase 3 study. *Lancet Gastroenterol. Hepatol.* **2022**, *7*, 648–657. [CrossRef]

114. Sandborn, W.J.; Baert, F.; Danese, S.; Krznarić, Ž.; Kobayashi, T.; Yao, X.; Chen, J.; Rosario, M.; Bhatia, S.; Kisfalvi, K.; et al. Efficacy and Safety of Vedolizumab Subcutaneous Formulation in a Randomized Trial of Patients With Ulcerative Colitis. *Gastroenterology* 2020, *158*, 562–572.e12. [CrossRef] [PubMed]
115. Sands, B.E.; Peyrin-Biroulet, L.; Loftus, E.V., Jr.; Danese, S.; Colombel, J.-F.; Törüner, M.; Jonaitis, L.; Abhyankar, B.; Chen, J.; Rogers, R.; et al. Vedolizumab versus Adalimumab for Moderate-to-Severe Ulcerative Colitis. *N. Engl. J. Med.* 2019, *381*, 1215–1226. [CrossRef] [PubMed]
116. Lasa, J.S.; Olivera, P.A.; Danese, S.; Peyrin-Biroulet, L. Efficacy and safety of biologics and small molecule drugs for patients with moderate-to-severe ulcerative colitis: A systematic review and network meta-analysis. *Lancet Gastroenterol. Hepatol.* 2022, *7*, 161–170. [CrossRef]
117. Vermeire, S.; D'Haens, G.; Baert, F.; Danese, S.; Kobayashi, T.; Loftus, E.V.; Bhatia, S.; Agboton, C.; Rosario, M.; Chen, C.; et al. Efficacy and Safety of Subcutaneous Vedolizumab in Patients With Moderately to Severely Active Crohn's Disease: Results From the VISIBLE 2 Randomised Trial. *J. Crohn's Colitis* 2022, *16*, 27–38. [CrossRef]
118. Hibi, T.; Motoya, S.; Ashida, T.; Sai, S.; Sameshima, Y.; Nakamura, S.; Maemoto, A.; Nii, M.; Sullivan, B.A.; Gasser, R.A., Jr.; et al. Efficacy and safety of abrilumab, an α4β7 integrin inhibitor, in Japanese patients with moderate-to-severe ulcerative colitis: A phase II study. *Intest. Res.* 2019, *17*, 375–386. [CrossRef]
119. Sandborn, W.J.; Mattheakis, L.C.; Modi, N.B.; Pugatch, D.; Bressler, B.; Lee, S.; Bhandari, R.; Kanwar, B.; Shames, R.; D'Haens, G.; et al. PTG-100, an Oral α4β7 Antagonist Peptide: Preclinical Development and Phase 1 and 2a Studies in Ulcerative Colitis. *Gastroenterology* 2021, *161*, 1853–1864.e10. [CrossRef]
120. Peyrin-Biroulet, L.; Hart, A.; Bossuyt, P.; Long, M.; Allez, M.; Juillerat, P.; Armuzzi, A.; Loftus, E.V.; Ostad-Saffari, E.; Scalori, A.; et al. Etrolizumab as induction and maintenance therapy for ulcerative colitis in patients previously treated with tumour necrosis factor inhibitors (HICKORY): A phase 3, randomised, controlled trial. *Lancet Gastroenterol. Hepatol.* 2022, *7*, 128–140. [CrossRef]
121. Danese, S.; Colombel, J.-F.; Lukas, M.; Gisbert, J.P.; D'Haens, G.; Hayee, B.; Panaccione, R.; Kim, H.-S.; Reinisch, W.; Tyrrell, H.; et al. Etrolizumab versus infliximab for the treatment of moderately to severely active ulcerative colitis (GARDENIA): A randomised, double-blind, double-dummy, phase 3 study. *Lancet Gastroenterol. Hepatol.* 2022, *7*, 118–127. [CrossRef]
122. Sandborn, W.J.; Vermeire, S.; Tyrrell, H.; Hassanali, A.; Lacey, S.; Tole, S.; Tatro, A.R. The Etrolizumab Global Steering Committee Etrolizumab for the Treatment of Ulcerative Colitis and Crohn's Disease: An Overview of the Phase 3 Clinical Program. *Adv. Ther.* 2020, *37*, 3417–3431. [CrossRef] [PubMed]
123. Schreiner, P.; Neurath, M.F.; Ng, S.C.; El-Omar, E.M.; Sharara, A.I.; Kobayashi, T.; Hisamatsu, T.; Hibi, T.; Rogler, G. Mechanism-Based Treatment Strategies for IBD: Cytokines, Cell Adhesion Molecules, JAK Inhibitors, Gut Flora, and More. *Inflamm. Intest. Dis.* 2019, *4*, 79–96. [CrossRef] [PubMed]
124. Binder, M.-T.; Becker, E.; Wiendl, M.; Schleier, L.; Fuchs, F.; Leppkes, M.; Atreya, R.; Neufert, C.; Atreya, I.; Neurath, M.F.; et al. Similar Inhibition of Dynamic Adhesion of Lymphocytes From IBD Patients to MAdCAM-1 by Vedolizumab and Etrolizumab-s. *Inflamm. Bowel Dis.* 2018, *24*, 1237–1250. [CrossRef] [PubMed]
125. Roosenboom, B.; van Lochem, E.G.; Meijer, J.; Smids, C.; Nierkens, S.; Brand, E.C.; van Erp, L.W.; Kemperman, L.G.; Groenen, M.J.; Horje, C.S.H.T.; et al. Development of Mucosal PNAd+ and MAdCAM-1+ Venules during Disease Course in Ulcerative Colitis. *Cells* 2020, *9*, 891. [CrossRef] [PubMed]
126. Reinisch, W.; Sandborn, W.J.; Danese, S.; Hébuterne, X.; Kłopocka, M.; Tarabar, D.; Vaňásek, T.; Greguš, M.; Hellstern, P.A.; Kim, J.S.; et al. Long-term Safety and Efficacy of the Anti-MAdCAM-1 Monoclonal Antibody Ontamalimab [SHP647] for the Treatment of Ulcerative Colitis: The Open-label Study TURANDOT II. *J. Crohn's Colitis* 2021, *15*, 938–949. [CrossRef]
127. Taftaf, R.; Liu, X.; Singh, S.; Jia, Y.; Dashzeveg, N.K.; Hoffmann, A.D.; El-Shennawy, L.; Ramos, E.K.; Adorno-Cruz, V.; Schuster, E.J.; et al. ICAM1 initiates CTC cluster formation and trans-endothelial migration in lung metastasis of breast cancer. *Nat. Commun.* 2021, *12*, 4867. [CrossRef]
128. Scarozza, P.; Schmitt, H.; Monteleone, G.; Neurath, M.F.; Atreya, R. Oligonucleotides—A Novel Promising Therapeutic Option for IBD. *Front. Pharmacol.* 2019, *10*, 314. [CrossRef]
129. Greuter, T.; Vavricka, S.R.; Biedermann, L.; Pilz, J.; Borovicka, J.; Seibold, F.; Sauter, B.; Rogler, G. Alicaforsen, an Antisense Inhibitor of Intercellular Adhesion Molecule-1, in the Treatment for Left-Sided Ulcerative Colitis and Ulcerative Proctitis. *Dig. Dis.* 2018, *36*, 123–129. [CrossRef]
130. Sokol, C.L.; Luster, A.D. The Chemokine System in Innate Immunity. *Cold Spring Harb. Perspect. Biol.* 2015, *7*, a016303. [CrossRef]
131. Singh, U.P.; Singh, N.P.; Murphy, E.A.; Price, R.L.; Fayad, R.; Nagarkatti, M.; Nagarkatti, P.S. Chemokine and cytokine levels in inflammatory bowel disease patients. *Cytokine* 2016, *77*, 44–49. [CrossRef]
132. Marafini, I.; Monteleone, I.; Dinallo, V.; Di Fusco, D.; De Simone, V.; Laudisi, F.; Fantini, M.C.; Di Sabatino, A.; Pallone, F.; Monteleone, G. CCL20 Is Negatively Regulated by TGF-β1 in Intestinal Epithelial Cells and Reduced in Crohn's Disease Patients With a Successful Response to Mongersen, a Smad7 Antisense Oligonucleotide. *J. Crohn's Colitis* 2017, *11*, 603–609. [CrossRef]
133. Kulkarni, N.; Meitei, H.T.; Sonar, S.A.; Sharma, P.K.; Mujeeb, V.R.; Srivastava, S.; Boppana, R.; Lal, G. CCR6 signaling inhibits suppressor function of induced-Treg during gut inflammation. *J. Autoimmun.* 2018, *88*, 121–130. [CrossRef] [PubMed]
134. Meitei, H.T.; Jadhav, N.; Lal, G. CCR6-CCL20 axis as a therapeutic target for autoimmune diseases. *Autoimmun. Rev.* 2021, *20*, 102846. [CrossRef] [PubMed]
135. Chen, W.; Fan, H.; Liang, R.; Zhang, R.; Zhang, J.; Zhu, J. Taraxacum officinale extract ameliorates dextran sodium sulphate—Induced colitis by regulating fatty acid degradation and microbial dysbiosis. *J. Cell. Mol. Med.* 2019, *23*, 8161–8172. [CrossRef]

136. Cho, H.-S.; Shin, H.M.; Haberstock-Debic, H.; Xing, Y.; Owens, T.D.; Funk, J.O.; Hill, R.J.; Bradshaw, J.M.; Berg, L.J. A Small Molecule Inhibitor of ITK and RLK Impairs Th1 Differentiation and Prevents Colitis Disease Progression. *J. Immunol.* **2015**, *195*, 4822–4831. [CrossRef]
137. Bassolas-Molina, H.; Raymond, E.; Labadia, M.; Wahle, J.; Ferrer-Picón, E.; Panzenbeck, M.; Zheng, J.; Harcken, C.; Hughes, R.; Turner, M.; et al. An RORγt Oral Inhibitor Modulates IL-17 Responses in Peripheral Blood and Intestinal Mucosa of Crohn's Disease Patients. *Front. Immunol.* **2018**, *9*, 2307. [CrossRef]
138. Sandborn, W.J.; Colombel, J.-F.; Ghosh, S.; Sands, B.E.; Dryden, G.; Hébuterne, X.; Leong, R.W.; Bressler, B.; Ullman, T.; Lakatos, P.L.; et al. Eldelumab [Anti-IP-10] Induction Therapy for Ulcerative Colitis: A Randomised, Placebo-Controlled, Phase 2b Study. *J. Crohn's Colitis* **2016**, *10*, 418–428. [CrossRef] [PubMed]
139. Sandborn, W.J.; Rutgeerts, P.; Colombel, J.F.; Ghosh, S.; Petryka, R.; Sands, B.E.; Mitra, P.; Luo, A. Eldelumab [anti-interferon-γ-inducible protein-10 antibody] Induction Therapy for Active Crohn's Disease: A Randomised, Double-blind, Placebo-controlled Phase IIa Study. *J. Crohn's Colitis* **2017**, *11*, 811–819. [CrossRef]
140. Polosukhina, D.; Singh, K.; Asim, M.; Barry, D.P.; Allaman, M.M.; Hardbower, D.M.; Piazuelo, M.B.; Washington, M.K.; Gobert, A.P.; Wilson, K.T.; et al. CCL11 exacerbates colitis and inflammation-associated colon tumorigenesis. *Oncogene* **2021**, *40*, 6540–6546. [CrossRef]
141. Sands, B.E. Leukocyte Anti-Trafficking Strategies: Current Status and Future Directions. *Dig. Dis.* **2017**, *35*, 13–20. [CrossRef]
142. Cappenberg, A.; Kardell, M.; Zarbock, A. Selectin-Mediated Signaling—Shedding Light on the Regulation of Integrin Activity in Neutrophils. *Cells* **2022**, *11*, 1310. [CrossRef] [PubMed]
143. Ajdukovic, J.; Salamunic, I.; Hozo, I.; Despalatovic, B.R.; Simunic, M.; Bonacin, D.; Puljiz, Z.; Trgo, G.; Sundov, Z.; Tonkic, A. Soluble P-selectin glycoprotein ligand—A possible new target in ulcerative colitis. *Bratisl. Lek. List.* **2015**, *116*, 147–149. [CrossRef] [PubMed]
144. Bravo, F.; Macpherson, J.A.; Slack, E.; Despalatovic, B.R.; Simunic, M.; Bonacin, D.; Puljiz, Z.; Trgo, G.; Sundov, Z.; Tonkic, A. Prospective Validation of CD-62L (L-Selectin) as Marker of Durable Response to Infliximab Treatment in Patients with Inflammatory Bowel Disease: A 5-Year Clinical Follow-up. *Clin. Transl. Gastroenterol.* **2021**, *12*, e00298. [CrossRef] [PubMed]
145. Nielsen, O.H.; Li, Y.; Johansson-Lindbom, B.; Coskun, M. Sphingosine-1-Phosphate Signaling in Inflammatory Bowel Disease. *Trends Mol. Med.* **2017**, *23*, 362–374. [CrossRef] [PubMed]
146. Sandborn, W.J.; Feagan, B.G.; D'Haens, G.; Wolf, D.C.; Jovanovic, I.; Hanauer, S.B.; Ghosh, S.; Petersen, A.; Hua, S.Y.; Lee, J.H.; et al. Ozanimod as Induction and Maintenance Therapy for Ulcerative Colitis. *N. Engl. J. Med.* **2021**, *385*, 1280–1291. [CrossRef]
147. Sandborn, W.J.; Feagan, B.G.; Hanauer, S.; Vermeire, S.; Ghosh, S.; Liu, W.J.; Petersen, A.; Charles, L.; Huang, V.; Usiskin, K.; et al. Long-Term Efficacy and Safety of Ozanimod in Moderately to Severely Active Ulcerative Colitis: Results From the Open-Label Extension of the Randomized, Phase 2 TOUCHSTONE Study. *J. Crohn's Colitis* **2021**, *15*, 1120–1129. [CrossRef]
148. Feagan, B.G.; Sandborn, W.J.; Danese, S.; Wolf, D.C.; Liu, W.J.; Hua, S.Y.; Minton, N.; Olson, A.; D'Haens, G. Ozanimod induction therapy for patients with moderate to severe Crohn's disease: A single-arm, phase 2, prospective observer-blinded endpoint study. *Lancet Gastroenterol. Hepatol.* **2020**, *5*, 819–828. [CrossRef]
149. Sandborn, W.J.; Peyrin-Biroulet, L.; Zhang, J.; Chiorean, M.; Vermeire, S.; Lee, S.D.; Kühbacher, T.; Yacyshyn, B.; Cabell, C.H.; Naik, S.U.; et al. Efficacy and Safety of Etrasimod in a Phase 2 Randomized Trial of Patients With Ulcerative Colitis. *Gastroenterology* **2020**, *158*, 550–561. [CrossRef]
150. Vermeire, S.; Chiorean, M.; Panés, J.; Peyrin-Biroulet, L.; Zhang, J.; Sands, B.E.; Lazin, K.; Klassen, P.; Naik, S.U.; Cabell, C.H.; et al. Long-term Safety and Efficacy of Etrasimod for Ulcerative Colitis: Results from the Open-label Extension of the OASIS Study. *J. Crohn's Colitis* **2021**, *15*, 950–959. [CrossRef]
151. Shimano, K.; Maeda, Y.; Kataoka, H.; Murase, M.; Mochizuki, S.; Utsumi, H.; Oshita, K.; Sugahara, K. Amiselimod (MT-1303), a novel sphingosine 1-phosphate receptor-1 functional antagonist, inhibits progress of chronic colitis induced by transfer of CD4+CD45RBhigh T cells. *PLoS ONE* **2019**, *14*, e0226154. [CrossRef]
152. D'Haens, G.; Danese, S.; Davies, M.; Watanabe, M.; Hibi, T. A phase II, Multicentre, Randomised, Double-Blind, Placebo-controlled Study to Evaluate Safety, Tolerability, and Efficacy of Amiselimod in Patients with Moderate to Severe Active Crohn's Disease. *J. Crohn's Colitis* **2022**, *16*, 746–756. [CrossRef]
153. Abdalla, M.I.; Levesque, B.G. Progress in Corticosteroid Use in the Era of Biologics With Room for Improvement. *Am. J. Gastroenterol.* **2021**, *116*, 1187–1188. [CrossRef] [PubMed]
154. Targownik, L.E.; Bernstein, C.N.; Benchimol, E.I.; Kaplan, G.G.; Singh, H.; Tennakoon, A.; Nugent, Z.; Coward, S.B.; Kuenzig, M.E.; Murthy, S.K. Trends in Corticosteroid Use During the Era of Biologic Therapy: A Population-Based Analysis. *Am. J. Gastroenterol.* **2021**, *116*, 1284–1293. [CrossRef] [PubMed]
155. D'Haens, G.R. Top-down therapy for IBD: Rationale and requisite evidence. *Nat. Rev. Gastroenterol. Hepatol.* **2010**, *7*, 86–92. [CrossRef] [PubMed]
156. Atreya, R.; Neurath, M.F. IL-23 Blockade in Anti-TNF Refractory IBD: From Mechanisms to Clinical Reality. *J. Crohn's Colitis* **2022**, *16* (Suppl. S2), ii54–ii63. [CrossRef] [PubMed]
157. Turner, D.; Ricciuto, A.; Lewis, A.; D'Amico, F.; Dhaliwal, J.; Griffiths, A.M.; Bettenworth, D.; Sandborn, W.J.; Sands, B.E.; Reinisch, W.; et al. STRIDE-II: An Update on the Selecting Therapeutic Targets in Inflammatory Bowel Disease (STRIDE) Initiative of the International Organization for the Study of IBD (IOIBD): Determining Therapeutic Goals for Treat-to-Target strategies in IBD. *Gastroenterology* **2021**, *160*, 1570–1583. [CrossRef]

158. Siegel, C.A. Refocusing IBD Patient Management: Personalized, Proactive, and Patient-Centered Care. *Am. J. Gastroenterol.* **2018**, *113*, 1440–1443. [CrossRef] [PubMed]
159. Wu, T. The Importance of Adopting Leadership Concepts in Communicating Medicinal Culture of Chinese Medicine in the Western World. *Chin. Med. Cult.* **2021**, *4*, 58–65. [CrossRef]
160. Li, H.; Wei, W.; Xu, H. Drug discovery is an eternal challenge for the biomedical sciences. *Acta Mater. Med.* **2022**, *1*, 1–3. [CrossRef]

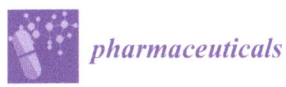

Review

Pharmacological Therapy in Inflammatory Bowel Diseases: A Narrative Review of the Past 90 Years

Marcello Imbrizi [1,*], Fernando Magro [2] and Claudio Saddy Rodrigues Coy [1]

1. Department of Surgery, Faculty of Medical Sciences, University of Campinas, Cidade Universitária Zeferino Vaz-Barão Geraldo, Campinas 13083-970, SP, Brazil
2. Unit of Pharmacology and Therapeutics, Department of Biomedicine, Faculty of Medicine, University of Porto, 4200-450 Porto, Portugal
* Correspondence: marcelloimbrizi@gmail.com

Abstract: Inflammatory Bowel Diseases had their first peak in incidence in countries in North America, Europe, and Oceania and are currently experiencing a new acceleration in incidence, especially in Latin America and Asia. Despite technological advances, 90 years after the development of the first molecule for the treatment of IBD, we still do not have drugs that promote disease remission in a generalized way. We carried out a narrative review on therapeutic advances in the treatment of IBD, the mechanisms of action, and the challenges facing the therapeutic goals in the treatment of IBD. Salicylates are still used in the treatment of Ulcerative Colitis. Corticosteroids have an indication restricted to the period of therapeutic induction due to frequent adverse events, while technologies with less systemic action have been developed. Most immunomodulators showed a late onset of action, requiring a differentiated initial strategy to control the disease. New therapeutic perspectives emerged with biological therapy, initially with anti-TNF, followed by anti-integrins and anti-interleukins. Despite the different mechanisms of action, there are similarities between the general rates of effectiveness. These similar results were also evidenced in JAK inhibitors and S1p modulators, the last therapeutic classes approved for the treatment of IBD.

Keywords: Crohn's disease; ulcerative colitis; 5-ASA; corticosteroid; immunomodulator; biological therapy; JAK; s1P

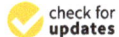

Citation: Imbrizi, M.; Magro, F.; Coy, C.S.R. Pharmacological Therapy in Inflammatory Bowel Diseases: A Narrative Review of the Past 90 Years. *Pharmaceuticals* **2023**, *16*, 1272. https://doi.org/10.3390/ph16091272

Academic Editor: Angel Josabad Alonso-Castro

Received: 10 July 2023
Revised: 23 August 2023
Accepted: 4 September 2023
Published: 8 September 2023

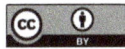

Copyright: © 2023 by the authors. Licensee MDPI, Basel, Switzerland. This article is an open access article distributed under the terms and conditions of the Creative Commons Attribution (CC BY) license (https:// creativecommons.org/licenses/by/ 4.0/).

1. Introduction

The history of medicine and the emergence of diseases is intertwined with the history of humanity. The development of sanitary techniques, with the subsequent knowledge of antibiotic therapies, led to a partial decline in infectious and contagious diseases, especially in terms of mortality. Parallel to this event, the socio-environmental changes that occurred after the first and second industrial revolutions contributed to the occurrence of immunological and metabolic changes in individuals, and since the 20th century, we have observed an exponential increase in many diseases, among them, immune-mediated disorders [1,2].

Naturally, a continuous and balanced inflammatory process is observed in the digestive tract, a barrier organ. The interaction between the microbiota and the immune response (especially innate) is harmonious and self-limiting [3]. An imbalance that occurs in genetically prone individuals (genome), exposed to a propitious environment (interactome) causes the modification of the intestinal microbiota (microbiome) and an uncontrolled immune response (immunome) leading to the emergence of Ulcerative Colitis (UC) and Crohn's Disease (CD): Inflammatory Bowel Diseases (IBD) [4–8].

Until the 1930s, no therapy of proven efficacy was used for the treatment of Inflammatory Bowel Diseases. In the first half of the twentieth century, knowledge of these diseases was as scarce as therapeutic options (Figure 1). The first step towards the attempt to control IBD with medication was taken by Nanna Svartz with the development of Sulfasalazine and until the 90's, other therapeutic classes were developed: glucocorticoids and immunomodulators. This set of therapeutic modalities is currently called "conventional therapies". From the 1990s onwards, the development of monoclonal antibodies, which were already used in other diseases, (e.g., rheumatologic, and oncologic), showed efficacy in IBD. The first approved monoclonal antibodies were TNF-alpha antagonists (anti-TNF), followed by integrin antagonists (anti-integrins) and more recently interleukin antagonists (anti-IL). The use of monoclonal antibodies in IBD are called "biological therapies". In the 2010s, there was the development of new synthetic technologies, called "small molecules", where efficacy was observed in Janus Kinase inhibitors (anti-JAK) and sphingosine-1-phosphate modulators (S1p modulators) [4,6,9].

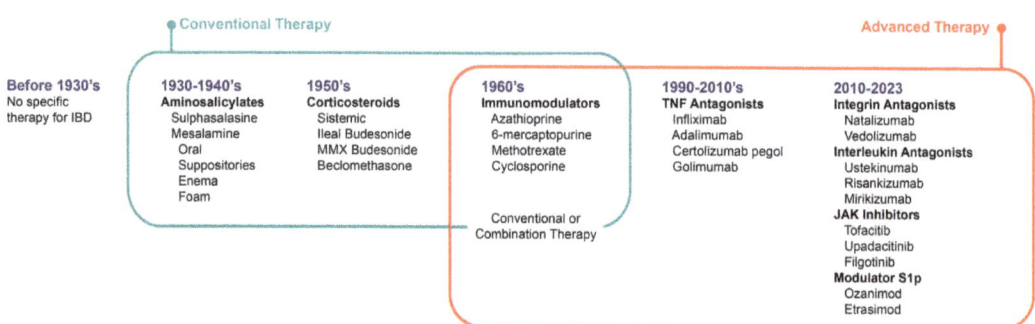

Figure 1. Timeline: development of IBD therapies by decade. IBD: Inflammatory Bowel Disease. MMX: Multi-matrix system. TNF: tumor necrosis factor. JAK: Janus Kinase. S1p: Sphingosine-1-phosphate.

In the field of IBD in pediatrics, the scenario changes due to the longer time to include this population in clinical trials and, consequently, its on-label indication. In advanced therapies, although only some anti-TNF are formally indicated, other therapies, such as integrin antagonists or anti-interleukin, are routinely used pending the completion of pivotal studies in this population [10–12]. Another differential concerns the greater knowledge of dietary therapies such as the Exclusive Enteral Diet and the CD Exclusion Diet [10,13,14].

Considering almost a century of evolution in drug therapies for IBD, we still observe an insurmountable therapeutic ceiling for the drugs approved so far, and we note some discrepancies between the therapeutic objectives in clinical trials and in clinical practice [15–18]. Based on this statement, the main objective of this review is to approach in a narrative way the mechanisms of action of each therapeutic class and their results when tested in controlled studies. At the same time, we critically evaluated the changes in the main outcomes in clinical trials and the lack of data consistent with clinical practice. Thus, we intend to point out to IBD professionals, in an objective and contemporaneous way, the indications and therapeutic differentials proposed for the treatment of Crohn's Disease and Ulcerative Colitis.

2. Methodology

A non-systematic review of the literature was carried out with the objective of exploring, analyzing, and synthesizing the existing knowledge about the different lines of drug treatment for IBD. A bibliographic search was carried out in the databases: PubMed, Scopus and Web of Science using specific keywords: IBD, Crohn's Disease, Ulcerative Colitis, treatment, and drugs. We use studies of relevance and notorious knowledge, as well as the use of cross-references. Review, cohort, cross-sectional studies, and clinical trials were included. Considering the mandatory nature of clinical trials since the advent of biological therapy, these were the studies selected to address the main outcomes related to biological therapy and small molecules, as well as address methodological advances and their shortcomings.

Once the studies have been selected, we analyze and summarize their results in a narrative and linear way, providing an overview and evolutionary view of therapies, therapeutic results, therapeutic indications, and gaps that still exist in the literature.

3. Therapies and Therapeutic Goals

Therapies aimed at the treatment of IBD, as well as the concepts about therapeutic objectives, are relatively recent. Although the first therapies date back to the first half of the 20th century, the first blind and randomized trials to assess therapeutic efficacy date back to the 1990s [19–21]. The drugs recommended for the treatment of IBD are shown in Table 1. Therapeutic studies demonstrated that the absence of symptoms was not capable of preventing the natural progression of IBD, thus, studies with an emphasis on clinical outcomes. Among numerous proposals, the proposal of the International Organization for IBD (IOIBD) is considered among the most relevant, which proposes target-directed therapy (Treat to Target—T2T) considering the short-term objectives (such as clinical response), medium-term (such as reduction in inflammatory markers), and long-term (such as mucosal healing) [16,22]. The same institution also proposes continuous care to patients with the proposal of the SPIRIT consensus, which warns about care in the different manifestations of the disease, even after controlling the inflammatory activity [23].

Table 1. Drugs recommended in the treatment of IBD [24–30].

Class	Drug	Disease	Dose		
			Induction	Maintenance	Dose Optimization
Aminosalicylates [26,28,30]	Sulfasalazine	UC	≥3 g/d	≥2 g/d	-
	5-ASA	UC	Distal colitis: rectal 5-ASA ≥ 1 g/d Extensive colitis: rectal 5-ASA ≥ 1 g/d + oral 5-ASA ≥ 2 g/d	≥1 g/d >2 g/d	>4 g/d
Glucocorticoids [26–29,31,32]	Prednisolone	CD, UC	0.5–0.75 mg/kg (maximum daily dose 60 mg)	-	-
	Budesonide	CD	9 mg/day 2–3 months	-	-
	Budesonide MMX	UC	9 mg/day 2–3 months	-	-
Immunomodulators [26–30,33]	Azathioprine	CD, UC	1.5–2.5 mg/kg/d		-
	6-Mercaptopurine	CD, UC	1–1.5 mg/kg/d		-
	Cyclosporine	UC	2 mg/kg/d IV	5 mg/kg/d (up to 3 months)	-
	Methotrexate	CD	25 mg/w SC or IM (12w)	15 mg/w SC or IM	-
Anti-TNF	Infliximab [34–37]	CD, UC	5 mg/kg IV at 0, 2 and 6 w	5 mg/kg IV every 8w 120 mg SC every 2w from w6	10 mg/kg IV every 8w (label) or 5 mg/kg every 4w (off-label)
	Adalimumab [38–40]	CD, UC	160 mg, then 80 mg after 2w SC	40 mg SC every 2w	80 mg SC every 2w or 40 mg SC weekly
	Certolizumab pegol [41,42]	CD	400 mg SC at weeks 0, 2 and 4	400 mg every 4w	-
	Golimumab [43,44]	UC	200 mg, then 100 mg after 2w SC	50–100 mg SC every 4w	<80 kg using 50 mg: 100 mg every 4w

Table 1. Cont.

Class	Drug	Disease	Dose		Dose Optimization
			Induction	Maintenance	
Anti-Integrin	Natalizumab [45]	CD	300 mg IV every 4w		
	Vedolizumab [46–48]	CD, UC	300 mg IV at weeks 0, 2 and 6. CD: an additional dose at w10 may be indicated	300 mg IV every 8w 108 mg SC every 2w	300 mg IV every 4w -
Anti-Interleukin	Ustekinumab [49,50]	CD, UC	<55 kg: 260 mg, 55–85 kg: 390 mg, >85 kg: 520 mg IV single dose.	90 mg SC every 12 or 8w	90 mg SC every 4w (off-label)
	Risankizumab [51,52]	CD	600 mg IV at weeks 0, 4 and 8	360 mg SC at w12 and then every 8w	-
	Mirikizumab * [53]	UC	300 mg IV every 4w for 12w	200 mg IV every 4w	
JAK-inhibitors	Tofacitinib [54]	UC	10 mg BID PO 8–12w	5 mg PO BID	In loss of response, consider new induction
	Filgotinib [55]	UC	200 mg PO OD 10w	100–200 mg PO OD	-
	Upadacitinib [56,57]	CD, UC	UC: 45 mg PO OD 8w CD: 45 mg PO OD 12w	15–30 mg PO OD	-
S1p modulators	Ozanimod [58]	UC	Day 1–4: 0.92 mg PO Day 5–7: 0.46 mg PO	0.92 mg PO	-
	Etrasimod * [59]	UC	2 mg PO OD		

Doses referring to the treatment of IBD in adults. * Doses used in phase 3 studies. 5-ASA: 5-aminosalicylates. MMX: multi-matrix system. PO: orally. SC: subcutaneous. IV: intravenous. D: day. W: week.

4. Amino Salicylates

The first medication directed at the treatment of IBD was sulfasalazine (SSZ), which consists of binding sulphapyridine (active metabolite responsible for most adverse events related to the use of SSZ) and the 5-ASA portion, which is responsible for the anti-inflammatory action [6]. Since then, isolated portions of 5-ASA have been developed, such as mesalamine, olasalazine, and balsalazide [60,61]. The mechanism of action of the medication is partially known and is presented in Figure 2.

The use of salicylates is currently only recommended for the treatment of UC [26–29]. The meta-analysis performed by Nikfar and colleagues comparing SSZ with 5-ASA showed no differences in efficacy in the treatment of UC [60]. In addition to the effect of salicylates on UC, their action in the prevention of colorectal cancer has been highlighted, although more studies are needed to identify the exact effect on cancer and to identify an ideal model of chemoprevention [62].

Most patients with UC will have mild to moderate manifestations of the disease and tend to respond to 5-ASA treatment. Patients with distal disease may benefit from the use of topical mesalamine therapies alone, while oral therapy is recommended in extensive disease, preferably in combination with the suppository or enema formulations [63]. A systematic review and meta-analysis in the network corroborate these data but point out that there is more evidence that high doses of 5-ASA have more evidence of its effectiveness than combined therapy in left or extensive UC [64]. However, formulations that require a greater number of doses or oral and topical associations reduce therapeutic adherence in approximately 40% of patients. Single daily doses are proven to be better adhered to, even interfering in the reduction in surgeries and hospitalizations [65].

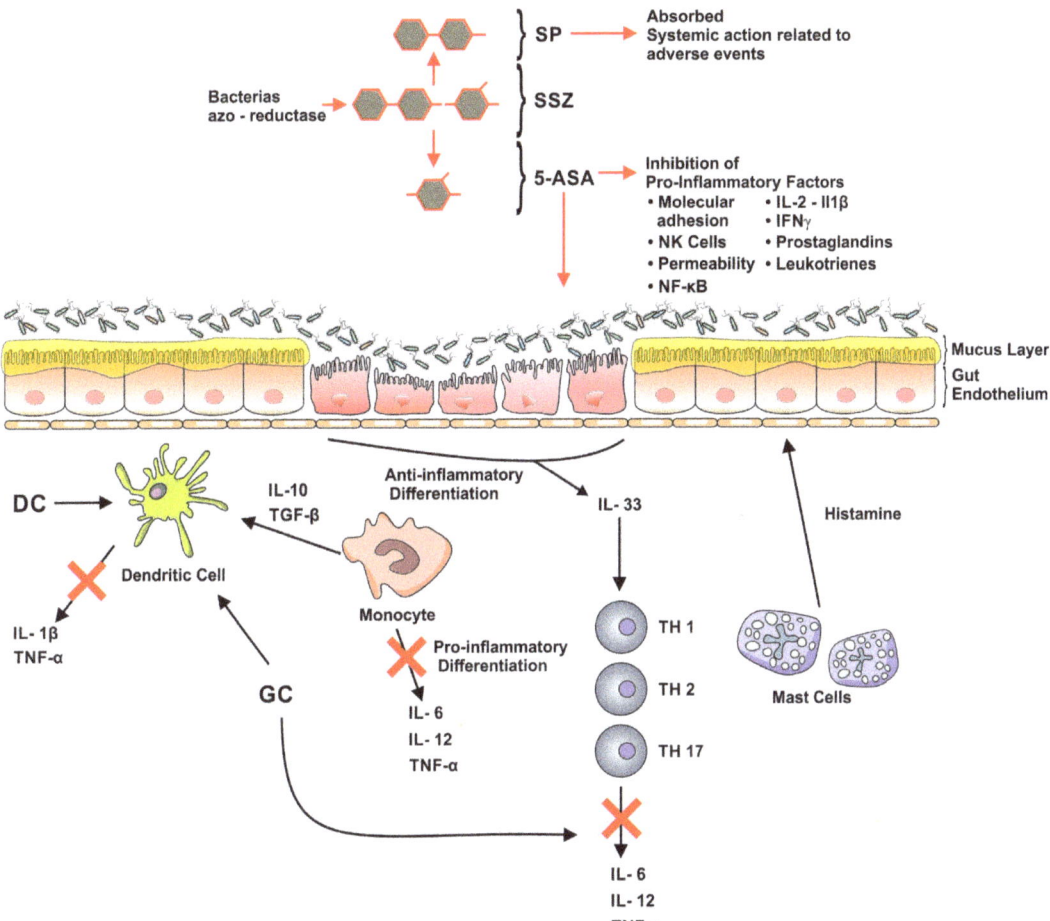

Figure 2. Action of salicylates and glucocorticoids in IBD. 5-ASA acts on pro-inflammatory factors such as molecular adhesion, Natural Killer cell activation, intestinal permeability, nuclear factor kappa B activation, IL-1β, IL-2, Interferon gamma, prostaglandins, and leukotrienes. Sulfasalazine is converted by bacterial azo-reductases into 5-ASA, the UC-acting moiety, and into Sulphapyridine, which is absorbed and is generally associated with adverse events. Glucocorticoids downregulate the inflammatory cascade by reducing cytokines (represented by the red crosses) such as IL-1 beta, IL-6, IL-12, TNF-alpha, in addition to allowing the release of regulatory cytokines such as IL-10. DC: Dendritic cell. GC: glucocorticoids. IL: interleukin. IFN: interferon. *NF-κB*: nuclear factor kappa B. NK: Natural Killer cells. SP: sulfapyridine. SSZ: sulfasalazine. TGF-β: transforming growth factor beta. TH: T helper. TNF: tumor necrosis factor. 5-ASA: 5-aminosalicylate.

The IMPACT, a phase 4 non-interventional study, evaluated the use of oral prolonged-release mesalamine in patients with mild to moderate UC in a Dutch cohort and found that mesalamine is effective in inducing clinical and endoscopic remission, regardless of the extent of the disease and is associated with low recurrence rates [66].

Most recommendations suggest the use of oral 5-ASA at a dose greater than or equal to 2 g daily, and high doses of mesalamine (greater than or equal to 4g daily) may be used in diseases with greater inflammatory activity and during therapeutic induction. The recommended topical dose (suppository or enema) is usually 1 g daily [26,28].

5. Glucocorticoids

Corticosteroids were the second therapeutic class developed that demonstrated efficacy in the treatment of IBD. [67]. This class is effective for therapeutic induction and quick disease control in situations of clinical flares; however, long-term use is not recommended because it is the class with the highest potential for adverse events [28,29].

Glucocorticoids (GC) are endogenous hormones which began to be produced synthetically in the mid-twentieth century. Inflammatory stimuli are one of the mechanisms that stimulate endogenous GC secretion to regulate inflammatory activity. GCs operate in genomic and non-genomic pathways in both the innate and adaptive immune systems. The genomic action acts on genes responsible for pro-inflammatory mediators, such as activator protein-1 and nuclear factor kappa B. Among the non-genomic actions, GC can delay the inflammatory process by generating secondary intracellular transmissions and signal transduction cascades [68]. Figure 2 exemplifies some of the GC action movements.

The first generation of GC is the most used, and the main representatives are prednisone, methylprednisolone, and hydrocortisone [28,29]. There is a consensus among international recommendations that doses equivalent to 1 mg/kg of prednisone, not exceeding 40–60 mg daily, are effective for the treatment of IBD [28,29].

Aiming to reduce the severity of adverse events from glucocorticoids, the second generation of this class was developed to concentrate its action in the gastrointestinal tract and reduce its systemic action [32,69]. Examples of this generation are ileally acting budesonide, budesonide multi-matrix system, and beclomethasone dipropionate. Although the effectiveness of this class does not parallel that of systemic therapy, some phenotypes of CD (e.g., mild to moderately active ileal Crohn's disease) and UC (e.g., mild to moderate ulcerative colitis unresponsive to 5-ASA) show benefit in the use of this therapy [26,28,70]. The classic study by Campieri et al. compared the action of ileal budesonide with prednisone in ileal CD or ileum and right colon CD, demonstrating similarity in achieving clinical remission with lower rates of adverse events in the budesonide group [71]. The CORE II study randomized, double-blind, double-dummy, placebo-controlled, and parallel-group evaluation of the efficacy of Budesonide MMX using combined clinical and endoscopic remission as the primary endpoint. The results of budesonide MMX and its comparators, the group using ileal budesonide and the placebo group were 17.4%, 12.6%, and 4.5%, the statistical difference being present only in the comparison between budesonide MMX and placebo. Interestingly, the study found that although oral budesonide is a locally acting corticosteroid with poor bioavailability, both ileally acting budesonide and MMX affected baseline cortisol when compared to placebo [31].

6. Immunomodulators: Thiopurines and Methotrexate

The first immunomodulatory drugs with the possibility of long-term use, in order to maintain the remission of patients' refractory to 5-ASA or corticosteroid-dependent or corticosteroid-refractory, were azathioprine, 6-mercaptopurine, and methotrexate, classically named immunomodulators (Figure 1) [6,72]. Immunomodulators have a slow onset of action and should not be used as monotherapy in therapeutic induction [61].

The mechanism of action of thiopurines (azathioprine and 6-mercaptopurine) in IBD is complex and knowledge is incomplete, where several metabolites are involved in several immunosuppressive and cytotoxic mechanisms. Telm et al. mention three more relevant mechanisms: I. The incorporation of 6-thioguanine to DNA or RNA, inhibiting replication, DNA repair, and protein synthesis; II. the metabolite 6-thioinosine $5'$-monophosphate causes inhibition of de novo purine synthesis, altering replication; III. apoptosis of T cells via mitochondrial pathway activated by 6-thioguanosine $5'$-triphosphate. Several other mechanisms are studied as well as their genetic and metabolic differentials [73].

Thiopurines show efficacy in monotherapy in maintaining remission, they can be used in the prevention of postoperative recurrence, and in association with biological therapies. Studies indicate that the effectiveness of this class is directly related to the levels of 6-thioguanine (6-TGN) [29]. There is less data in the literature on the use of methotrexate in IBD when compared to thiopurines. It is shown to be effective in maintaining remission in Crohn's disease, and there are few data that suggest its effectiveness in reducing the formation of anti-drug antibodies [74,75].

The OPTIC study was a prospective, randomized, double-blind, placebo-controlled trial that evaluated the efficacy of mercaptopurine in maintaining clinical, endoscopic, and histologic remission following corticosteroid induction. With a total of 59 participants, the 29 patients in the mercaptopurine group had at the end of 52 weeks, rates of 48.3%, 51.7%, and 41.4% of clinical, endoscopic, and histological remission, respectively, while only 10%, 13.3%, and 16.7% of the placebo group achieved the same results [33].

Some considerations about immunomodulators should be remembered. In general, they are safe drugs. However, methotrexate should not be used in pregnant women because it is teratogenic, and the use of thiopurines increases the risk of lymphoma, especially in young men, in both sexes over 50 years old, and individuals that have never been infected by Epstein Barr virus, if they present the first infection [28,29].

7. Biological Therapy

In the 1990s, the advent of immunobiological therapies reached the IBD therapeutic panel. Infliximab ushered in the era of biologics, medications that achieve higher rates of disease remission when compared to conventional therapies and that have reduced the rate of hospitalizations and resections over the past two decades. Technology accompanied the development of these medications, starting from a chimeric molecule to the development of humanized and fully human molecules. Three classes of biological therapies are currently used in the treatment of IBD: (I) anti-TNF, (II) anti-integrins, and (III) anti-interleukins [6,35]. Figure 3 exemplifies an inflammatory process in the intestinal mucosa and the main sites of action of these therapies. We will cite the efficacy results of each therapy preferably in the naive population of biological therapies or small molecules, according to the main outcomes of the pivotal studies.

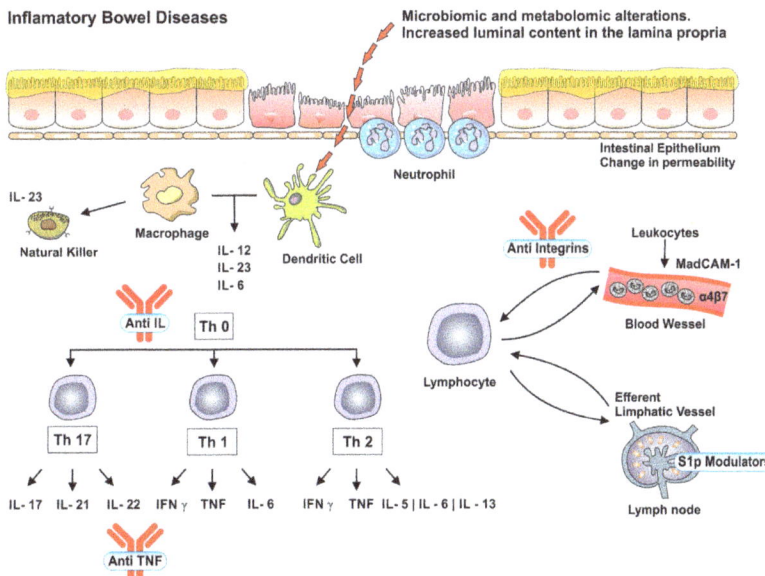

Figure 3. Inflammatory pathways in IBD and areas of action of biological therapies and S1p modulators. IL: Interleukin. Th: T helper. INF: Interferon. TNF: Tumor Necrosis Factor. MadCAM-1: Mucosal vascular addressin cell adhesion molecule 1. S1p: Sphingosine-1-phosphate.

8. Anti-TNF

TNFα is part of a wide network of proteins and receptors involved in immune regulation. This protein is involved in many inflammatory manifestations, such as fever, activation of T cells, and granulocytes. In IBD, this mediator can recruit inflammatory cells, causing edema, angiogenesis, and hypervascularization, activating the coagulation cascade, among others. Specifically in CD, acting in the formation of granuloma [76–78].

Infliximab (IFX) is a chimeric mAb (75% human and 25% murine) with high affinity and specificity for TNFα. The ACCENT 1 study demonstrated its efficacy in CD by assessing clinical response at week 2 (achieved by 58% of patients) and clinical remission at week 30 (39%) and loss of response at week 54, which was low in the group with the standard dose of IFX [34]. ACCENT 2 indicated its action in perianal CD with fistulas, where therapeutic response and remission were observed in 46% and 36% of patients [36]. The SONIC trial showed an increase in the effectiveness of IFX when associated with AZA both in clinical remission and in mucosal healing (44% × 56% and 30% × 43% in monotherapy or combined therapy, respectively) [79]. The REACH study showed efficacy and safety of the drug in the pediatric population with CD [80].

In UC, the action of IFX was demonstrated through clinical response and mucosal healing by the ACT 1 and ACT 2 trials. In ACT 1, the clinical response was 69%, 52%, and 45%, and mucosal healing was 62%, 50%, and 45% at weeks 8, 30, and 54. In ACT 2, the clinical response was 64% and 47%, and mucosal healing was 60% and 46% at weeks 8 and 30, respectively [81].

In 2021, a study proved the effectiveness of the subcutaneous formulation of infliximab in the maintenance of therapy in IBD, as well as the safety in switching from the intravenous to the subcutaneous formulation in patients on remission [37,82].

Adalimumab (ADA) is a fully human recombinant immunoglobulin G1 mAb with high affinity and specificity to TNFα. The CLASSIC I and II trials demonstrated the efficacy of ADA in CD reaching 36% clinical remission at week 4 and 79% at the end of 56 weeks (however, with a small number of patients at the end of the study) [38]. The CHARM study evaluated the efficacy of ADA in maintaining response and remission in CD, achieving remission rates of 40% and 36% at weeks 26 and 56, respectively [83].

The action of ADA on UC was evidenced by studies ULTRA 1 and 2. In the ULTRA 1, a clinical response rate to ADA at week 8 of 54.6% was observed with 18.5% of patients in clinical remission [40]. Subsequently, ULTRA 2 showed response and clinical remission at week 52 of 34.6% and 17.3% [40]. The phase 3, double-blind, randomized, multicenter study entitled SERENE UC researched if high doses of Adalimumab in induction and maintenance would increase the UC remission rate. However, high doses did not increase significantly in the therapeutic response rate [84].

Certolizumab pegol is a human monoclonal antibody Fab' conjugated with polyethylene glycol (PEG), an inert 40-kDa macromolecule. The PRECISE 1 and 2 studies evaluated the effectiveness of Certolizumab pegol in Crohn's Disease. The studies indicate a clinical response rate of 40% in the bio naive population at week 6. The clinical remission rate at week 6, including patients with previous use of IFX, was 22% [41]. PRECISE-2 evaluated the response rate and clinical remission up to week 26 in a population containing 24% of patients with previous use of IFX. Of responders at week 6, 62% maintained clinical response at week 26. The clinical remission rate at week 26 was 48% in an Intention-to-Treat assessment [42].

Golimumab is a fully human IgG1 kappa monoclonal antibody, which binds to TNF-α bound to the membrane and soluble developed through the technique of producing transgenic human antibodies and has brought several clinical gains, such as greater affinity for TNF-α and lower immunogenicity. The action of Golimumab on UC was demonstrated by PURSUIT SC (induction) and PURSUIT-M (maintenance). Clinical response and remission were seen in 51% and 17.8% of patients at week 6 [43]. Maintenance of clinical response at week 54 occurred in 47% of patients while the clinical remission rate was 23.2% [44].

9. Anti-Integrin

Anti-integrins are molecules expressed by leukocytes that bind to adhesion molecules (CAM) and allow the trafficking of these cells [85]. The first drug of this class was Natalizumab (anti-alpha4), intended for the treatment of CD; however, as it lacks specificity for the digestive tract, it was associated with the development of progressive multifocal leukoencephalopathy, and its use is limited or restricted in most countries [86,87]. The ENCORE trial showed a response and clinical remission rate of 60% and 38% on week 8 [45].

Vedolizumab (VEDO) is a humanized mAb capable of specifically blocking the α4β7 heterodimer causing a selective inhibition of intestinal lymphocyte traffic without interfering with traffic to the central nervous system (as occurred with Natalizumab). The α4β7 integrin, located on the leukocyte surface (B and T lymphocytes) specifically interacts with the adhesion molecule CAM-1 (MAdCAM-1) which is predominantly expressed in the vascular endothelium of the digestive tract [88].

The GEMINI 2 and 3 trials showed the effectiveness of Vedolizumab in the treatment of CD. In GEMINI 2, a clinical response and remission rate of 31.4% and 14.5% was observed at week 6. It is important to consider that 67.7% of patients had already used one or more anti-TNF. At the end of 54 weeks, patients using the standard dose of VEDO achieved 43.5% clinical response and 39% clinical remission [46]. GEMINI 3 separates the population into anti-TNF failed and anti-TNF naïve, demonstrating the same clinical response at week 6 (39.2%) but with a higher rate of clinical remission in the anti-TNF naive population (31.4% × 15.2% in those exposed to anti-TNF) [89].

In the GEMINI 1 trial, where the efficacy of VEDO in UC was tested, 47.1% of response and 16.9% of clinical remission were observed at week 6. At the end of 52 weeks, 56.6% and 41.8% of patients were in the response or remission clinic, respectively [47]. The effectiveness of Vedolizumab in UC patients undergoing proctocolectomy with ileal-pouch anastomosis with the subsequent development of pouchitis was evaluated in a phase 4, multicenter, double-blind, randomized, placebo-controlled trial for 34 weeks. The primary outcome was the remission of the disease assessed by the Modified Pouchitis Disease Activity Index (mPDAI). Remission was reached by 31% and 35% of patients using Vedolizumab in weeks 14 and 34, while the placebo group reached 10% and 18%, respectively [90].

Recently, the VISIBLE studies demonstrated the efficacy and safety of the subcutaneous formulation of Vedolizumab in achieving and maintaining clinical remission after induction with intravenous doses [48,91].

10. Anti-Interleukin

Interleukins play a prominent role in the pathogenesis of immune-mediated diseases. Specifically, in IBD, interleukins 12 and 23, produced mainly by dendritic cells and macrophages, are involved in lymphocyte differentiation with Th1 and Th17 responses, respectively [92].

Ustekinumab (UST) is a human monoclonal antibody that binds to the p40 subunit of interleukin-12 and interleukin-23. The UNITI-1 trial evaluated the effectiveness of UST in CD patients who had failed previous biological therapy, while the UNITI-2 trial used a bio naive population. Response and clinical remission rates at week 6 were 33.7% and 18.5% in the UNITI-1 and 55.5% and 34.9% in the UNITI-2. At the end of 44 weeks, clinical remission was observed in 41.1% and 62.5% of patients in the UNITI 1 and 2, respectively, who received doses every 8 weeks [49].

UNIFI Induction demonstrated the efficacy of UST in UC, achieving 52% and 62% clinical response and 14% and 24% clinical remission at week 8, in populations exposed to biological therapy and bio naives, respectively. Maintenance of clinical response was observed in 70% and 78%, while clinical remission rates reached 41% and 49% of the population previously exposed or naive to biological therapy at the end of week 44, according to data from the UNIFI Maintenance trial [50].

Risankizumab (RIZA) is an anti-interleukin 23 Mab directed against its p19 subunit. The ADVANCE AND MOTIVATE studies evaluated the efficacy of therapeutic induction of

RIZA in CD. The difference between the studies was that in ADVANCE 42% of patients were bio naive while in MOTIVATE all patients had already been treated with some biological therapy. The primary endpoints in the studies were clinical remission and endoscopic response in week 12. In ADVANCE, 47% and 37% of bio-naive or bio-failure patients achieved clinical remission, while 43% and 23% demonstrated endoscopic response at week 12. In MOTIVATE, 40% achieved clinical remission and 34% endoscopic response [51].

The assessment of therapeutic maintenance of RIZA in CD was studied in FORTIFY. In total, 64% of bio-naive and 48% of bio-failures patients experienced clinical remission at week 52, while endoscopic response was achieved in 53% and 44% in the respective groups [52].

Mirikizumab is a p19-driven antibody against interleukin-23. Its efficacy and safety in the treatment of UC were evaluated in the LUCENT-1 (induction) and LUCENT-2 (maintenance) studies. Clinical remission after 12 and 52 weeks using Mirikizumab was 24.2% and 49.9% against 13.3% and 25.1 in the placebo group, respectively [53].

11. Small Molecules

The high rate of non-responders to biologic therapy has prompted research into novel signaling pathway blocks, including Janus Kinases (JAK) blockers, DNA transcription activation and transduction signaling (STAT) blockers, and sphingosine-1-phosphate (S1p) modulators. Because they are synthetic molecules, but with greater immunomodulatory potential than conventional therapies, this latest therapeutic generation was called "small molecules" [93].

12. JAK Inhibitors

The JAK family is composed of JAK 1, JAK 2, JAK 3, and tyrosine kinase 2 (TKY2). An extracellular signal (cytokine) can bind to these receptors and induce their activation and, consequently, auto-phosphorylation, and/or transphosphorylation with subsequent interaction of the family composed of seven STATs (STAT 1, 2, 3, 4, 5A, and 5B) with subsequent translocation of information to the cell nucleus. JAK signaling occurs in pairs, with different combinations of commands capable of activating and regulating biological processes, such as apoptosis, cell proliferation and differentiation, among others [94]. Figure 4.

Tofacitinib was the first small molecule released for the treatment of UC, it is a molecule that acts on all JAK, mainly on JAK 1 and 3. The OCTAVE 1 and 2 studies evaluated the ability to induce clinical remission at week 8. Previous exposure to anti-TNF occurred in 52% and 53% of groups 1 and 2 and clinical remission was achieved by 18.5% and 16.6% of patients, respectively [54]. Assessment of maintenance of response was assessed by the OCTAVE Sustain trial in which clinical remission at week 52 was the primary endpoint and was achieved by 40.6% of patients not using the standard dose of tofacitinib [54].

Filgotinib is a preferred inhibitor of JAK 1 (blocking potency over JAK 1 five times greater than the others) and has been evaluated in the treatment of UC through the SELECTION trials. Unlike most IBD therapies, there are no differences in induction or maintenance doses. Clinical remission in week 10 was achieved by 26.1% of bio-naive patients and 11.5% of bio-experienced patients. At the end of 58 weeks, 37.2% of patients (both groups) achieved clinical remission [55].

Upadacitinib (UPA) is a selective JAK-1 inhibitor molecule that had its action on the UC evaluated by the U-ACHIVE and U-ACCOMPLISH trials, and the main outcome was clinical remission. Induction of clinical remission was assessed by UC 1 and 2, where 53% and 50% of the population was previously exposed to biological therapy. Clinical remission at week 8 was 26% and 33% in the respective trials. In the maintenance study, 42% of patients using UPA 15mg daily and 52% of patients using UPA 30mg daily achieved clinical remission at the end of 52 weeks [56]. More recently UPA received its regulatory approval for the treatment of CD based on the results of the U-EXCEL and U-EXCEED studies for therapeutic induction, with clinical remission of 49.5% and 38.9% (versus placebo 29.1%

and 21.1%), respectively, and U-ENDURE for the maintenance phase achieved clinical remission rates of 37.3% and 47.6% with the 15mg and 30mg doses compared to 15.1% in the placebo group [57].

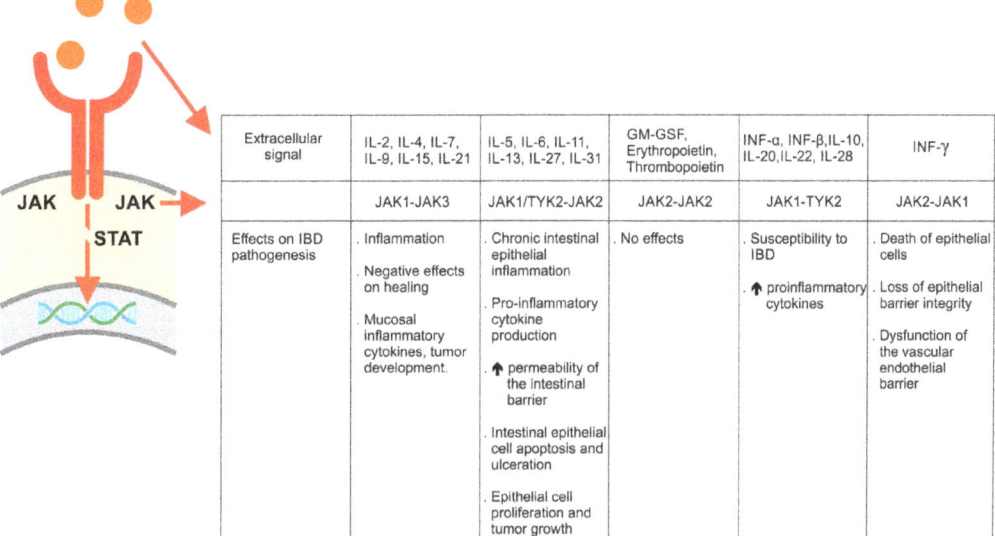

Figure 4. Mechanism of action of JAK inhibitors in IBD [95]. JAK blockade occurs in pairs involving five different inhibition scenarios interrupting STAT-mediated extracellular-nuclear communication. IL: Interleukin; JAK: Janus Kinase; GM-GSF: Granulocyte-macrophage colony-stimulating factor; INF: STAT: Signal transducer and activator of transcription proteins; INF: Interferon. Adapted with permission from Pippis, Elleni J; Yacyshyn, Bruce R, Inflammatory Bowel Diseases; published by Oxford University Press, 2020.

13. S1p Modulators

S1p modulators act as functional antagonists in lymphocytic receptors, inhibiting lymphocytes dependent on this receptor from leaving secondary lymph nodes for peripheral blood, reducing the circulating number of these cells. There are five variants of the S10 receptor (1, 2, 3, 4, and 5) with different actions, and the action of this therapeutic class will depend on the extent of the blockade [94].

Ozanimod is an oral S1p1 and S1p5 agonist that induces lymphocyte sequestration by peripheral lymph nodes, potently reducing the number of activated lymphocytes circulating to the gastrointestinal tract. The TOUCHSTONE study evaluated the effectiveness of this drug in UC. A total of 19% of the patients in the group using the standard dose had previously been treated with biological drugs. The primary end point was clinical remission, achieved at week 8 by 16% of patients and at the end of 32 weeks (maintenance) by 21% [58].

The ELEVATE UC 12 and ELEVATE UC 52 studies, respectively, evaluated the efficacy of Etrasimod in inducing clinical remission in patients with UC at weeks 12 and 52. At week 12, 25% of Etrasimod users achieved clinical remission, compared to 15% of the placebo group. At week 52, 32% of the patients on etrasimod and 7% of the placebo group achieved clinical remission [59].

14. Advances in the Safety of Immunosuppressive Therapies

With the advent of conventional immunosuppressants and later biological therapy and small molecules, concerns have arisen, especially related to infectious events and neoplasms.

In an evaluation of clinical studies on the safety of azathioprine and 6-mercaptopurine in the treatment of IBD, it was observed that the therapies are safe if patients are regularly monitored for side effects, especially hepatotoxicity and leukopenia. Although rare, the incidence of non-melanoma skin cancer is increased in users of these immunosuppressants, especially when taken in high doses [96]. Methotrexate has been associated with an increase in respiratory tract infections and is contraindicated in women intending to become pregnant or pregnant women due to its teratogenic effects [97].

Regarding biologicals, the use of anti-TNF agents has revolutionized the treatment of IBD, demonstrating significant benefits in most patients. Although therapeutic risks such as infections, malignancies, and infusion reactions exist, the more than 20 years of use of anti-TNF in IBD and in other immune-mediated diseases have shown that they are safer drugs even than conventional immunosuppression [98]. The most prominent serious adverse events are the risk for tuberculosis disease or latent tuberculosis, the worsening of cardiac functional status in patients previously diagnosed with heart failure and the onset of immune-mediated or demyelinating diseases. The most common adverse events of biologic therapy are injection site reactions and mild infections, such as colds and flu [98–100]. The classic combination of infliximab and azathioprine proved to be more effective than the use of the biologic alone, moderately reducing therapeutic safety [79]. Vedolizumab has a selective immunosuppressive action on the gastrointestinal tract and stands out in terms of safety [48,101,102]. Similarly, long-term studies of ustekinumab have shown no increase in the rate of serious infections, as well as no correlation with malignancies [103]. Initial data for risankizumab point to the same safety profile, although long-term studies in the IBD population are needed [104,105].

JAK inhibitors have a lower initial safety profile, although more long-term studies in patients with IBD are needed to corroborate information from other populations, especially those with Rheumatoid Arthritis (RA). A large retrospective cohort involving RA patients using JAK inhibitors showed a significant increase in the risk of lung cancer and lymphoma [95,106–108]. These results were not observed in studies involving patients with IBD. Differently, population data of patients with RA using tofacitinib increased the risk of cardiovascular and thromboembolic events and the risk of thrombosis was also evidenced in patients with CD using the same medication, in addition to serious infections and death. These risks, although greater than in the general population, are still low and the therapeutic benefits are greater. It is prudent that patients with this therapeutic indication be carefully selected and monitored [56,107,109,110]. Some regulatory agencies in some countries advise that JAK inhibitors be recommended only in case of failure of a previous biological therapy [111].

Although S1p modulators have shown efficacy in reducing IBD inflammation, there are concerns regarding the long-term safety of these drugs [112]. Studies addressing the safety of S1p modulators in the treatment of IBD are still scarce. Although headache, nasopharyngitis, and elevated liver enzymes were the most common adverse events in the True North studies, viral infections, especially Herpes zoster, were important events [58]. In addition, the medication is contraindicated in patients with heart failure or a recent history of acute myocardial infarction or stroke, patients with cardiac arrhythmias, patients with severe obstructive sleep apnea, or in use of monoamine oxidase inhibitor [113–115].

Care with the risks associated with the therapy deserves to be adopted, as these are a major concern for patients, but the therapeutic benefits outweigh the risks of the therapy, especially the risks related to the disease [116,117]. As well as the evaluation of therapeutic efficacy, the evaluation of safety is dynamic and changes according to the time of use of each drug and the continuity of observation of patients included in clinical trials (generally incorporated into extension studies) and publications of cohorts of the real world. Therefore, one must consider that the more recent the drugs, the lower the safety data. From this point of view, a recent review of biologics and small molecules used in IBD points to JAK inhibitors and S1p modulators as drugs with a greater safety profile than TNF antagonists, especially considering drugs with greater selectivity [118]. Individualized prescribing can select the best therapy for each individual. Figure 5 outlines that, except for corticosteroids, immunosuppressive therapies go beyond the line of efficacy and therapeutic safety in the treatment of IBD, although safety differs between classes.

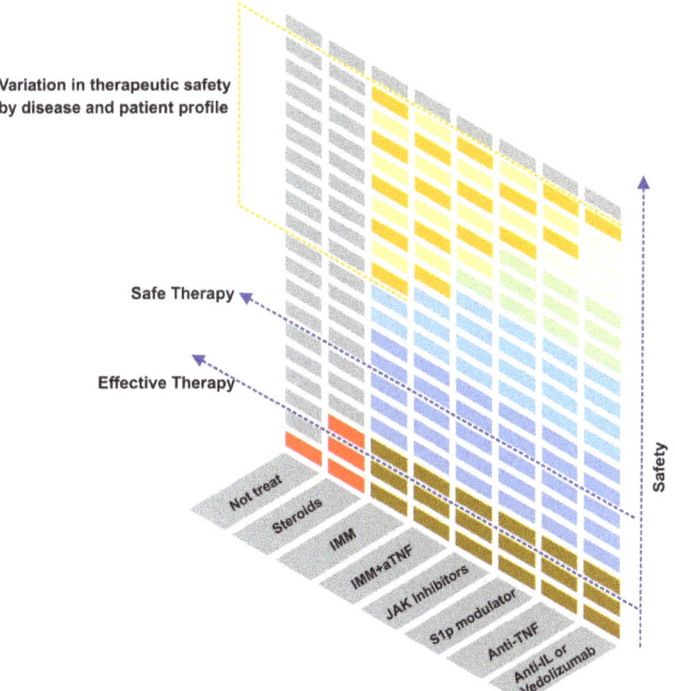

Figure 5. Immunosuppressive therapies for the treatment of inflammatory bowel diseases. The therapies currently proposed for treatment are safe and effective, except for corticosteroids, which in the long term have benefits that are outweighed by the risks. The graph demonstrates a lower to higher safety profile, considering the authors' opinion. We consider newly approved therapies to be at a disadvantage in this review due to fewer studies addressing long-term safety. Safety between therapies varies by therapeutic class or combination. More importantly, safety varies by subgroup of patient (characteristics such as age and comorbidities) and disease (characteristics such as phenotypes and systemic manifestations) (variation represented by the yellow blocks). The use of safe therapies that are not ideal for the characteristics of the patient's disease is also a therapeutic risk factor. S1p: Sphingosine 1-Phosphate; JAK: Janus Kinases; IMM: immunomodulators; aTNF: anti-Tumor Necrosis Factor; IL: Interleukins.

15. Future Perspectives

The development of new molecules is a reality both for previously approved classes and for new therapeutic classes with different targets. As for TNF antagonists, oral formulations such as AVX-470 and OPRX-106 stand out [119].

While the HIBISCUS and GARDENIA trials found that although Etrolizumab (an anti-integrin monoclonal antibody that binds to the β7 subunit of α4β7 and αEβ7 integrins) was effective in inducing but ineffective in maintaining clinical remission, further analysis identified that microRNAs expressed in patients with UC may indicate patients with a better outcome to this drug [119,120]. Other drugs that act on leukocyte trafficking are under study, such as PN-943, an orally administered α4β7 antagonist, and PF-00547659, a human mAb that binds to a mucosal cell adhesion molecule (MadCAM) [119].

In the class of interleukin blockers, Guselkumab has shown good results in CD treatment in published analyzes of the GALAXI studies [121].

Among small molecules, new therapies with greater selectivity to JAK 1 such as Izencitinib and Peficitinib are under study, in addition to JAK/TYK2 combinations such as Brepocitinib [119].

As for the new mechanisms of action with greater progress in the tests, Phosphodiesterase 4 Inhibitors stand out, where Apremilast has been shown to cause a cyclic adenosine monophosphate breakdown, leading to the activation of the nuclear factor kappa B (responsible for the upregulation of proinflammatory cytokines) [122]. Cobitolimode, a representative Toll-Like Receptor 9 (TLR9) agonist, has demonstrated the ability to induce the expression of IL-1 and type 1 interferon (INF). Currently, Cobitolimode is undergoing phase 3 testing in the CONCLUDE trial [123].

Considering the large number of patients refractory to IBD therapies, the therapeutic combination of biologics and small molecules has been used and disseminated through small real-life studies. In general, the association between different mechanisms of action is chosen [124,125]. The VEGA study evaluated the association of the combination of Golimumab associated with Guselkumab compared to the two drugs in monotherapy with the main objective of evaluating clinical response at week 12, which was achieved by 83%, 61%, and 75% of the groups of combination therapy, Golimumab and Guselkumab, respectively [126]. This therapeutic combination is being evaluated in the DUET studies.

It seems that the therapeutical ceiling in IBD is a reality. This may be due to (i) the inability of novel biologics agents to increase the efficacy of older drugs, (ii) the result of substandard reporting of clinical outcomes in clinical trials designed to adequately test the efficacy, (iii) the result of a wrong strategy when compared to treat-to-target or tight control. Indeed, we need to test new therapeutic strategies such as therapeutic drug monitoring (TDM), intensive treatment based on inflammatory markers, adjusting drug sequencing, use of bispecific antibodies, preventing drug resistance and immune escape, or combination of drugs with different targets, particularly in induction. While the drug combination shows promising efficacy during induction, further investigation is needed to determine if monotherapy during the maintenance phase will be sufficient. Hence, there is a pressing need for innovative strategies that go beyond the development of new drugs, focusing on the identification of effective interventions with similar safety profiles and the establishment of precise biomarkers to closely monitor disease burden in inflammatory bowel disease. These strategies should aim to identify effective targets and strive for achieving disease clearance. Moreover, exploring new and more ambitious targets, such as urgency in ulcerative colitis and quality of life in IBD, is essential to meet the needs felt by the patient.

The limitations of this narrative review of the literature occur due to the authors' option to describe the launches of therapies for IBD in a linear, temporal way associated with the mechanism of action. In this way, we involved drugs developed before and after the era of clinical trials, making a comparative review of results impossible. Compiling cross-analyses was not intended either.

16. Conclusions

The advancement of therapeutic development for IBD has accelerated in the last two decades, but conventional therapies are still widely used, with emphasis on 5-ASA, the first therapeutic class developed, remaining with an important position in the treatment of mild to moderate UC. Despite the different mechanisms of action already released for the treatment of CD and UC, many patients remain unable to achieve remission. The wide phenotypic variation of these diseases may prevent us from identifying individualized actions of each drug for each phenotype since, so far, few trials have been conducted for specific IBD phenotypes. The main outcomes of clinical trials are still focused on clinical remission, while therapy guidelines guide the search for a short-term clinical response and medium- and long-term clinical remission and mucosal healing. Although biological therapies are proven to be safe and effective, the development of small molecules assumes the combination of similar effectiveness with the therapeutic convenience of oral administration. Finally, the development of new therapeutic classes, as well as tests aimed at the combination of biological agents and small molecules, promise to occupy a prominent position in the publications of the next decade. Advances in other therapeutic modalities, such as stem cell transplantation and therapies directed at the microbiota, combined with the introduction of artificial intelligence, can change the scenario of IBD therapy at the end of this century of innovations.

Funding: This research received no external funding.

Institutional Review Board Statement: Not applicable.

Informed Consent Statement: Not applicable.

Data Availability Statement: Data sharing is not applicable.

Acknowledgments: We thank Mario Moreira da Silva and Bruno de Jorge for their great dedication in preparing the images for this review.

Conflicts of Interest: MI reports personal fees from AbbVie, Ferring, Nestle, Janssen, Takeda and Pfizer. F Magro severd as speaker for: Abbvie, Arena, Biogen, Bristol-Myers Squibb, Falk, Ferring, Hospira, Janssen, Laboratórios Vitoria, Pfizer, Lilly, Merck Sharp & Dohme, Sandoz, Takeda, UCB, Vifor.

References

1. Celebi Sozener, Z.; Ozdel Ozturk, B.; Cerci, P.; Turk, M.; Gorgulu Akin, B.; Akdis, M.; Altiner, S.; Ozbey, U.; Ogulur, I.; Mitamura, Y.; et al. Epithelial Barrier Hypothesis: Effect of the External Exposome on the Microbiome and Epithelial Barriers in Allergic Disease. *Allergy* **2022**, *77*, 1418–1449. [CrossRef]
2. Barrett, B.; Charles, J.W.; Temte, J.L. Climate Change, Human Health, and Epidemiological Transition. *Prev. Med.* **2015**, *70*, 69–75. [CrossRef]
3. Colella, M.; Charitos, I.A.; Ballini, A.; Cafiero, C.; Topi, S.; Palmirotta, R.; Santacroce, L. Microbiota Revolution: How Gut Microbes Regulate Our Lives. *World J. Gastroenterol.* **2023**, *29*, 4368–4383. [CrossRef]
4. Ananthakrishnan, A.N. Epidemiology and Risk Factors for IBD. *Nat. Rev. Gastroenterol. Hepatol.* **2015**, *12*, 205–217. [CrossRef]
5. Gearry, R.B. IBD and Environment: Are There Differences between East and West. *Dig. Dis.* **2016**, *34*, 84–89. [CrossRef]
6. Actis, G.C.; Pellicano, R.; Fagoonee, S.; Ribaldone, D.G. History of Inflammatory Bowel Diseases. *J. Clin. Med.* **2019**, *8*, 1970. [CrossRef]
7. Agrawal, M.; Jess, T. Implications of the Changing Epidemiology of Inflammatory Bowel Disease in a Changing World. *United Eur. Gastroenterol. J.* **2022**, *10*, 1113–1120. [CrossRef]
8. Padoan, A.; Musso, G.; Contran, N.; Basso, D. Inflammation, Autoinflammation and Autoimmunity in Inflammatory Bowel Diseases. *Curr. Issues Mol. Biol.* **2023**, *45*, 5534–5557. [CrossRef]
9. Jefremow, A.; Neurath, M.F. Novel Small Molecules in IBD: Current State and Future Perspectives. *Cells* **2023**, *12*, 1730. [CrossRef]
10. Ashton, J.J.; Beattie, R.M. Inflammatory Bowel Disease: Recent Developments. *Arch. Dis. Child.* **2023**, 325668. [CrossRef]
11. Lomazi, E.A.; Oba, J.; Rodrigues, M.; Marmo, M.C.D.R.; Sandy, N.S.; Sdepanian, V.L.; Imbrizi, M.; Baima, J.P.; Magro, D.O.; Albuquerque, I.C.D.; et al. Brazilian Consensus on the Management of Inflammatory Bowel Diseases in Pediatric Patients: A Consensus of the Brazilian Organization for Crohn's Disease and Colitis (GEDIIB). *Arq. Gastroenterol.* **2023**, *59*, 85–124. [CrossRef]
12. Van Rheenen, P.F.; Aloi, M.; Assa, A.; Bronsky, J.; Escher, J.C.; Fagerberg, U.L.; Gasparetto, M.; Gerasimidis, K.; Griffiths, A.; Henderson, P.; et al. The Medical Management of Paediatric Crohn's Disease: An ECCO-ESPGHAN Guideline Update. *J. Crohns Colitis* **2021**, *15*, 171–194. [CrossRef]
13. Gkikas, K.; Gerasimidis, K.; Milling, S.; Ijaz, U.Z.; Hansen, R.; Russell, R.K. Dietary Strategies for Maintenance of Clinical Remission in Inflammatory Bowel Diseases: Are We There Yet? *Nutrients* **2020**, *12*, 2018. [CrossRef]
14. Albenberg, L. The Role of Diet in Pediatric Inflammatory Bowel Disease. *Gastroenterol. Clin. N. Am.* **2023**, *52*, 565–577. [CrossRef]
15. Raine, T.; Danese, S. Breaking Through the Therapeutic Ceiling: What Will It Take? *Gastroenterology* **2022**, *162*, 1507–1511. [CrossRef] [PubMed]
16. Turner, D.; Ricciuto, A.; Lewis, A.; D'Amico, F.; Dhaliwal, J.; Griffiths, A.M.; Bettenworth, D.; Sandborn, W.J.; Sands, B.E.; Reinisch, W.; et al. STRIDE-II: An Update on the Selecting Therapeutic Targets in Inflammatory Bowel Disease (STRIDE) Initiative of the International Organization for the Study of IBD (IOIBD): Determining Therapeutic Goals for Treat-to-Target Strategies in IBD. *Gastroenterology* **2021**, *160*, 1570–1583. [CrossRef]
17. Liu, J.; Di, B.; Xu, L. Recent Advances in the Treatment of IBD: Targets, Mechanisms and Related Therapies. *Cytokine Growth Factor Rev.* **2023**, *71–72*, 1–12. [CrossRef]

18. Parigi, T.L.; D'Amico, F.; Abreu, M.T.; Dignass, A.; Dotan, I.; Magro, F.; Griffiths, A.M.; Jairath, V.; Iacucci, M.; Mantzaris, G.J.; et al. Difficult-to-Treat Inflammatory Bowel Disease: Results from an International Consensus Meeting. *Lancet Gastroenterol. Hepatol.* **2023**, *8*, 853–859. [CrossRef]
19. Dubois-Camacho, K.; Ottum, P.A.; Franco-Muñoz, D.; De la Fuente, M.; Torres-Riquelme, A.; Díaz-Jiménez, D.; Olivares-Morales, M.; Astudillo, G.; Quera, R.; Hermoso, M.A. Glucocorticosteroid Therapy in Inflammatory Bowel Diseases: From Clinical Practice to Molecular Biology. *World J. Gastroenterol.* **2017**, *23*, 6628–6638. [CrossRef] [PubMed]
20. Grevenitis, P.; Thomas, A.; Lodhia, N. Medical Therapy for Inflammatory Bowel Disease. *Surg. Clin. N. Am.* **2015**, *95*, 1159–1182. [CrossRef]
21. Bonovas, S.; Nikolopoulos, G.K.; Lytras, T.; Fiorino, G.; Peyrin-Biroulet, L.; Danese, S. Comparative Safety of Systemic and Low-Bioavailability Steroids in Inflammatory Bowel Disease: Systematic Review and Network Meta-Analysis: Comparative Safety of Steroids in IBD. *Br. J. Clin. Pharmacol.* **2018**, *84*, 239–251. [CrossRef] [PubMed]
22. Dignass, A.; Rath, S.; Kleindienst, T.; Stallmach, A. Review Article: Translating STRIDE-II into Clinical Reality—Opportunities and Challenges. *Aliment. Pharmacol. Ther.* **2023**, *58*, 492–502. [CrossRef] [PubMed]
23. Le Berre, C.; Peyrin-Biroulet, L.; Sandborn, W.J.; Colombel, J.-F.; Rubin, D.; Chowers, Y.; Reinisch, W.; Schreiber, S.; Allez, M.; D'Haens, G.; et al. Selecting End Points for Disease-Modification Trials in Inflammatory Bowel Disease: The SPIRIT Consensus From the IOIBD. *Gastroenterology* **2021**, *160*, 1452–1460.e21. [CrossRef] [PubMed]
24. Feuerstein, J.D.; Ho, E.Y.; Shmidt, E.; Singh, H.; Falck-Ytter, Y.; Sultan, S.; Terdiman, J.P.; Sultan, S.; Cohen, B.L.; Chachu, K.; et al. AGA Clinical Practice Guidelines on the Medical Management of Moderate to Severe Luminal and Perianal Fistulizing Crohn's Disease. *Gastroenterology* **2021**, *160*, 2496–2508. [CrossRef]
25. Feuerstein, J.D.; Isaacs, K.L.; Schneider, Y.; Siddique, S.M.; Falck-Ytter, Y.; Singh, S.; Chachu, K.; Day, L.; Lebwohl, B.; Muniraj, T.; et al. AGA Clinical Practice Guidelines on the Management of Moderate to Severe Ulcerative Colitis. *Gastroenterology* **2020**, *158*, 1450–1461. [CrossRef] [PubMed]
26. Raine, T.; Bonovas, S.; Burisch, J.; Kucharzik, T.; Adamina, M.; Annese, V.; Bachmann, O.; Bettenworth, D.; Chaparro, M.; Czuber-Dochan, W.; et al. ECCO Guidelines on Therapeutics in Ulcerative Colitis: Medical Treatment. *J. Crohn's Colitis* **2022**, *16*, 2–17. [CrossRef]
27. Torres, J.; Bonovas, S.; Doherty, G.; Kucharzik, T.; Gisbert, J.P.; Raine, T.; Adamina, M.; Armuzzi, A.; Bachmann, O.; Bager, P.; et al. ECCO Guidelines on Therapeutics in Crohn's Disease: Medical Treatment. *J. Crohn's Colitis* **2020**, *14*, 4–22. [CrossRef]
28. Baima, J.P.; Imbrizi, M.; Ribas, A.; Andrade, L.; Costa, M.; Freitas, N.S.; Azevedo, M.F.C.; de Magalhães, M.H.; Brito, R.d.S. Second Brazilian Consensus on the Management of Ulcerative Colitis in Adults: A Consensus of the Brazilian Organization for Crohn's Disease and Colitis (GEDIIB). *Arq. Gastroenterol.* **2023**, *59*, 51–84. [CrossRef]
29. Imbrizi, M.; Baima, J.P.; Azevedo, M.F.C.; Ribas, A.; Freitas, N.S.; Andrade, L.; Costa, M.; Yukie, L.; Serafim, R.; Botelho, A.; et al. Second Brazilian Consensus on the Management of Crohn's Disease in Adults: A Consensus of the Brazilian Organization for Crohn's Disease and Colitis (GEDIIB). *Arq. Gastroenterol.* **2023**, *59*, 20–50. [CrossRef]
30. Juliao-Baños, F.; Grillo-Ardila, C.F.; Alfaro, I.; Andara-Ramírez, M.T.; Avelar-Escobar, O.; Barahona-Garrido, J.; Bautista-Martínez, S.; Bosques-Padilla, F.J.; De Paula, J.A.; Ernest-Suárez, K.; et al. Update of the PANCCO Clinical Practice Guidelines for the Treatment of Ulcerative Colitis in the Adult Population. *Rev. Gastroenterol. M. Engl. Ed.* **2022**, *87*, 342–361. [CrossRef]
31. Travis, S.P.L.; Danese, S.; Kupcinskas, L.; Alexeeva, O.; D'Haens, G.; Gibson, P.R.; Moro, L.; Jones, R.; Ballard, E.D.; Masure, J.; et al. Once-Daily Budesonide MMX in Active, Mild-to-Moderate Ulcerative Colitis: Results from the Randomised CORE II Study. *Gut* **2014**, *63*, 433–441. [CrossRef] [PubMed]
32. Edsbacker, S.; Andersson, T. Pharmacokinetics of Budesonide (Entocort EC) Capsules for Crohn's Disease. *Clin. Pharmacokinet.* **2004**, *43*, 803–821. [CrossRef] [PubMed]
33. Löwenberg, M.; Volkers, A.; Van Gennep, S.; Mookhoek, A.; Montazeri, N.; Clasquin, E.; Duijvestein, M.; Van Bodegraven, A.; Rietdijk, S.; Jansen, J.; et al. Mercaptopurine for the Treatment of Ulcerative Colitis: A Randomized Placebo-Controlled Trial. *J. Crohn's Colitis* **2023**, *17*, 1055–1065. [CrossRef] [PubMed]
34. Hanauer, S.B.; Feagan, B.G.; Lichtenstein, G.R.; Mayer, L.F.; Schreiber, S.; Colombel, J.F.; Rachmilewitz, D.; Wolf, D.C.; Olson, A.; Bao, W.; et al. Maintenance Infliximab for Crohn's Disease: The ACCENT I Randomised Trial. *Lancet* **2002**, *359*, 1541–1549. [CrossRef] [PubMed]
35. Van Dullemen, H.M.; van Deventer, S.J.H.; Hommes, D.W.; Bijl, H.A.; Jansen, J.; Tytgat, G.N.J.; Woody, J. Treatment of Crohn's Disease with Anti-Tumor Necrosis Factor Chimeric Monoclonal Antibody (CA2). *Gastroenterology* **1995**, *109*, 129–135. [CrossRef]
36. Sands, B.E.; Anderson, F.H.; Bernstein, C.N.; Chey, W.Y.; Feagan, B.G.; Fedorak, R.N.; Kamm, M.A.; Korzenik, J.R.; Lashner, B.A.; Onken, J.E.; et al. Infliximab Maintenance Therapy for Fistulizing Crohn's Disease. *N. Engl. J. Med.* **2004**, *350*, 876–885. [CrossRef]
37. Buisson, A.; Nachury, M.; Reymond, M.; Yzet, C.; Wils, P.; Payen, L.; Laugie, M.; Manlay, L.; Mathieu, N.; Pereira, B.; et al. Effectiveness of Switching from Intravenous to Subcutaneous Infliximab in Patients with Inflammatory Bowel Diseases: The REMSWITCH Study. *Clin. Gastroenterol. Hepatol.* **2022**, *21*, 2338–2346.e3. [CrossRef]
38. Hanauer, S.B.; Sandborn, W.J.; Rutgeerts, P.; Fedorak, R.N.; Lukas, M.; MacIntosh, D.; Panaccione, R.; Wolf, D.; Pollack, P. Human Anti–Tumor Necrosis Factor Monoclonal Antibody (Adalimumab) in Crohn's Disease: The CLASSIC-I Trial. *Gastroenterology* **2006**, *130*, 323–333. [CrossRef]

39. Sandborn, W.J.; Hanauer, S.B.; Rutgeerts, P.; Fedorak, R.N.; Lukas, M.; MacIntosh, D.G.; Panaccione, R.; Wolf, D.; Kent, J.D.; Bittle, B.; et al. Adalimumab for Maintenance Treatment of Crohn's Disease: Results of the CLASSIC II Trial. *Gut* **2007**, *56*, 1232–1239. [CrossRef]
40. Reinisch, W.; Sandborn, W.J.; Hommes, D.W.; D'Haens, G.; Hanauer, S.; Schreiber, S.; Panaccione, R.; Fedorak, R.N.; Tighe, M.B.; Huang, B.; et al. Adalimumab for Induction of Clinical Remission in Moderately to Severely Active Ulcerative Colitis: Results of a Randomised Controlled Trial. *Gut* **2011**, *60*, 780–787. [CrossRef]
41. Sandborn, W.J.; Honiball, P.J.; Bloomfield, R.; Schreiber, S. Certolizumab Pegol for the Treatment of Crohn's Disease. *N. Engl. J. Med.* **2007**, *357*, 228–238. [CrossRef] [PubMed]
42. Schreiber, S.; Thomsen, O.Ø.; McColm, J. Maintenance Therapy with Certolizumab Pegol for Crohn's Disease. *N. Engl. J. Med.* **2007**, *357*, 239–250. [CrossRef] [PubMed]
43. Sandborn, W.J.; Feagan, B.G.; Marano, C.; Zhang, H.; Strauss, R.; Johanns, J.; Adedokun, O.J.; Guzzo, C.; Colombel, J.-F.; Reinisch, W.; et al. Subcutaneous Golimumab Induces Clinical Response and Remission in Patients with Moderate-to-Severe Ulcerative Colitis. *Gastroenterology* **2014**, *146*, 85–95. [CrossRef]
44. Sandborn, W.J.; Feagan, B.G.; Marano, C.; Zhang, H.; Strauss, R.; Johanns, J.; Adedokun, O.J.; Guzzo, C.; Colombel, J.; Reinisch, W.; et al. Subcutaneous Golimumab Maintains Clinical Response in Patients with Moderate-to-Severe Ulcerative Colitis. *Gastroenterology* **2014**, *146*, 96–109.e1. [CrossRef] [PubMed]
45. Targan, S.R.; Feagan, B.G.; Fedorak, R.N.; Lashner, B.A.; Panaccione, R.; Present, D.H.; Spehlmann, M.E.; Rutgeerts, P.J.; Tulassay, Z.; Volfova, M.; et al. Natalizumab for the Treatment of Active Crohn's Disease: Results of the ENCORE Trial. *Gastroenterology* **2007**, *132*, 1672–1683. [CrossRef]
46. Sandborn, W.J.; Feagan, B.G.; Rutgeerts, P.; Hanauer, S.; Colombel, J.-F.; Sands, B.E.; Lukas, M.; Fedorak, R.N.; Lee, S.; Bressler, B.; et al. Vedolizumab as Induction and Maintenance Therapy for Crohn's Disease. *N. Engl. J. Med.* **2013**, *369*, 711–721. [CrossRef] [PubMed]
47. Feagan, B.G.; Rutgeerts, P.; Sands, B.E.; Hanauer, S.; Colombel, J.-F.; Sandborn, W.J.; Van Assche, G.; Axler, J.; Kim, H.-J.; Danese, S.; et al. Vedolizumab as Induction and Maintenance Therapy for Ulcerative Colitis. *N. Engl. J. Med.* **2013**, *369*, 699–710. [CrossRef]
48. Vermeire, S.; D'Haens, G.; Baert, F.; Danese, S.; Kobayashi, T.; Loftus, E.V.; Bhatia, S.; Agboton, C.; Rosario, M.; Chen, C.; et al. Efficacy and Safety of Subcutaneous Vedolizumab in Patients with Moderately to Severely Active Crohn's Disease: Results from the VISIBLE 2 Randomised Trial. *J. Crohn's Colitis* **2022**, *16*, 27–38. [CrossRef]
49. Feagan, B.G.; Sandborn, W.J.; Gasink, C.; Jacobstein, D.; Lang, Y.; Friedman, J.R.; Blank, M.A.; Johanns, J.; Gao, L.-L.; Miao, Y.; et al. Ustekinumab as Induction and Maintenance Therapy for Crohn's Disease. *N. Engl. J. Med.* **2016**, *375*, 1946–1960. [CrossRef]
50. Sands, B.E.; Sandborn, W.J.; Panaccione, R.; O'Brien, C.D.; Zhang, H.; Johanns, J.; Adedokun, O.J.; Li, K.; Peyrin-Biroulet, L.; Van Assche, G.; et al. Ustekinumab as Induction and Maintenance Therapy for Ulcerative Colitis. *N. Engl. J. Med.* **2019**, *381*, 1201–1214. [CrossRef]
51. D'Haens, G.; Panaccione, R.; Baert, F.; Bossuyt, P.; Colombel, J.-F.; Danese, S.; Dubinsky, M.; Feagan, B.G.; Hisamatsu, T.; Lim, A.; et al. Risankizumab as Induction Therapy for Crohn's Disease: Results from the Phase 3 ADVANCE and MOTIVATE Induction Trials. *Lancet* **2022**, *399*, 2015–2030. [CrossRef] [PubMed]
52. Ferrante, M.; Panaccione, R.; Baert, F.; Bossuyt, P.; Colombel, J.-F.; Danese, S.; Dubinsky, M.; Feagan, B.G.; Hisamatsu, T.; Lim, A.; et al. Risankizumab as Maintenance Therapy for Moderately to Severely Active Crohn's Disease: Results from the Multicentre, Randomised, Double-Blind, Placebo-Controlled, Withdrawal Phase 3 FORTIFY Maintenance Trial. *Lancet* **2022**, *399*, 2031–2046. [CrossRef] [PubMed]
53. D'Haens, G.; Dubinsky, M.; Kobayashi, T.; Irving, P.M.; Howaldt, S.; Pokrotnieks, J.; Krueger, K.; Laskowski, J.; Li, X.; Lissoos, T.; et al. Mirikizumab as Induction and Maintenance Therapy for Ulcerative Colitis. *N. Engl. J. Med.* **2023**, *388*, 2444–2455. [CrossRef]
54. Sandborn, W.J. Tofacitinib as Induction and Maintenance Therapy for Ulcerative Colitis. *N. Engl. J. Med.* **2017**, *376*, 1723–1736. [CrossRef]
55. Feagan, B.G.; Danese, S.; Loftus, E.V.; Vermeire, S.; Schreiber, S.; Ritter, T.; Fogel, R.; Mehta, R.; Nijhawan, S.; Kempiński, R.; et al. Filgotinib as Induction and Maintenance Therapy for Ulcerative Colitis (SELECTION): A Phase 2b/3 Double-Blind, Randomised, Placebo-Controlled Trial. *Lancet* **2021**, *397*, 2372–2384. [CrossRef]
56. Danese, S.; Vermeire, S.; Zhou, W.; Pangan, A.L.; Siffledeen, J.; Greenbloom, S.; Hébuterne, X.; D'Haens, G.; Nakase, H.; Panés, J.; et al. Upadacitinib as Induction and Maintenance Therapy for Moderately to Severely Active Ulcerative Colitis: Results from Three Phase 3, Multicentre, Double-Blind, Randomised Trials. *Lancet* **2022**, *399*, 2113–2128. [CrossRef] [PubMed]
57. Loftus, E.V.; Panés, J.; Lacerda, A.P.; Peyrin-Biroulet, L.; D'Haens, G.; Panaccione, R.; Reinisch, W.; Louis, E.; Chen, M.; Nakase, H.; et al. Upadacitinib Induction and Maintenance Therapy for Crohn's Disease. *N. Engl. J. Med.* **2023**, *388*, 1966–1980. [CrossRef]
58. Sandborn, W.J.; Feagan, B.G.; Wolf, D.C.; D'Haens, G.; Vermeire, S.; Hanauer, S.B.; Ghosh, S.; Smith, H.; Cravets, M.; Frohna, P.A.; et al. Ozanimod Induction and Maintenance Treatment for Ulcerative Colitis. *N. Engl. J. Med.* **2016**, *374*, 1754–1762. [CrossRef]
59. Sandborn, W.J.; Vermeire, S.; Peyrin-Biroulet, L.; Dubinsky, M.C.; Panes, J.; Yarur, A.; Ritter, T.; Baert, F.; Schreiber, S.; Sloan, S.; et al. Etrasimod as Induction and Maintenance Therapy for Ulcerative Colitis (ELEVATE): Two Randomised, Double-Blind, Placebo-Controlled, Phase 3 Studies. *Lancet* **2023**, *401*, 1159–1171. [CrossRef]
60. Nikfar, S.; Rahimi, R.; Rezaie, A.; Abdollahi, M. A Meta-Analysis of the Efficacy of Sulfasalazine in Comparison with 5-Aminosalicylates in the Induction of Improvement and Maintenance of Remission in Patients with Ulcerative Colitis. *Dig. Dis. Sci.* **2009**, *54*, 1157–1170. [CrossRef]

61. Magro, F.; Cordeiro, G.; Dias, A.M.; Estevinho, M.M. Inflammatory Bowel Disease—Non-Biological Treatment. *Pharmacol. Res.* **2020**, *160*, 105075. [CrossRef] [PubMed]
62. Słoka, J.; Madej, M.; Strzalka-Mrozik, B. Molecular Mechanisms of the Antitumor Effects of Mesalazine and Its Preventive Potential in Colorectal Cancer. *Molecules* **2023**, *28*, 5081. [CrossRef] [PubMed]
63. Le Berre, C.; Honap, S.; Peyrin-Biroulet, L. Ulcerative Colitis. *Lancet* **2023**, *402*, 571–584. [CrossRef] [PubMed]
64. Barberio, B.; Segal, J.P.; Quraishi, M.N.; Black, C.J.; Savarino, E.V.; Ford, A.C. Efficacy of Oral, Topical, or Combined Oral and Topical 5-Aminosalicylates, in Ulcerative Colitis: Systematic Review and Network Meta-Analysis. *J. Crohn's Colitis* **2021**, *15*, 1184–1196. [CrossRef]
65. Chibbar, R.; Moss, A.C. Mesalamine in the Initial Therapy of Ulcerative Colitis. *Gastroenterol. Clin. N. Am.* **2020**, *49*, 689–704. [CrossRef]
66. West, R.; Russel, M.; Bodelier, A.; Kuijvenhoven, J.; Bruin, K.; Jansen, J.; Van Der Meulen, A.; Keulen, E.; Wolters, L.; Ouwendijk, R.; et al. Lower Risk of Recurrence with a Higher Induction Dose of Mesalazine and Longer Duration of Treatment in Ulcerative Colitis: Results from the Dutch, Non-Interventional, IMPACT Study. *J. Gastrointest. Liver Dis.* **2022**, *31*, 18–24. [CrossRef]
67. Kisner, J.B.; Palmer, W.L. Ulcerative Colitis: Therapeutic Effects of Corticotropin (ACTH) and Cortisone in 120 Patients. *J. Lab Clin. Med.* **1950**, *41*, 232–250. [CrossRef]
68. Bruscoli, S.; Febo, M.; Riccardi, C.; Migliorati, G. Glucocorticoid Therapy in Inflammatory Bowel Disease: Mechanisms and Clinical Practice. *Front. Immunol.* **2021**, *12*, 691480. [CrossRef]
69. Lichtenstein, G.R. Budesonide Multi-Matrix for the Treatment of Patients with Ulcerative Colitis. *Dig. Dis. Sci.* **2016**, *61*, 358–370. [CrossRef]
70. Hoy, S.M. Budesonide MMX®: A Review of Its Use in Patients with Mild to Moderate Ulcerative Colitis. *Drugs* **2015**, *75*, 879–886. [CrossRef]
71. Campieri, M.; Ferguson, A.; Doe, W.; Persson, T.; Nilsson, L.-G. Oral Budesonide Is as Efective as Oral Prednisolone in Active Crohn's Disease. *Gut* **1997**, *41*, 209–214. [CrossRef] [PubMed]
72. Brooke, B.N.; Swarbrick, E.T. Azathioprine for Crohn's Disease. *Lancet* **1969**, *294*, 612–614. [CrossRef] [PubMed]
73. Teml, A.; Schaeffeler, E.; Herrlinger, K.R.; Klotz, U.; Schwab, M. Thiopurine Treatment in Inflammatory Bowel Disease. *Clin. Pharmacokinet.* **2007**, *46*, 187–208. [CrossRef]
74. Estevinho, M.M.; Afonso, J.; Rosa, I.; Lago, P.; Trindade, E.; Correia, L.; Dias, C.C.; Magro, F.; On behalf GEDII [Portuguese IBD Group]. A Systematic Review and Meta-Analysis of 6-Thioguanine Nucleotide Levels and Clinical Remission in Inflammatory Bowel Disease. *J. Crohn's Colitis* **2017**, *11*, 1381–1392. [CrossRef]
75. Pariente, B.; Laharie, D. Review Article: Why, When and How to de-Escalate Therapy in Inflammatory Bowel Diseases. *Aliment. Pharmacol. Ther.* **2014**, *40*, 338–353. [CrossRef] [PubMed]
76. Van Deventer, S.J. Tumour Necrosis Factor and Crohn's Disease. *Gut* **1997**, *40*, 443–448. [CrossRef]
77. Papadakis, K.A.; Targan, S.R. Role of Cytokines in the Pathogenesis of Inflammatory Bowel Disease. *Annu. Rev. Med.* **2000**, *51*, 289–298. [CrossRef]
78. Neurath, M.F. Cytokines in Inflammatory Bowel Disease. *Nat. Rev. Immunol.* **2014**, *14*, 329–342. [CrossRef]
79. Colombel, J.F.; Mantzaris, G.J.; Rachmilewitz, D.; Diamond, R.H. Infliximab, Azathioprine, or Combination Therapy for Crohn's Disease. *N. Engl. J. Med.* **2010**, *362*, 1383–1395. [CrossRef]
80. Hyams, J.; Crandall, W.; Kugathasan, S.; Griffiths, A.; Olson, A.; Johanns, J.; Liu, G.; Travers, S.; Heuschkel, R.; Markowitz, J.; et al. Induction and Maintenance Infliximab Therapy for the Treatment of Moderate-to-Severe Crohn's Disease in Children. *Gastroenterology* **2007**, *132*, 863–873. [CrossRef]
81. Rutgeerts, P.; Sandborn, W.J.; Feagan, B.G.; Reinisch, W.; Olson, A.; Johanns, J.; Suzanne, T.; Rachmilewitz, D.; Hanauer, S.B.; Lichtenstein, G.R.; et al. Infliximab for Induction and Maintenance Therapy for Ulcerative Colitis. *N. Engl. J. Med.* **2006**, *353*, 2462–2476. [CrossRef] [PubMed]
82. Schreiber, S.; Ben-Horin, S.; Leszczyszyn, J.; Dudkowiak, R.; Lahat, A.; Gawdis-Wojnarska, B.; Pukitis, A.; Horynski, M.; Farkas, K.; Kierkus, J.; et al. Randomized Controlled Trial: Subcutaneous vs. Intravenous Infliximab CT-P13 Maintenance in Inflammatory Bowel Disease. *Gastroenterology* **2021**, *160*, 2340–2353. [CrossRef] [PubMed]
83. Colombel, J.; Sandborn, W.J.; Rutgeerts, P.; Enns, R.; Hanauer, S.B.; Panaccione, R.; Schreiber, S.; Byczkowski, D.; Li, J.; Kent, J.D.; et al. Adalimumab for Maintenance of Clinical Response and Remission in Patients with Crohn's Disease: The CHARM Trial. *Gastroenterology* **2007**, *132*, 52–65. [CrossRef] [PubMed]
84. Panés, J.; Colombel, J.-F.; D'Haens, G.R.; Schreiber, S.; Panaccione, R.; Peyrin-Biroulet, L.; Loftus, E.V.; Danese, S.; Tanida, S.; Okuyama, Y.; et al. Higher vs. Standard Adalimumab Induction and Maintenance Dosing Regimens for Treatment of Ulcerative Colitis: SERENE UC Trial Results. *Gastroenterology* **2022**, *162*, 1891–1910. [CrossRef]
85. Gubatan, J.; Keyashian, K.; Rubin, S.J.; Wang, J.; Buckman, C.; Sinha, S. Anti-Integrins for the Treatment of Inflammatory Bowel Disease: Current Evidence and Perspectives. *Clin. Exp. Gastroenterol.* **2021**, *14*, 333–342. [CrossRef]
86. Ghosh, S.; Malchow, H.A.; Rutgeerts, P.; Palmer, T.; Donoghue, S. Natalizumab for Active Crohn's Disease. *N. Engl. J. Med.* **2003**, *348*, 24–32. [CrossRef]
87. Hellwig, K.; Gold, R. Progressive Multifocal Leukoencephalopathy and Natalizumab. *J. Neurol.* **2011**, *258*, 1920–1928. [CrossRef]
88. McLean, L.P.; Shea-Donohue, T.; Cross, R.K. Vedolizumab for the Treatment of Ulcerative Colitis and Crohn's Disease. *Immunotherapy* **2012**, *4*, 883–898. [CrossRef]

89. Sands, B.E.; Feagan, B.G.; Rutgeerts, P.; Colombel, J.-F.; Sandborn, W.J.; Sy, R.; D'Haens, G.; Ben-Horin, S.; Xu, J.; Rosario, M.; et al. Effects of Vedolizumab Induction Therapy for Patients with Crohn's Disease in Whom Tumor Necrosis Factor Antagonist Treatment Failed. *Gastroenterology* **2014**, *147*, 618–627.e3. [CrossRef]
90. Travis, S.; Silverberg, M.S.; Danese, S.; Gionchetti, P.; Löwenberg, M.; Jairath, V.; Feagan, B.G.; Bressler, B.; Ferrante, M.; Hart, A.; et al. Vedolizumab for the Treatment of Chronic Pouchitis. *N. Engl. J. Med.* **2023**, *388*, 1191–1200. [CrossRef]
91. Sandborn, W.J.; Baert, F.; Danese, S.; Krznarić, Ž.; Kobayashi, T.; Yao, X.; Chen, J.; Rosario, M.; Bhatia, S.; Kisfalvi, K.; et al. Efficacy and Safety of Vedolizumab Subcutaneous Formulation in a Randomized Trial of Patients with Ulcerative Colitis. *Gastroenterology* **2020**, *158*, 562–572.e12. [CrossRef] [PubMed]
92. Moschen, A.R.; Tilg, H.; Raine, T. IL-12, IL-23 and IL-17 in IBD: Immunobiology and Therapeutic Targeting. *Nat. Rev. Gastroenterol. Hepatol.* **2019**, *16*, 185–196. [CrossRef] [PubMed]
93. Al-Bawardy, B.; Shivashankar, R.; Proctor, D.D. Novel and Emerging Therapies for Inflammatory Bowel Disease. *Front. Pharmacol.* **2021**, *12*, 651415. [CrossRef] [PubMed]
94. Imbrizi, M.; Coy, C.S.R. Tratado de Doença Inflamatória Intestinal. In *Pequenas Moléculas*, 1st ed.; Saad-Hosne, R., Sassaki, L.Y., Eds.; Atheneu: Rio de Janeiro, Brazil, 2023; Volume 1.
95. Pippis, E.J.; Yacyshyn, B.R. Clinical and Mechanistic Characteristics of Current JAK Inhibitors in IBD. *Inflamm. Bowel Dis.* **2021**, *27*, 1674–1683. [CrossRef]
96. Chaparro, M.; Ordás, I.; Cabré, E.; Garcia-Sanchez, V.; Bastida, G.; Peñalva, M.; Gomollón, F.; García-Planella, E.; Merino, O.; Gutiérrez, A.; et al. Safety of Thiopurine Therapy in Inflammatory Bowel Disease: Long-Term Follow-up Study of 3931 Patients. *Inflamm. Bowel Dis.* **2013**, *19*, 1404–1410. [CrossRef]
97. Nielsen, O.H.; Steenholdt, C.; Juhl, C.B.; Rogler, G. Efficacy and Safety of Methotrexate in the Management of Inflammatory Bowel Disease: A Systematic Review and Meta-Analysis of Randomized, Controlled Trials. *EClinicalMedicine* **2020**, *20*, 100271. [CrossRef]
98. Holmer, A.; Singh, S. Overall and Comparative Safety of Biologic and Immunosuppressive Therapy in Inflammatory Bowel Diseases. *Expert Rev. Clin. Immunol.* **2019**, *15*, 969–979. [CrossRef]
99. Click, B.; Regueiro, M. Managing Risks with Biologics. *Curr. Gastroenterol. Rep.* **2019**, *21*, 1. [CrossRef]
100. Peyrin-Biroulet, L.; Rahier, J.-F.; Kirchgesner, J.; Abitbol, V.; Shaji, S.; Armuzzi, A.; Karmiris, K.; Gisbert, J.P.; Bossuyt, P.; Helwig, U.; et al. I-CARE, a European Prospective Cohort Study Assessing Safety and Effectiveness of Biologics in Inflammatory Bowel Disease. *Clin. Gastroenterol. Hepatol.* **2023**, *21*, 771–788.e10. [CrossRef]
101. Singh, S.; Kim, J.; Luo, J.; Paul, P.; Rudrapatna, V.; Park, S.; Zheng, K.; Syal, G.; Ha, C.; Fleshner, P.; et al. Comparative Safety and Effectiveness of Biologic Therapy for Crohn's Disease: A CA-IBD Cohort Study. *Clin. Gastroenterol. Hepatol.* **2022**, *21*, 2359–2369.e5. [CrossRef]
102. Pugliese, D.; Privitera, G.; Crispino, F.; Mezzina, N.; Castiglione, F.; Fiorino, G.; Laterza, L.; Viola, A.; Bertani, L.; Caprioli, F.; et al. Effectiveness and Safety of Vedolizumab in a Matched Cohort of Elderly and Nonelderly Patients with Inflammatory Bowel Disease: The IG-IBD LIVE Study. *Aliment. Pharmacol. Ther.* **2022**, *56*, 95–109. [CrossRef] [PubMed]
103. Sandborn, W.J.; Rebuck, R.; Wang, Y.; Zou, B.; Adedokun, O.J.; Gasink, C.; Sands, B.E.; Hanauer, S.B.; Targan, S.; Ghosh, S.; et al. Five-Year Efficacy and Safety of Ustekinumab Treatment in Crohn's Disease: The IM-UNITI Trial. *Clin. Gastroenterol. Hepatol.* **2022**, *20*, 578–590.e4. [CrossRef] [PubMed]
104. Ferrante, M.; Feagan, B.G.; Panés, J.; Baert, F.; Louis, E.; Dewit, O.; Kaser, A.; Duan, W.R.; Pang, Y.; Lee, W.-J.; et al. Long-Term Safety and Efficacy of Risankizumab Treatment in Patients with Crohn's Disease: Results from the Phase 2 Open-Label Extension Study. *J. Crohn's Colitis* **2021**, *15*, 2001–2010. [CrossRef]
105. Singh, S.; Murad, M.H.; Fumery, M.; Sedano, R.; Jairath, V.; Panaccione, R.; Sandborn, W.J.; Ma, C. Comparative Efficacy and Safety of Biologic Therapies for Moderate-to-Severe Crohn's Disease: A Systematic Review and Network Meta-Analysis. *Lancet Gastroenterol. Hepatol.* **2021**, *6*, 1002–1014. [CrossRef] [PubMed]
106. Ytterberg, S.R.; Bhatt, D.L.; Mikuls, T.R.; Koch, G.G.; Fleischmann, R.; Rivas, J.L.; Germino, R.; Menon, S.; Sun, Y.; Wang, C.; et al. Cardiovascular and Cancer Risk with Tofacitinib in Rheumatoid Arthritis. *N. Engl. J. Med.* **2022**, *386*, 316–326. [CrossRef] [PubMed]
107. McLornan, D.P.; Pope, J.E.; Gotlib, J.; Harrison, C.N. Current and Future Status of JAK Inhibitors. *Lancet* **2021**, *398*, 803–816. [CrossRef]
108. Sivaraman, P.; Cohen, S.B. Malignancy and Janus Kinase Inhibition. *Rheum. Dis. Clin. N. Am.* **2017**, *43*, 79–93. [CrossRef]
109. Queiroz, N.S.F.; Regueiro, M. Safety Considerations with Biologics and New Inflammatory Bowel Disease Therapies. *Curr. Opin. Gastroenterol.* **2020**, *36*, 257–264. [CrossRef]
110. Sandborn, W.J.; Peyrin-Biroulet, L.; Quirk, D.; Wang, W.; Nduaka, C.I.; Mukherjee, A.; Su, C.; Sands, B.E. Efficacy and Safety of Extended Induction with Tofacitinib for the Treatment of Ulcerative Colitis. *Clin. Gastroenterol. Hepatol.* **2022**, *20*, 1821–1830.e3. [CrossRef]
111. Kragstrup, T.W.; Glintborg, B.; Svensson, A.L.; McMaster, C.; Robinson, P.C.; Deleuran, B.; Liew, D.F. Waiting for JAK Inhibitor Safety Data. *RMD Open* **2022**, *8*, e002236. [CrossRef]
112. Verstockt, B.; Vetrano, S.; Salas, A.; Nayeri, S.; Duijvestein, M.; Vande Casteele, N.; Alimentiv Translational Research Consortium (ATRC); Danese, S.; D'Haens, G.; Eckmann, L.; et al. Sphingosine 1-Phosphate Modulation and Immune Cell Trafficking in Inflammatory Bowel Disease. *Nat. Rev. Gastroenterol. Hepatol.* **2022**, *19*, 351–366. [CrossRef] [PubMed]

113. Solitano, V.; Facciorusso, A.; Jess, T.; Ma, C.; Hassan, C.; Repici, A.; Jairath, V.; Armuzzi, A.; Singh, S. Comparative Risk of Serious Infections with Biologic Agents and Oral Small Molecules in Inflammatory Bowel Diseases: A Systematic Review and Meta-Analysis. *Clin. Gastroenterol. Hepatol.* **2023**, *21*, 907–921.e2. [CrossRef]
114. Sattler, L.; Hanauer, S.B.; Malter, L. Immunomodulatory Agents for Treatment of Patients with Inflammatory Bowel Disease (Review Safety of Anti-TNF, Anti-Integrin, Anti IL-12/23, JAK Inhibition, Sphingosine 1-Phosphate Receptor Modulator, Azathioprine/6-MP and Methotrexate). *Curr. Gastroenterol. Rep.* **2021**, *23*, 30. [CrossRef] [PubMed]
115. Andrew, B.; Srinivasan, A.; Zhou, A.; Vasudevan, A. Letter: Elderly Onset Inflammatory Bowel Disease—Treat to Target Approach Is Still Warranted. *Aliment. Pharmacol. Ther.* **2023**, *58*, 556–557. [CrossRef] [PubMed]
116. Almario, C.V.; Keller, M.S.; Chen, M.; Lasch, K.; Ursos, L.; Shklovskaya, J.; Melmed, G.Y.; Spiegel, B.M.R. Optimizing Selection of Biologics in Inflammatory Bowel Disease: Development of an Online Patient Decision Aid Using Conjoint Analysis. *Am. J. Gastroenterol.* **2018**, *113*, 58–71. [CrossRef]
117. Rubin, D.T.; Sninsky, C.; Siegmund, B.; Sans, M.; Hart, A.; Bressler, B.; Bouhnik, Y.; Armuzzi, A.; Afzali, A. International Perspectives on Management of Inflammatory Bowel Disease: Opinion Differences and Similarities Between Patients and Physicians from the IBD GAPPS Survey. *Inflamm. Bowel Dis.* **2021**, *27*, 1942–1953. [CrossRef]
118. Bhat, S.; Click, B.; Regueiro, M. Safety and Monitoring of Inflammatory Bowel Disease Advanced Therapies. *Inflamm. Bowel Dis.* **2023**, izad120. [CrossRef]
119. Zurba, Y.; Gros, B.; Shehab, M. Exploring the Pipeline of Novel Therapies for Inflammatory Bowel Disease; State of the Art Review. *Biomedicines* **2023**, *11*, 747. [CrossRef]
120. Dai, B.; Hackney, J.A.; Ichikawa, R.; Nguyen, A.; Elstrott, J.; Orozco, L.D.; Sun, K.-H.; Modrusan, Z.; Gogineni, A.; Scherl, A.; et al. Dual Targeting of Lymphocyte Homing and Retention through A4β7 and AEβ7 Inhibition in Inflammatory Bowel Disease. *Cell Rep. Med.* **2021**, *2*, 100381. [CrossRef]
121. Sandborn, W.J.; D'Haens, G.R.; Reinisch, W.; Panés, J.; Chan, D.; Gonzalez, S.; Weisel, K.; Germinaro, M.; Frustaci, M.E.; Yang, Z.; et al. Guselkumab for the Treatment of Crohn's Disease: Induction Results from the Phase 2 GALAXI-1 Study. *Gastroenterology* **2022**, *162*, 1650–1664.e8. [CrossRef]
122. Danese, S.; Neurath, M.F.; Kopoń, A.; Zakko, S.F.; Simmons, T.C.; Fogel, R.; Siegel, C.A.; Panaccione, R.; Zhan, X.; Usiskin, K.; et al. Effects of Apremilast, an Oral Inhibitor of Phosphodiesterase 4, in a Randomized Trial of Patients with Active Ulcerative Colitis. *Clin. Gastroenterol. Hepatol.* **2020**, *18*, 2526–2534.e9. [CrossRef]
123. Atreya, R.; Peyrin-Biroulet, L.; Klymenko, A.; Augustyn, M.; Bakulin, I.; Slankamenac, D.; Mihellér, P.; Gasbarrini, A.; Hébuterne, X.; Arnesson, K.; et al. Cobitolimod for Moderate-to-Severe, Left-Sided Ulcerative Colitis (CONDUCT): A Phase 2b Randomised, Double-Blind, Placebo-Controlled, Dose-Ranging Induction Trial. *Lancet Gastroenterol. Hepatol.* **2020**, *5*, 1063–1075. [CrossRef]
124. Vuyyuru, S.K.; Kedia, S.; Ahuja, V. Considerations When Starting Patients on Multiple Biologics and Small Molecules. *Curr. Opin. Gastroenterol.* **2022**, *38*, 562–569. [CrossRef] [PubMed]
125. Balderramo, D. Role of the Combination of Biologics and/or Small Molecules in the Treatment of Patients with Inflammatory Bowel Disease. *World J. Gastroenterol.* **2022**, *28*, 6743–6751. [CrossRef] [PubMed]
126. Feagan, B.G.; Sands, B.E.; Sandborn, W.J.; Germinaro, M.; Vetter, M.; Shao, J.; Sheng, S.; Johanns, J.; Panés, J.; Tkachev, A.; et al. Guselkumab plus Golimumab Combination Therapy versus Guselkumab or Golimumab Monotherapy in Patients with Ulcerative Colitis (VEGA): A Randomised, Double-Blind, Controlled, Phase 2, Proof-of-Concept Trial. *Lancet Gastroenterol. Hepatol.* **2023**, *8*, 307–320. [CrossRef] [PubMed]

Disclaimer/Publisher's Note: The statements, opinions and data contained in all publications are solely those of the individual author(s) and contributor(s) and not of MDPI and/or the editor(s). MDPI and/or the editor(s) disclaim responsibility for any injury to people or property resulting from any ideas, methods, instructions or products referred to in the content.

MDPI
St. Alban-Anlage 66
4052 Basel
Switzerland
www.mdpi.com

Pharmaceuticals Editorial Office
E-mail: pharmaceuticals@mdpi.com
www.mdpi.com/journal/pharmaceuticals

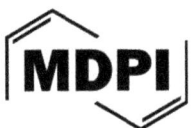

Disclaimer/Publisher's Note: The statements, opinions and data contained in all publications are solely those of the individual author(s) and contributor(s) and not of MDPI and/or the editor(s). MDPI and/or the editor(s) disclaim responsibility for any injury to people or property resulting from any ideas, methods, instructions or products referred to in the content.

www.ingramcontent.com/pod-product-compliance
Lightning Source LLC
LaVergne TN
LVHW070725100526
838202LV00013B/1171